W9-BXO-853

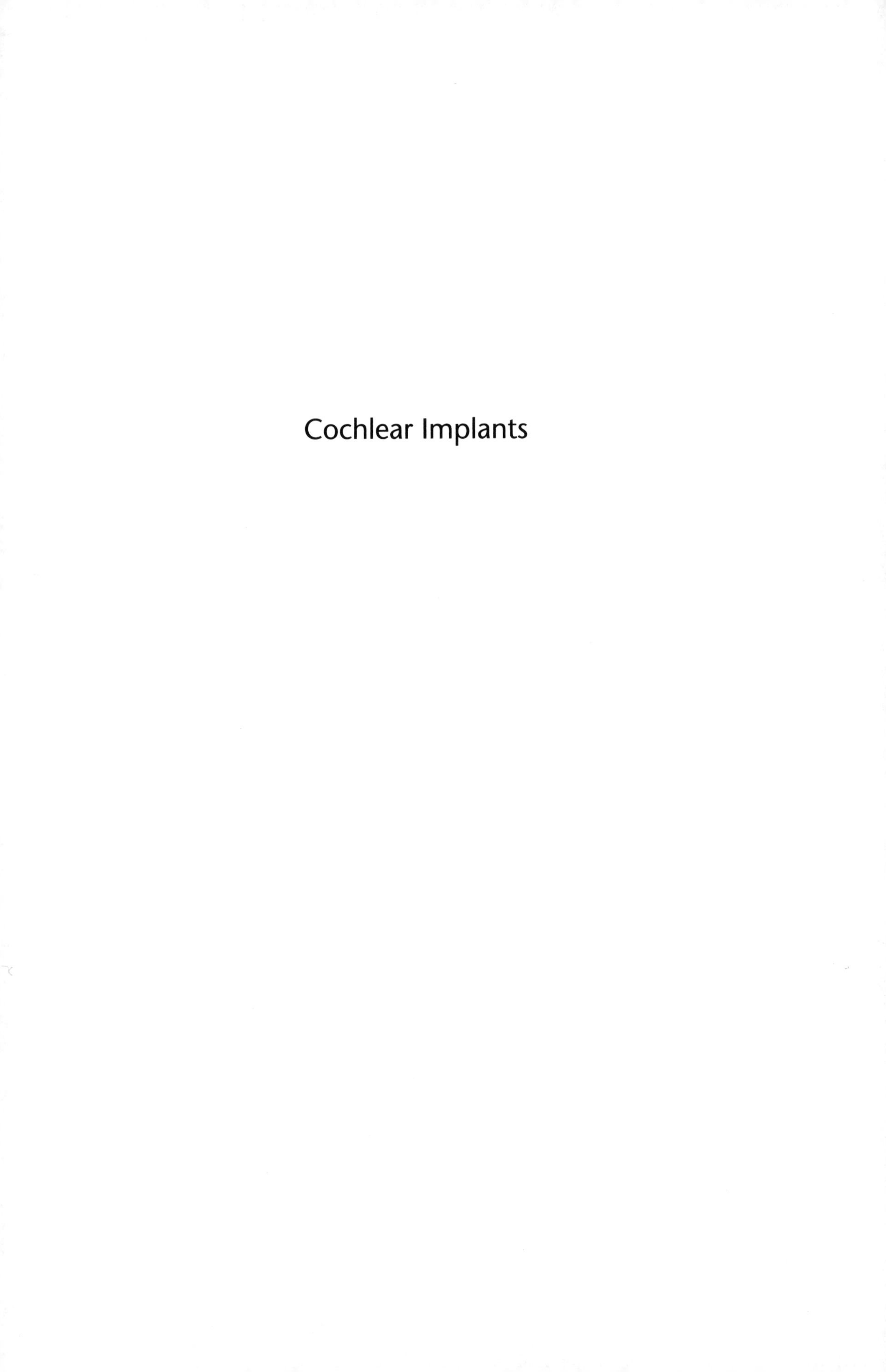

Cochlear Implants

COCHLEAR IMPLANTS
Evolving Perspectives

Raylene Paludneviciene
Irene W. Leigh
Editors

Gallaudet University Press
Washington, DC

MW

Gallaudet University Press
Washington, DC 20002
http://gupress.gallaudet.edu

Printed in the United States of America

Library of Congress Cataloging-in-Publication Data

Cochlear implants : evolving perspectives / Raylene Paludneviciene, Irene W. Leigh, editors.
p.; cm.
Includes bibliographical references and index.
ISBN-13: 978-1-56368-503-3 (hard cover : alk. paper)
ISBN-10: 1-56368-503-5 (hard cover : alk. paper)
ISBN-13: 978-1-56368-504-0 (e-book)
ISBN-10: 1-56368-504-3 (e-book)
1. Cochlear implants. 2. Cochlear implants—Social aspects. 3. Deafness—Psychology.
I. Paludneviciene, Raylene. II. Leigh, Irene.
[DNLM: 1. Cochlear Implants. 2. Hearing Impaired Persons—psychology. WV 274]
RF305.C622 2011
617.8′9—dc23

2011021026

∞ The paper used in this publication meets the minimum requirements of American National Standard for Information Sciences—Permanence of Paper for Printed Library Materials, ANSI Z39.48–1984.

3/12/12

CONTENTS

INTRODUCTION

Irene W. Leigh and Raylene Paludneviciene

For many members of the Deaf community, the issue of cochlear implants has been fraught with trepidation, anger, frustration, and outright rejection of the concept that surgical insertion of an auditory device is required to restore a sense that is "missing." A good number of these members saw it as an attack on a "visual way of living" and on their signed languages. They also feared the loss of their culture, a culture that has been around for centuries, one that was only formally acknowledged as a bona fide culture in the latter half of the 20th century.

It took decades of struggle before culturally Deaf adults who decided on cochlear implantation began to be viewed by opponents of the procedure no longer as automatic traitors, guilty of betraying their Deaf culture values but rather as individuals who wanted exposure to different sensory experiences, in this case auditory stimulation, while holding on to the use of their signed language. Perspectives on pediatric cochlear implantation, viewed by many Deaf individuals as an ethical affront that took away a child's right to decide on the surgery and an auditory way of life, are very gradually giving way to a more nuanced view on the part of those Deaf community members, who recognize that the number of children with cochlear implants is growing exponentially. This gradual change in perspective seems to be giving substance to Jay Innes' observation that "the deaf community is strong enough and mature enough to tolerate a full range of opinions on the topic of cochlear implants" (Christiansen & Leigh, 2002/2005, p. 288).

We, Raylene Paludneviciene and Irene W. Leigh, the editors of this book, have been interested observers of the maelstrom surrounding the debate on cochlear implants, in particular pediatric cochlear implants. Both of us are members of the Department of Psychology at Gallaudet University, the world's only liberal arts university for deaf students. As both of us are deaf and interact with the Deaf community, we come to this book from these vantage points. Disclosure: Neither of us are cochlear implant users, but we have extensive experience with the topic.

Irene W. Leigh previously served as a consulting psychologist in the cochlear implant program at the former Manhattan Eye, Ear, and Throat Hospital in New York City. She later participated in a research project with John B. Christiansen that involved interviewing 57 sets of parents who decided on cochlear implants for their children and obtaining their perspectives (Christiansen & Leigh, 2002/2005). In general, findings indicated that a good number of the parents labeled the Deaf community as being misinformed about the merits of cochlear implants and not understanding or respecting the parents' perspectives. These parents did not necessarily deny the importance of Deaf culture. Rather, they felt the cochlear implants provided additional options for expanding the world of their deaf children. Since then, Leigh has had many interactions with individuals who have gotten the implant and remained a part of their Deaf community.

Raylene Paludneviciene is a native user of American Sign Language and a member of a multigenerational Deaf family immersed in the Deaf community. She became interested in the cochlear implant debate after several of her friends opted to receive cochlear implants about a decade ago. In professional settings, she sought out opportunities to work with pediatric and adult cochlear implant users to broaden her understanding of how cochlear implants work and the effects on the individual and environment. After several members of her family received cochlear implants, her direct experiences with the medical establishment, educational agencies, and members of the Deaf community provided the original impetus for this book.

We felt that it was important to substantiate Innes' perspective by illustrating the diversity of perspectives and the world of possibilities espoused by the authors who contributed chapters to this book. A good number of these contributors are themselves cochlear implant users. Nonetheless, we do not take a position on cochlear implants. We know cochlear implants are here to stay until some other technological advancement comes along. We recognize the presence of an inherent contradiction between the focus on auditory languages as exemplified by messages about the value of cochlear implants and the focus on vision as exemplified by visual languages/signed languages. For quite some time, it has appeared that following one of these focuses has traditionally negated the other focus. However, the assumption that the two cannot coexist is now being challenged with the emergence of programs that incorporate both approaches in facilitating the learning of languages. This movement from a solely auditory focus for pediatric users of cochlear implants to a focus that presents the possibility of combining auditory and visual approaches in the education of these children has gained traction since not all of these children fully master age appropriate receptive and expressive spoken language, although a good number do. In this vein, we have included authors who present information and research findings so that readers can come to their own conclusions regarding the interface between cochlear implants and the Deaf community, and between auditory and visual approaches to the mastery of both spoken and signed languages.

The first part of this book starts with an introduction to cochlear implants and the Deaf community. It includes an in-depth examination of the issues that influence perceptions of cochlear implants. Raylene Paludneviciene and Raychelle Harris bring a unique perspective to the debate, as they are deaf researchers with relatives who are cochlear implant users. The next chapter provides an overview of genetic research, bioethical issues, and cochlear implants as these affect the Deaf community. Jane Dillehay, a deaf biologist and cochlear implant user, reports on the rapid advancement of technology related to genetic information and hearing enhancement. In view of this, she affirms the importance of involving Deaf community members in assessing the implications of each new technology development that potentially impacts the lives of deaf people. The succeeding chapter by John Christiansen, who has a cochlear implant, and Irene W. Leigh examines the impact of cochlear implants on the Deaf community. Going beyond the general, they compare perspectives on cochlear implants expressed by members of the Gallaudet University community in 2000 and again in 2008 in the process of assessing the extent of changes in attitudes.

Next, three cochlear implant users, Khadijat Rashid, Poorna Kushalnagar, and Raja Kushalnagar, report on a survey of how deaf adult signers experience implants. Since the perception is positive for the most part, the authors feel that an increasing number of signing deaf adults have moved beyond the battle against cochlear implantation. The next chapter, by Julie Mitchiner and Marilyn Sass-Lehrer, reinforces this perspective. Mitchiner is a deaf educator who initially professed skepticism about the effectiveness of cochlear implants. After recognizing that deaf parents were beginning to implant their deaf children, she developed a research project that involved interviewing three deaf mothers about their decision to implant their children and their perspectives on how American Sign Language and spoken English can coexist. The findings that the authors report provide illuminating food for thought.

Lastly, Irene W. Leigh and Deborah Maxwell-McCaw, who is also a cochlear implant user, examine the relationship between having a cochlear implant and one's identity development. They explore the concept of identity and how it evolves, what deaf-related identities are all about, and the various perceptions of cochlear implants and their role in psychosocial/identity development.

The second part examines the nature of visual and auditory processing of languages. Donna A. Morere has spent years in the study of language processing and is the mother of a deaf son with a cochlear implant. She presents evidence of the effectiveness of bimodal processing and demonstrates the importance not only of audition but also of vision, including the role of gesture, in enhancing the development of spoken language. She argues for the need to study the neurological foundations for the simultaneous development of spoken and signed languages, considering that many deaf individuals use a combination of signs and speech. Ellen A. Rhoades, a cochlear implant user who is also a certified Auditory-Verbal therapist, provides a treatise on how Auditory-Verbal therapy can benefit children who use some form of signing. In so doing, she also reviews the literature on select unimodal and bimodal bilingual findings regarding language development.

Building on this research foundation, part III covers educational approaches for cochlear implant users that involve efforts at integrating spoken and signed languages within the classroom. Debra Berlin Nussbaum and Susanne M. Scott provide their perspectives on effective educational practices for children with cochlear implants. Considering that the path to developing spoken language will vary depending on the nature of the child, they advocate a program that includes both spoken and signed languages. Their chapter addresses the complex considerations for designing effective, comprehensive programs for children with cochlear implants. Following this, Maribel Gárate presents techniques for educating children with cochlear implants in an American Sign Language/English bilingual classroom. Her goal is that of developing social and academic language proficiency in both languages so that Deaf and hard of hearing children benefit from the affective, cognitive, and academic advantages of bilingualism. Next, Jill Duncan explains how teachers of the deaf can incorporate Auditory-Verbal strategies within a signed communication education context. She presents the case history of a child who is dealing with two different spoken languages in addition to the signed language of the educational setting.

In the final part of the book, we present two chapters that challenge the readers to reframe the context of the cochlear implant debate. Joseph Michael Valente, Benjamin Bahan, and H-Dirksen Bauman highlight the role of sensory politics in the various ways our senses are perceived in different cultures. They note how Western culture has emphasized the primacy of audition to the detriment of the other senses and recommend a reframing so that individuals can understand that there are various ways of being that are equally valid. More to the point, they argue that signed language based on sight is a modality that is as much a biological norm as speech. Finally, Josh Swiller, also a cochlear implant user, reviews the stressors faced by the Deaf community, specifically demographic, political, technological, and ultimately financial. He argues that if the Deaf community is to survive, it needs to transform itself in ways that connect with the world at large and in ways that reinforce economic independence. He provides suggestions for how this transformation can be accomplished.

It is our hope that this book takes you, the reader, in a different direction from the directions that are most often expressed in treatises on cochlear implantation and provides you with a broader understanding of what may work for individuals with cochlear implants. We anticipate that you may come away with a different perspective on how the Deaf community is adjusting to the presence of cochlear implants in its midst. Reframing the meanings of cochlear implantation may also provide a means for moving into the future in ways that emphasize the value of both vision and audition in the development of any one deaf individual.

This book is a direct outcome of our experiences with the cochlear implant debate. Raylene Paludneviciene would like to thank her family members and friends with cochlear implants for pushing the boundaries of what it means to be part of the Deaf community. Professionals in the educational and medical fields spent hours of their time in discussing with her the functions of cochlear implants and envisioning the optimal educational and social environments for deaf children with cochlear implants.

Irene W. Leigh owes a debt of gratitude to Patricia Chute, former director of the Manhattan Eye, Ear, and Throat Hospital cochlear implant program, who graciously invited her to be a consulting psychologist. This provided Leigh with the opportunity to meet with parents and children who were investigating the possibility of cochlear implantation. She also owes a huge debt of gratitude to John B. Christiansen for inviting her to join him in the development of the cochlear implant research project that culminated in the book *Cochlear implants in children: Ethics and choices*. And finally, she acknowledges all the parents and cochlear implant users who taught her about life with cochlear implants.

References

Christiansen, J. B., & Leigh, I. W. (2002/2005). *Cochlear implants in children: Ethics and choices*. Washington, DC: Gallaudet University Press.

PART I

The Deaf Community and Cochlear Implants

1

IMPACT OF COCHLEAR IMPLANTS ON THE DEAF COMMUNITY

Raylene Paludneviciene and Raychelle L. Harris

Due to recent improvements in cochlear implant (CI) technology and the trend toward early implantation in infants as young as 6 months of age, how deaf children acquire spoken language has changed significantly. Recent research has demonstrated the dramatic improvement in spoken language for many of these children, essentially because of increased auditory access to spoken language (e.g., Sorkin, 2010). This in turn has created a generation of deaf children with CIs who in some ways are markedly different from previous generations in terms of educational and social experiences. The rapid changes in CI technology have resulted in evolving perspectives of CIs by professionals and members of the Deaf community. Even though deaf people have long used hearing assistance technology, no specific technology has caused the type of repercussions within the Deaf[1] community and professionals the way the development of the CI has.

Functions and Benefits of Cochlear Implants

Many members of the Deaf community wear hearing aids, which provide a wide range of benefit ranging from access to spoken language to environmental sound awareness. Since CIs also result in similar benefits, depending on individual attributes such as age at implantation and ability to learn the meaning of sound input among others, some may wonder why CIs have become the recommended hearing assistive technology for many deaf children and adults. The way sound is accessed differs based on the different technological functions of hearing aids and CIs.

The main difference between CIs and hearing aids is in how sound is conveyed to the brain. Hearing aids are designed to amplify sound, although digital hearing aids can be programmed to dampen specific sounds (e.g., very loud

For clarity, we use lowercase "d" to include all deaf people, regardless of level of involvement in the deaf community or fluency in a signed language.

background noise) while amplifying another kind of sound (e.g., human voices). Their effectiveness depends on the nature of the user's residual hearing. In contrast, the surgically implanted internal part of the CI converts sound to electrical impulses, which are then sent to the auditory nerve and from there to the auditory centers of the brain. These impulses can be manipulated through the use of a computer program capable of translating sounds that the user can learn to recognize. This is a process technically known as "mapping." CIs do not amplify sound nor do they depend on the residual hearing of the individual since the electrodes inserted in the cochlea send impulses directly to the auditory nerve. CIs do not make a child or adult hard of hearing, contrary to assumptions that some may have, although they may be viewed as functioning like hard of hearing persons. These individuals are still deaf and still have to learn what the sounds they hear mean.

Profoundly deaf individuals typically are candidates for cochlear implantation, given that the auditory nerve is still functioning. The possibility that they will derive significant benefits from CIs is a real one, especially if they are implanted at a young age. Changes in surgical procedures and improvement in the equipment (e.g., making the inner coil less rigid, causing less damage during insertion into the cochlea) have made it possible to preserve residual hearing in some patients (Niparko, 2009). The practical aspects of preserving residual hearing in this case include providing CI users with the option of utilizing their residual hearing in certain situations (e.g., listening to music).

Age of implantation is the single most important factor affecting the success rate of acquisition of spoken English (Sorkin, 2010), although multiple other factors also come into play. For example, in one study, deaf children who received a CI at 13 months of age had similar vocabulary levels as hearing peers of the same age, whereas deaf children who received their CIs later performed more poorly (Indiana University School of Medicine, 2010). The recent increase in the prevalence of bilateral CIs, meaning that each ear is implanted with a CI, has resulted in an increase in positive benefits for deaf children. Tait et al. (2010) compared 42 unilaterally implanted and 27 bilaterally implanted children and found that bilaterally implanted children were significantly more likely to vocalize and to use audition when interacting vocally without looking while conversing with an adult.

For children, the path to cochlear implantation starts shortly after birth. To date, 42 states provide newborn hearing screening, which is critical for early identification of hearing loss and subsequent intervention (King, 2010). Prior to newborn hearing screenings, age of identification of hearing loss averaged around 36 months (King, 2010). This essentially meant that two years of communication access and remediation were lost. Currently, more than 95% of newborns nationally are screened for hearing loss (King, 2010). In states with newborn hearing screening, typically upon identification of hearing loss the audiologist providing the hearing screening refers the family for further testing. Unfortunately, 50% on average do not follow up postidentification, although efforts are being made to address this issue (Centers for Disease Control and Prevention, 2003). During follow-up, if the hearing loss is confirmed, audiologists and otologists provide information about various services, including cochlear implantation. It is up to the family to choose whether and how they wish to follow up on specific recommendations.

Several factors impede successful intervention. Not all deaf children who can benefit from CIs have access to this technology. In the United States, most children who have CIs come from families who have health insurance coverage or are able to pay for it (see Christiansen & Leigh, 2005 for examples). Basically, access to CIs relies greatly on socioeconomical factors, including access to hearing intervention programs and government funding if one qualifies for Medicaid coverage. Specifically, socioeconomical factors might prevent families from obtaining hearing aids or CIs (e.g., Kuntze, 2004), especially if health insurance coverage is limited or unavailable. The costs of the surgery and CI equipment are usually covered by Medicaid; nevertheless, Chang, Ko, Murray, Arnold, and Megerian (2010) documented that patients from lower socioeconomic backgrounds had higher rates of complications associated with CI surgery, worse follow-up compliance, and lower rates of bilateral implantation.

Several factors might impede compliance with follow-up appointments, which are critical for success with CIs and mapping purposes. At some hospitals, preoperative requirements to determine one's eligibility prior to CI surgery include results from auditory brainstem response audiometry, computed tomography scan, audiology and speech-language testing, psychological evaluation, and hearing aid trials. As these procedures may be required before the client becomes eligible for CI surgery, related preoperative appointments before their child can undergo CI surgery can seem daunting for parents with limited resources.

Meeting the minimum candidacy requirements for CI surgery requires a significant time commitment, possibly including being able to afford time off from work, insurance coverage, and transportation to appointments. Transportation and inflexibility in scheduling due to competing priorities such as childcare and work obligations might also impede families with limited resources from obtaining the best possible care for their child with CIs.

In addition to the expenses of surgery itself, the rehabilitation process can be expensive as well as time consuming. On top of all that, maintenance of the equipment and replacement of broken parts (which occurs frequently with young children) need to be taken into account. Niparko et al. (2010) documented that children from higher socioeconomic backgrounds had the best results with CIs, as their parents are better positioned to deal with the complexities of the process in getting their children implanted, managing appropriate follow-up, and caring for the equipment.

In summary, factors that impede access to CI technology include socioeconomic factors such as family income, health insurance coverage, ability to gather information, transportation, and availability of newborn hearing screening. Many of these factors are unique to the United States, where only 55% of eligible children receive CIs (Bradham & Jones, 2008). When the parents are deaf and part of the Deaf community, misinformation about CIs and fear of rejection by their community are factors that may prevent them from deciding to implant their deaf children (Mitchiner & Sass-Lehrer, this volume).

The Deaf Community

Members of the Deaf community have a long history of dealing with auditory equipment. They also have experience with a variety of methods that have been used to teach speech and listening skills to deaf children. As a result of this history, which includes many negative experiences, advances in hearing enhancement technology may be met with skepticism and resistance from some within the Deaf community. Many deaf adults remember an era during which all deaf children, regardless of ability to access spoken English via residual hearing and/or listening devices/hearing aids, were forced to try to learn through oral methods. Oralism is an educational approach used with deaf children that focuses on instruction provided via spoken English, speechreading, and the use of residual hearing (Moores, 2001). This approach has historically discouraged the use of a visual language such as American Sign Language ([ASL] Branson & Miller, 2002). As a result of this history, deaf adults who grew up with limited access to communication and hearing assistance equipment that provided limited or no access to spoken English view the return of "oralism" and promotion of CIs as returning to a dark era in deaf history.

An important concern among deaf adults and stakeholders in deaf education is that too much attention is focused on auditory/speech training at the expense of overall cognitive development, resulting in language delays, often on top of delayed identification of hearing loss, especially if a visually based language foundation is lacking (Cummins, 2006; Grosjean, 2001; Harris, 2011; Johnson, Liddell, & Erting, 1989; Vygotsky, 1986). In addition to recommendations that some deaf people see as depriving deaf children of a visually based language that is fully accessible, the publicized risks associated with CIs are often a frequent visual reminder to members of the Deaf community about the dangers of CIs.

The death of some deaf children after cochlear implantation due to meningitis and the lack of appropriate preventive vaccination (Biernath et al., 2006) sent shock waves throughout the Deaf community and gave rise to fears that CIs could cause more deaths. Many felt that access to spoken language was not worth the perceived risk. Beyond these, there were more issues that were of concern for many individuals.

In addition to the reported deaths, CI surgery resulted in partial temporary facial paralysis for some deaf patients (Fayad, Wanna, Micheletto, & Parisier, 2003). Contributing to the fears expressed by some deaf people, a person with partial facial paralysis attributed to CI surgery appeared in the video *Audism Unveiled* (Bahan, Bauman, & Montenegro, 2008). This video discussed the oppression of deaf people through the practice of "audism," a term that reflects a system of advantage based on hearing ability (Bauman, 2004). Using vlogs (videos uploaded on the Internet), Deaf adults have shared stories of how, as teenagers, they were forced by their parents to undergo CI surgery against their will. There are also vlogs reporting frequent severe and debilitating headaches and vertigo, in addition to large visible scars from the surgery. Some people who are deaf have since refused to wear their CI processors for a variety of reasons; for some CI recipients, the processors provided very limited benefit.

The deaths, facial paralysis, splitting headaches, and large scars are some of the factors that have reinforced the resistance of some in the Deaf community to embracing this new technology for deaf children. Although attitudes of some of the members in the Deaf community have changed over time regarding adults who choose CIs for themselves, their perception of parents choosing implants for their children reflects comparatively less acceptance (Christiansen & Leigh, this volume; Rashid, Kushalnagar, & Kushalnagar, this volume). Another facet of the resistance by some in the Deaf community toward CIs for children, in addition to the risks of CI surgery, is the fear that parents would not allow their children to learn sign language and to become members of the Deaf community.

Perceptions of Signed Languages

After centuries of suppression of signed languages and subsequent efforts to educate the general public about signed languages, only recently have signed languages begun to experience a renaissance. Amid a climate of greater acceptance of signed languages as bona fide languages and efforts to include signed languages in all aspects of the Deaf community, the presence and the message of CIs seem to negate the viability of visual languages. If deaf children can hear, then why use a signed language when these children now have improved access to spoken languages?

Amid this climate of change, the Center for American Sign Language and English Bilingual Education and Research (CAEBER), previously funded by grant money from the U.S. Department of Education Office of Special Education and Rehabilitative Services under the Research and Innovation to Improve Services and Results for Children with Disabilities (Nover, Andrews, Baker, Everhart, & Bradford, 2002), was established to explore the possibilities of ASL/English bilingualism. Several states have passed laws recognizing ASL as a language (States that recognize ASL, 2004). ASL/English bilingualism was recently incorporated into the mission statement of Gallaudet University, the world's only liberal arts university for deaf students (Gallaudet University, 2011). However, bilingualism within the Deaf community has typically been described as written English/ASL, rather than spoken English/ASL. CAEBER has included "oracy" as part of their studies of bilingualism (see Gárate, this volume). Gallaudet University's adoption of the word "bilingualism" in its mission statement tacitly implies written English/ASL, as there is no mention of how spoken English can be part of the concept of bilingualism used on its campus. On the other hand, however, the question remains regarding where sign language can be placed within the context of children with CIs who are able to access and use spoken English. In part III of this volume (Educational Approaches), authors address this issue by discussing how ASL can be part of the education of students with CIs.

Changes in Deaf Education

How has the advent of CIs impacted deaf education? To understand current changes, it helps to have a brief glimpse of how deaf education has evolved and how it is relevant to the Deaf community. Deaf education has its roots in the history of special education. In the United States, near the end of the 18th century, "different" populations began to be identified and categorized. In reaction to the categories and recognizing that the populations in these categories needed special attention, the typical course of action was to create institutions for these individuals for the ostensible purpose of housing them and educating them to fit into society. Thus, from the early 1800s onward, institutions were established for specific categories, including, for example, those who were categorized as having mental retardation or as blind. As a consequence of this movement, numerous institutions were established for deaf children, the first permanent one in 1817.

Because deaf children lived together on a regular and quasipermanent basis, a distinct culture was cemented in which sign language flourished. Through residential schools for those who are deaf, socialization patterns incorporating sign language and Deaf cultural ways of being became critical for one's identity as a deaf person (Leigh, 2009; Winzer, 1993). Since sign language was widely used and accepted within the residential schools, language and communication for deaf people in schools during this time was productive and accessible.

However, at the same time, proponents of the oral method, which had its inception in some European educational settings for deaf children, created a situation in which there were ongoing debates reflecting different levels of conflict over language and communication approaches (Branson & Miller, 2002; Burch, 2002; Moores, 2001). By the time of the 1800 International Congress on the

Education of the Deaf in Milan, Italy, the attendees were essentially confirming the spread of oral or spoken language education with their vote "to outlaw the use of sign language as a method for educating deaf children" (Gannon, 1981, p. 65).

Up to the 1960s, the focus on spoken language (oralism) was prevalent in deaf schools and deaf education programs. The use of sign language was frowned on, and deaf children who used sign language were punished (Branson & Miller, 2002). Many deaf people were embarrassed to use sign language in public (Lane, 1984) but used it freely in private.

The civil rights movement of the 1960s resulted in a focus on minorities fighting for their rights through marches, sit-ins, and protests, which in turn highlighted the importance of social justice for groups who felt disenfranchised, including groups of people with disabilities and deaf people. Moving forward, in the spirit of civil rights, new legislation and laws such as Section 504 of the Rehabilitation Act of 1973 and the Education for All Handicapped Children Act (1975), also known as PL 94–142, then later renamed Individuals with Disabilities Education Act, emerged (e.g., Marschark, Lang, & Albertini, 2002). Those new laws made Americans relatively more aware of the importance of equal access and opportunities for those who previously had to struggle for their rights to education available to the general public.

Although deaf people as a minority generally were bystanders in the civil rights movement, this movement helped deaf people begin to think and talk about their language and culture once again—not only that, but other seminal events were also at work.

In 1965, a government report titled the Babbidge report declared oral deaf education to be a failure. This report created a forum whereby consideration of the possibility of using sign language as the mode of communication in the classroom over oralism increasingly became a topic of attention. At the same time, Stokoe, Casterline, and Croneberg (1965) published their *Dictionary of American Sign Language on Linguistic Principles,* which affirmed that the sign communication deaf people used was, in fact, a bona fide language equal to English and that deaf people were indeed members of a culture. In describing Stokoe's work, Chamot (2000) reported, "Before William Stokoe's groundbreaking research, ASL was erroneously viewed as a pantomime, a poor substitute for spoken speech. Now ASL is recognized as a language with its own syntax, morphology, and structure" (p. 1).

In the 1970s, a new philosophy of communication surfaced. This new approach was called "total communication" and comprised all forms of communication including gestures, sign language, speech, fingerspelling, lipreading, reading, and writing. The total communication philosophy quickly swept the field and was eagerly adopted by two thirds of schools for the deaf by 1976, supplanting the purely oral approach (Gannon, 1981). As a consequence, deaf people were finally able to point to the bona fide use of their language, ASL, smuggled in under the guise of total communication.

Despite the enthusiastic adoption of the total communication approach as well as sign supported speech in deaf education (Lane, Hoffmeister, & Bahan, 1996), in 1988 the Commission on the Education of the Deaf reported to the U.S. Congress that, yet again, the deaf education system had failed to provide proper education and literacy for deaf children who still demonstrated deficiencies in academic achievement (Marschark et al., 2002). The report discussed the "vital role" of ASL for deaf children and recommended that the U.S. Department of Education recognize ASL as one of the native languages for deaf children (Commission on the Education of the Deaf, 1988, p. 8). This report and the 1965 Babbidge report, both of which emphasized the overall failure of deaf education, may have helped open doors for the use of ASL within deaf schools and deaf education programs.

In 1989, the authors of *Unlocking the Curriculum,* claiming yet again that the current deaf education system was a failure, recommended early access to a natural sign language through competent models of sign language and a change from the paradigm of deaf children as inadequate based on a "defective model" to a view where they are perceived to be as normal as hearing children (Johnson et al., 1989, p. 18). This seminal manifesto may be credited as one that encouraged the consideration of bilingualism, conceptualized as the equal partnership of ASL and English, within school systems to address the academic achievement gap for deaf students.

Subsequently, beginning in 1990, educators of deaf children began to frame ASL/English bilingual education as a response to the educational needs of deaf students (Israelite, Ewoldt, & Hoffmeister, 1992; LaSasso & Lollis, 2003; Strong, 1995). The goal of ASL/English bilingual education programs is that of linguistic competency in both ASL and written English (and spoken English when appropriate) and academic achievement at or above grade level (Knight & Swanwick, 1999; Nover et al., 2002). The philosophical basis of ASL/English bilingual education programs is that ASL is acquired naturally and in similar developmental stages as other languages. Unlike spoken languages, ASL is a visual-gestural language that allows deaf children complete linguistic access to language easily and quickly (Baker, 2006; Johnson et al., 1989; Knight & Swanwick, 1999). The acquisition of second language literacy in English is built on a foundation of ASL literacy (Knight & Swanwick, 1999; Nover et al., 2002). This ASL/English bilingual philosophy is viewed as allowing deaf children access to educational content through a visual language.

Even as this ASL/English bilingual philosophy was being formulated, a different reality in deaf education sent a different message. Beginning at the end of World War II, there was a strong move toward education programs in local public schools that created the concept of mainstreaming students with disabilities, including deaf children, in regular classrooms (Moores, 2001). Mainstreaming was touted as a solution to the low standards in the field of deaf education, but there were issues with language and communication access for deaf children in integrated settings. Although some deaf children experienced academic success in these settings, many did not. In response to this, Ramsey (1997) argued that deaf children must receive education designed for them in sign language—and comprehensible—to alleviate difficulties in acquiring the basic skills needed in school. The values and attitudes of the teachers and "hearing" classmates indicated that equity in access to information was not the case. In integrated classes, teachers and hearing classmates treated deaf children as "mascots" and acted like "stern but benevolent caretakers" (Ramsey, 1997, p. 113). Ramsey argues that the goal for hearing teachers was not to educate the deaf pupils in their class but to meet the legal goal of integration.

Nonetheless, based on state mandates and the federal legislation mentioned earlier, enrollment at schools for deaf students plummeted, which meant fewer students were exposed to ASL, the language commonly associated with residential dormitories for deaf students (Lane et al., 1996; Moores, 2001). The number of deaf children attending residential schools continues to dwindle compared with rising numbers of mainstreamed deaf students with CIs (Gallaudet Research Institute, 2008; Marschark et al., 2002).

Residential state schools for deaf students were once and still are a place where sign language and Deaf culture are transmitted. With the downsizing and closure of some of these schools (see Swiller, this volume), many in the Deaf community are placing the blame not only on the laws mentioned earlier, which increased access to public education, but also on the increase in pediatric cochlear implantation and professionals recommending mainstream education for cochlear-implanted children based on the need for auditory reinforcement to facilitate the utilization of spoken language. These deaf individuals view schools for the deaf as being uniquely designed to meet the needs of deaf students.

In contrast, many parents usually enroll their deaf children in public or private schools that do not incorporate the use of sign language, perhaps because of the distance (deaf schools are few and far between) or because of concerns regarding the development of spoken language if the school does not provide educational opportunities using spoken language. Most deaf schools do provide support for spoken languages, usually in the form of a few hourly sessions a week with a speech therapist, which is insufficient in itself for the acquisition of spoken language.

In public or private schools where sign language is not emphasized or used for deaf students, there are some educational opportunities that even children with optimal benefit from CIs might not be able to fully take advantage of, such as interactions in the school cafeteria or on the playground. These environments are not conductive to listening due to poor acoustics created by high ceilings, bare floors, and other factors that create a very high noise level. Children with CIs may miss out on important social interactions with hearing peers in noisy conditions, interactions that are critical for social development and lifelong adjustment (Spencer, 2009). Sign language is 100% accessible at all times for children with CIs, especially in these noisy situations, and that is a strong argument supporting why these children need sign language in addition to spoken language.

The fact of the matter is that if traditional schools for deaf students are to survive, they must adapt to meet the needs of students with CIs to preserve their numbers and their educational strengths. Contrary to popular belief, some specialized schools have developed strategies that facilitate the educational development of students with CIs in a primarily signing environment. For example, a couple of these schools that used to adopt a 100% sign language policy except for individual or group speech therapy are now starting to incorporate spoken English classes (e.g., the Maryland School for the Deaf). These classes are for hard of hearing students or students with CIs who are able to access academic information via spoken English with very little or no sign support, which is different from speech therapy sessions with a focus on improving speech skills (articulation, pronunciation, voice pitch control, etc). The Learning Center in Framingham, Massachusetts, one of the first schools to adopt a bilingual and bicultural education approach, was also the first to incorporate spoken English classes to meet the educational needs of the growing number of deaf children with CIs (Maguire, Angelini, & Grass, 2002). The addition of spoken English classes at a prominent bilingual-bicultural school has set a model for other deaf schools. The reader is directed to part III of this book for further discussion of detailed strategies.

Despite the best intentions of deaf schools incorporating spoken language in educational programming, there is still some controversy regarding whether sign language in itself would impede the acquisition of spoken language. This is an area that requires further research, but in the meantime, other questions remain. For example, what about those children who benefit from CIs to the extent that they can function in a spoken language environment with minimal support (i.e., an FM [frequency-modulated] system)? Can they truly benefit from attending specialized schools for deaf students? Can they truly benefit from sign language, considering the documented difficulties in noisy situations? We consider these concerns briefly in the next section.

Bimodal Bilingualism

There is much controversy about whether deaf infants should be exposed to a signed language before and after implantation. One side advocates full language access via visual means while deaf infants are learning how to interpret sound transmitted via hearing aids and CIs. The other side believes that sign language would impede successful acquisition of a spoken language. In Canada, parents are encouraged to choose from several educational options, such as ASL or spoken English, but there is no option for both ASL and spoken English in the same program (Malkowski, 2009). Malkowski reported that if parents choose the spoken language route, their children are not allowed to learn ASL and are asked to leave the program if they are caught signing or learning how to sign. This extreme reaction can be explained in part by the fear that learning sign language somehow impedes the child's ability to learn how to hear and speak.

Mounting theoretical and empirical evidence shows that bilingualism in general does not impair but instead enhances the linguistic and cognitive development of hearing children, even to the point that bilinguals perform better than monolinguals on cognitive tests (Diaz, 1985; Hakuta, 1986; Hakuta & Diaz, 1985; Jiminéz, García, & Pearson, 1996). These findings support the cognitive and linguistic value of ASL and its transfer to a second language, in this case English. In fact, in the past two decades, an increase in research on ASL/English bilingualism in deaf children has found a significant correlation between ASL proficiency and English proficiency (Hoffmeister, 2000; Kuntze, 2004; Mayberry, Lock, & Kazmi, 2002; Padden & Ramsey, 1998, 2000; Prinz & Strong, 1998; Singleton, Morgan, DiGello, Wiles, & Rivers, 2004; Singleton, Supalla, Litchfield, & Schley, 1998; Strong & Prinz, 1997, 2000). Studies of the impact of early sign language exposure on the future acquisition of spoken languages do not demonstrate that signing in and of itself impedes spoken language development (Spencer, 2009).

Deaf children with CIs who are exposed to both visual and auditory languages can be described as bimodal bilinguals—individuals who use two different languages in two different modes. Signed languages are visually based in that the hands and other features of the body are used to express meaning, whereas in spoken languages, sounds manipulated by the vocal chords and mouth express meaning through audition. As discussed in the literature, there are different types of bimodal bilinguals, such as hearing individuals who use ASL and spoken English and have deaf parents (Emmorey & McCullough, 2009) and deaf individuals who read English and use ASL (Kushalnagar, Hannay, & Hernandez, 2010). In the context of this book, we describe bimodal bilinguals as individuals who can communicate using a spoken (auditorily received) and a signed (visually received) language. This definition encompasses hearing users of a spoken and signed language but also deaf individuals who can communicate using a signed language and also wear CIs, which enable some of them to understand a spoken language using auditory means only. In that sense, bimodal bilingualism as defined here is not limited by auditory status but rather defined by language mode.

In addition to the effects of auditory experiences on brain functioning, the effects of sign language experience on brain organization have been documented in the areas of motion processing, mental rotation abilities, image generation, some aspects of face processing, and short-term memory capacity. Bavelier, Dye, and Hauser (2006) reviewed the literature for the effects of auditory deprivation on cortical functions, and Emmorey and McCullough (2009) documented sign language effects on cortical functions. Deafness and using a visual language have different observable effects on brain organization. As a result of deafness, the secondary auditory cortex and associative cortical areas are altered in deaf individuals (Bavelier et al., 2006).

However, much is still not fully understood. For example, is there evidence that early exposure to sign language permanently alters and limits auditory cortical functions, particularly in the first year of life? The consequence of bimodal bilingualism on brain organization and current research regarding functional reallocation of the auditory cortex due to deafness and sign language use remain a fertile area for further research, the results of which can lead to recommendations for language learning.

Some parents are encouraged not to sign to their deaf infants before implantation, based on a fear that cortical pathways would be permanently oriented to a visual mean of communication. However, the first 12 months of life is a fertile ground for language acquisition, and language deprivation during that time period may have negative consequences for the child (Johnson & Newport, 1989; Lenneberg, 1967; Newport, 1990). Currently, CI surgeries tend to take place when the deaf infant is 12 months old, which means the first 12 months would be deprived of any language input if sign language is not utilized. Also, after implantation, approximately one year is required for the deaf infant to become accustomed to the signals conveyed by the implant to the brain and to learn how to interpret these signals as meaningful information. That would mean about two years of language learning opportunities would be lost if the deaf infant is denied access to a visual and fully accessible language. Full communication access can be achieved via a signed language for deaf infants while simultaneously maintaining auditory areas via hearing aids prior to implantation to prevent language and communication delays while preserving cortical areas critical for the acquisition of auditory-based languages.

Conclusion

In this chapter we discussed some of the issues related to CIs and their impacts on the Deaf community. CIs bring new opportunities for deaf members of the community—and new challenges as well. With early hearing detection and intervention programs in place in most states and with access to technology, more deaf children receive CIs at a very early age, which facilitates the ability to acquire spoken language skills. The roles of sign language, deaf schools, and the Deaf community for CI users continue to be in flux. However, studying the cortical functions of bimodal bilinguals allow us to get a glimpse of the potential benefits of sign language for all children, regardless of hearing status. The Deaf community can provide support and understanding to CI users by sharing similar experiences and welcoming them into the community. The rest of the chapters in this volume will provide the reader with a sense of the possibilities, necessities, and concerns occasioned by the development of CIs.

REFERENCES

Babbidge, J. (1965). *The Babbidge committee report*. Washington, DC: Department of Health, Education, and Welfare. (ERIC Document Reproduction Service No. ED014188).

Bahan, B., Bauman, D., & Montenegro, F. (Writers/Directors/Producers). (2008). *Audism unveiled* [DVD]. Washington, DC: BlackMountain Films.

Baker, C. (2006). *Foundations of bilingual education and bilingualism* (4th ed.). Buffalo, NY: Multilingual Matters.

Bauman, H. (2004). Audism: Exploring the metaphysics of oppression. *Journal of Deaf Studies and Deaf Education, 9*(2), 239–246.

Bavelier, D., Dye, M. W. G., & Hauser, P. C. (2006). Do deaf individuals see better? *Trends in Cognitive Sciences, 10*(11), 512–518.

Biernath, K., Reefhuis, J., Whitney, C., Mann, E., Costa, P., Eichwald, J., et al. (2006). Bacterial meningitis among children with cochlear implants beyond 24 months after implantation. *Pediatrics, 117*(2), 284–289.

Bradham, T., & Jones, J. (2008). Cochlear implant candidacy in the United States: Prevalence in children 12 months to 6 years of age. *International Journal of Pediatric Otorhinolaryngology, 72*(7), 1023–1028.

Branson, J., & Miller, D. (2002). *Damned for their difference: The cultural construction of deaf people as disabled*. Washington, DC: Gallaudet University Press.

Burch, S. (2002). *Signs of resistance: American Deaf cultural history, 1900–1942*. New York: New York University Press.

Centers for Disease Control and Prevention. (2003). *Infants tested for hearing loss—United States, 1999–2001*. Retrieved March 30, 2011, from http://www.cdc.gov/ncbddd/ehdi/documents/mm5241.pdf

Chamot, J. (2000). *American Sign Language spoken here*. Retrieved March 30, 2011, from http://www.nsf.gov/discoveries/disc_summ.jsp?cntn_id=100168

Chang, D., Ko, A., Murray, G., Arnold, J., & Megerian, C. (2010). Lack of financial barriers to pediatric cochlear implantation: Impact of socioeconomic status on access and outcomes. *The Archives of Otolaryngology—Head & Neck Surgery, 136*(7), 648–657.

Christiansen, J. B., & Leigh, I. W. (2005). *Cochlear implants in children: Ethics and choices*. Washington, DC: Gallaudet University Press.

Commission on the Education of the Deaf. (1988). *Toward equality: A report to the president and Congress of the United States*. Washington, DC: Government Printing Office.

Cummins, J. (2006). *The relationship between American Sign Language proficiency and English academic development: A review of the research*. Retrieved March 30, 2011, from http://aslthinktank.com/files/CumminsASL-Eng.pdf

Diaz, R. (1985). Bilingual cognitive development: Addressing three gaps in current research. *Child Development, 56*, 1376–1388.

Emmorey, K., & McCullough, S. (2009). The bilingual brain: Effects of sign language experience. *Brain and Language, 109*(2–3), 124–132.

Fayad, J., Wanna, G., Micheletto, J., & Parisier, S. (2003). Facial nerve paralysis following cochlear implant surgery. *Laryngoscope, 113*(8), 1344–1346.

Gallaudet Research Institute. (2008, November). *Regional and national summary report of data from the 2007–2008 annual survey of deaf and hard of hearing children and youth.* Washington, DC: Author.

Gallaudet University. (2011). *Gallaudet University mission and goals.* Retrieved March 30, 2011, from http://aaweb.gallaudet.edu/About_Gallaudet/Mission_and_Goals.html

Gannon, J. R. (1981). *Deaf heritage: A narrative history of deaf America.* Silver Spring, MD: National Association of the Deaf.

Grosjean, F. (2001). *Right of the deaf child to grow up bilingual.* Washington, DC: Gallaudet University Press.

Hakuta, K. (1986). *Mirror of language: The debate on bilingualism.* New York: Basic Books.

Hakuta, K., & Diaz, R. (1985). The relationship between degree of bilingualism and cognitive ability: A critical discussion and some new longitudinal data. In K. Nelson (Ed.), *Children's language* (Vol. 5, pp. 319–344). Hillsdale, NJ: Erlbaum.

Harris, R. (2011). A case study of extended discourse in an ASL/English bilingual preschool classroom. Unpublished doctoral dissertation, Gallaudet University, Washington, DC.

Hoffmeister, R. (2000). A piece of the puzzle: ASL and reading comprehension in deaf children. In C. Chamberlain, J. Morford, & R. Mayberry (Eds.), *Language acquisition by eye* (pp. 143–163). Mahwah, NJ: Erlbaum.

Indiana University School of Medicine. (2010). Word learning better in deaf children who receive cochlear implants by age 13 months. *ScienceDaily.* Retrieved March 1, 2010, from http://www.sciencedaily.com/releases/2010/02/100221143158.htm

Israelite, N., Ewoldt, C., & Hoffmeister, R. (1992). *Bilingual/bicultural education for deaf and hard-of-hearing students: A review of the literature on the effective use of native sign language on the acquisition of a majority language by hearing-impaired students.* Toronto, Canada: MGS Publications Services.

Jiminéz, R., García, G., & Pearson, P. (1996). The reading strategies of bilingual Latina/o students who are successful English readers: Opportunities and obstacles. *Reading Research Quarterly, 31*(1), 90–112.

Johnson, J., & Newport, E. (1989). Critical period effects in second language learning: The influence of maturational state on the acquisition of English as a second language. *Cognitive Psychology, 21*(1), 60–99.

Johnson, R., Liddell, S., & Erting, C. (1989). *Unlocking the curriculum: Principles for achieving access in deaf education.* Washington, DC: Gallaudet Research Institute.

King, T. (2010, July). *Identification and management of children with hearing impairment in the medical home.* Paper presented at the Maryland Early Hearing Detection and Intervention Stakeholders meeting, Baltimore, MD.

Knight, P., & Swanwick, R. (1999). *Working with deaf pupils: Sign bilingual policy into practice.* London: David Fulton.

Kuntze, M. (2004). Literacy acquisition and deaf children: A study of the interaction between ASL and written English (Doctoral dissertation, Stanford University). *ProQuest Digital Dissertations database.* (AAT No. 3128664).

Kushalnagar, P., Hannay, J., & Hernandez, A. (2010). Bilingualism and attention: A study of balanced and unbalanced bilingual deaf users of American Sign Language and English. *Journal of Deaf Studies and Deaf Education, 15*(3), 263–273.

Lane, H. (1984). *When the mind hears.* New York: Random House.

Lane, H., Hoffmeister, R., & Bahan, B. (1996). *A journey into the Deaf-World.* San Diego, CA: DawnSignPress.

LaSasso, C., & Lollis, J. (2003). Survey of residential and day schools for deaf students in the United States that identify themselves as bilingual-bicultural programs. *Journal of Deaf Studies and Deaf Education, 8*(1), 79–91.

Leigh, I. W. (2009). *A lens on deaf identities.* New York: Oxford University Press.

Lenneberg, E. (1967). *Biological foundations of language.* New York: Wiley.

Maguire, N., Angelini, S., & Grass, W. (2002). The Learning Center for Deaf Children: Framingham and Randolph, Massachusetts. In D. Nussbaum, R. LaPorta, & J. Hinger (Eds.), *Cochlear implants and sign language: Putting it all together (Identifying Effective Practices for Educational Settings) April 11–12, 2002, conference proceedings* (pp. 56–62). Washington, DC: Gallaudet University.

Malkowski, G. (2009). The situation in Canada. *Deaf Studies Digital Journal,* (1). Retrieved March 30, 2011, from http://dsdj.gallaudet.edu

Marschark, M., Lang, H., & Albertini, J. (2002). *Educating deaf students.* New York: Oxford University Press.

Mayberry, R. I., Lock, E., & Kazmi, H. (2002). Linguistic ability and early language exposure. *Nature, 417*(6884), 38.

Moores, D. F. (2001). *Educating the deaf: Psychology, principles, and practices.* Boston: Houghton Mifflin.

Newport, E. (1990). Maturational constraints on language learning. *Cognitive Science, 14*(1), 11–28.

Niparko, J. (2009). *Cochlear implants: Principles & practices.* Philadelphia: Lippincott Williams & Wilkins.

Niparko, J., Tobey, E., Thai, D., Eisenberg, L., Wang, N., Quittner, A., et al. (2010). Spoken language development in children following cochlear implantation. *JAMA, 303*(15), 1498–1506.

Nover, S., Andrews, J., Baker, S., Everhart, V., & Bradford, M. (2002). *Critical pedagogy in deaf education: Bilingual methodology and staff development: Year 5 (2001–2002).* Santa Fe: New Mexico School for the Deaf.

Padden, C., & Ramsey, C. (1998). Reading ability in signing deaf children. *Topics in Language Disorders, 18*(4), 30–46.

Padden, C., & Ramsey, C. (2000). American Sign Language and reading ability in deaf children. In C. Chamberlain, J. Morford, & R. Mayberry (Eds.), *Language acquisition by eye* (pp. 165–189). Mahwah, NJ: Erlbaum.

Prinz, P., & Strong, M. (1998). ASL proficiency and English literacy within a bilingual deaf education model of instruction. *Topics in Language Disorders, 18*(4), 47–60.

Ramsey, C. (1997). *Deaf children in public schools: Placement, context and consequences.* Washington, DC: Gallaudet University Press.

Ramsey, C., & Padden, C. (1998). Natives and newcomers: Gaining access to literacy in a classroom for deaf children. *Anthropology & Education quarterly, 29*(1), 5–24.

Singleton, J., Morgan, D., DiGello, E., Wiles, J., & Rivers, R. (2004). Vocabulary use by low, moderate, and high ASL-proficient writers compared to hearing ESL and monolingual speakers. *Journal of Deaf Studies and Deaf Education, 9*(1), 86–103.

Singleton, J., Supalla, S., Litchfield, S., & Schley, S. (1998). From sign to word: Considering modality constraints in ASL/English bilingual education. *Topics in Language Disorders, 18*(4), 16–29.

Sorkin, D. (2010, July). *The role of early intervention professionals in cochlear implant outcomes.* Paper presented at the International Congress on the Education of the Deaf, Vancouver, British Columbia, Canada.

Spencer, P. (2009, April). *Research to practice.* Paper presented at the Cochlear Implants and Sign Language: Building Foundations for Effective Educational Practices conference, Washington, DC.

States That Recognize ASL. (2004). *States that recognize American sign language as a foreign language.* Retrieved March 30, 2011, from http://www.ncssfl.org/links/ASL.pdf

Stokoe, W., Casterline, D., Croneberg, C. (1965). *A dictionary of American Sign Language on linguistic principles.* Washington, DC: Gallaudet College Press.

Strong, M. (1995). A review of bilingual/bicultural programs for deaf children in North America. *American Annals of the Deaf, 140*(2), 84–94.

Strong, M., & Prinz, P. (1997). A study of the relationship between ASL and English literacy. *Journal of Deaf Studies and Deaf Education, 2*(1), 37–46.

Strong, M., & Prinz, P. (2000). Is American Sign Language skill related to English literacy? In C. Chamberlain, J. Morford, & R. Mayberry (Eds.), *Language acquisition by eye* (pp. 131–141). Mahwah, NJ: Erlbaum.

Tait, M., Nikolopoulos, T. P., De Raeve, L., Johnson, S., Datta, G., Karltorp, E., et al. (2010). Bilateral versus unilateral cochlear implantation in young children. *International Journal of Pediatric Otorhinolaryngology, 74*(2), 206–211.

Vygotsky, L. (1986). *Thought and language.* Cambridge: Massachusetts Institute of Technology Press.

Winzer, M. (1993). *The history of special education: From isolation to integration.* Washington, DC: Gallaudet University Press.

2

GENETIC RESEARCH, BIOETHICAL ISSUES, AND COCHLEAR IMPLANTS: AN OVERVIEW OF THE ISSUES AFFECTING THE DEAF COMMUNITY

Jane Dillehay

> *Not everything that is faced can be changed, but nothing can be changed until it is faced.*
>
> —*James Baldwin*

The Deaf community has always had flexibility and foresight in adapting to innovative developments in technology. The products of researchers and engineers from hearing aids to telecommunication devices to the Internet and vlogs have been rapidly incorporated into Deaf culture and used to strengthen the Deaf community. As the National Association of the Deaf (NAD) position paper on cochlear implants (2000) states,

> The NAD recognizes all technological advancements with the potential to foster, enhance, and improve the quality of life of all deaf and hard of hearing persons. During the past three decades, technological developments . . . have had an important role in leveling the playing field. The role of the cochlear implant is evolving and will certainly change in the future.

It remains to be seen whether the current and rapidly accelerating advances in genetics research and the steadily increasing frequency of cochlear implantations will improve or jeopardize the future of the Deaf community.

Consequences of the Human Genome Project

A genome is the total sum of DNA, or genetic material, in each cell of an organism. The goal of the Human Genome Project was to understand human genetics by sequencing human DNA to create a map of the approximately 25,000 genes that make up a person. The complete sequencing of the human genome was first achieved in 2003, and the genome information for an ever-increasing number of humans and other species was made available to all researchers through Internet databases. Current research efforts focus on when and how genes are activated to produce the cell machinery necessary for life (U.S. Department of Energy Office of Science, Human Genome Program, 2009).

While mapping the genomes of different species continues to be an important endeavor, the next step in understanding how an organism functions is at the level of the proteome, which is the complete set of proteins produced by each cell or organism. Studying the proteome is a far more complex process because the genome is reasonably constant over time but the proteome changes from cell to cell and from conception to maturity to death, depending on gene activities. Therefore deciphering the proteome, including the structure and function of each cell protein and the complex interaction of thousands of proteins within and among cells and tissues, will be the next important step for developing an understanding of normal human physiology and therapeutic strategies for various conditions.

In addition to the tremendous increase in genome databases, increasing sophistication in research tools—rapid-sequencing low-cost genomic technology, software analytic algorithms, selective breeding of mouse genetic models—to cite a few examples, have come together to create a synergistic explosion of knowledge with breakthroughs identifying genes for given conditions almost daily. Although some genomic applications for the treatment of genetic conditions have progressed to the stage of human clinical trials, this is not yet the case for genes and proteins that modulate hearing.

GENETICS OF HEARING LOSS

Estimates of the prevalence of hearing loss in the American population vary widely depending on the survey methodology used. One recent study estimates the prevalence for speech-frequency hearing loss in one or both ears at 29 million Americans and for high-frequency hearing loss at 55 million based on survey data from the National Health and Nutrition Examination Survey 1999–2004 (Agrawal, Platz, & Niparko, 2008). This relatively high incidence of hearing loss in comparison to other disabilities is a motivating factor for providing federal funding for research to understand how hearing works and ultimately to discover therapeutic approaches for people who desire a change in their hearing status. It should be noted that this survey does not distinguish among causes of hearing loss, whether genetic, environmental, or some combination of the two, or age of onset of hearing loss.

Nance (2003) notes that hearing loss is an extremely complex condition with multiple known causes, both genetic and environmental, due to the orchestration of the many physical and biochemical interactions required to accomplish the task of hearing, from the mechanical structures of the ear to the conversion of sound to nerve impulses conducted via the auditory nerve to the brain's auditory complex for interpretation. For the Deaf community, it is important to distinguish between early-onset deafness with severe to profound loss—often due to mutations in a single gene (Mendelian inheritance) and found in a significant number of deaf individuals—and late-onset milder and progressive hearing loss—due to interaction among genes and environmental factors (multifactorial inheritance) and found in greater frequency in the aging population (Arnos, 2008; Brownstein & Avraham, 2006).

Approximately 50% to 60% of the cases of severe to profound congenital deafness or early-onset deafness are due to genetic causes, with an estimated incidence of 126 per 100,000 at birth and a prevalence of 146 per 100,000 at 4 years of age (Morton & Nance, 2006), a rate of incidence that is much lower than the rates cited above from the National Health and Nutrition Examination Survey. Researchers in the past decades before the Human Genome Project identified more than 110 genes for deafness (Arnos, 2002; Hereditary Hearing Loss Homepage, 2008; Morton & Nance, 2006) and the genes for more than 40 have been cloned for research purposes (Deafness Gene Mutation Database, 2010).

Current Genetics Research in Deafness

Human genome research is now leading to a deeper understanding of the roles of specific genes and their products in the hearing process as well as an accelerated rate of success in the identification of additional genes and proteins. It is not possible to give a comprehensive report of findings because of the rapid pace of discovery, but representative examples can be cited.

To see examples of research into progressive hearing loss, see the July 2009 quarterly newsletter of hear-it.org, which briefly describes several gene mutations: the *KCNQ4* gene is associated with age-related hearing loss as well as with Jervell and Lange-Nielson syndrome, which causes profound congenital deafness (Van Eyken et al., 2006); the *HSP70* gene is associated with increased risk of noise-induced hearing loss (Konings et al., 2009); mutations of the *SLC17A8* gene are linked to congenital hearing loss with diminished ability to hear high-frequency sounds (Ruel et al., 2008); and the *TGBF1* gene is linked to hearing loss due to otosclerosis (Thys et al., 2007).

These examples may not be directly relevant to the concerns of the Deaf community; nevertheless, the interconnected nature of scientific research means that work in one area may ultimately affect other areas of more immediate concern. Therefore, being aware of genetic research on the function of the cochlea and inner ear is a wise strategy. For example, the identification of the genes cited above leads to the probability of locating mutations to be used for genetic screening, as has occurred for the *GJB2* and *SLC26A4* genes, which play a role in connexin 26 and Pendred syndromes, respectively (Nance, 2003; Smith & Robin, 2002).

Pendred syndrome is an example of early-onset deafness caused by mutation in a single gene and is considered relatively common, with an incidence of 3% of newborns screened for hearing (Morton & Nance, 2006). This is one example of the more than 300 forms of syndromic hearing loss that have been identified. Mutations in the *GJB2* gene, which affects cochlear function, are found in 20% to 30% of all cases of early-onset severe to profound deafness that are nonsyndromic (i.e., lacking identifying characteristics other than hearing loss; Arnos et al., 2008) and has a unique effect on the Deaf community, which will be discussed in a later section.

Other genomic studies have identified several genes, such as *ATOH1*, *POU4F3*, and *GFI1*, that are responsible for hair cell differentiation and maintenance (Pauley, Kopecky, Beisel, Soukup, & Fritszch, 2008). The sensory hair cells with their stereocilia extensions found in the cochlea of the inner ear are the machinery that translates the physical vibrations of sound waves into electrochemical pulses that in turn stimulate the auditory nerve. Proteomic research has identified at least two classes of proteins—cadherins and harmonins—that build "switches" in cell membranes. When the mechanical vibrations strike the stereocilia, these switches open channels in the membranes to permit the flow of ions, which in turn creates tiny electric currents to stimulate the auditory nerve (Grillet, Xiong et al., 2009). Continuing research is underway to study how these genes and their products function in hearing.

U. Mueller's lab searched for potential genes involved in progressive hearing loss by using a technique called "forward genetics" to create random mutations in mouse germ cells and test the resulting offspring for hearing loss (Grillet, Schwander et al., 2009). After several generations of breeding, they created a new strain of mice with a mutation in a previously uncharacterized gene identified as *loxhd1*. Mice with two copies of the mutation became profoundly deaf after birth. The researchers found that the *loxhd1* mutations did not affect fetal development of the stereocilia but impaired the subsequent function and maintenance of these structures, leading to progressive hearing loss. Mutations in the *loxhd1* gene have now been found in some families with hearing loss (Grillet, Schwandler et al., 2009). The lab is now attempting to identify therapeutic drugs to reverse the molecular damage to the stereocilia in the mouse strain.

Davis (2003) has reported that two neurotrophin proteins in the cochlea—brain-derived neurotrophic factor and neurotrophin-3—are important for the effective relay of sounds to the auditory cortex of the brain. Neurotrophins stimulate the growth of nerve cells in the brain, but in the cochlea, they change the sensory neurons into either fast-firing transmitters to carry high-pitched sound messages to the brain or slow-firing transmitters to carry lower pitched signals. The neurotrophins accomplish this at the molecular level in hair cells by regulating a newly discovered series of signaling proteins used to coordinate cell activities both in individual cells and among groups of cells.

K. B. Avraham's lab (Lilach et al., 2009) has studied microRNAs, single-stranded RNA molecules that regulate gene expression and control the production of proteins. The healthy ear begins with 15,000 hair cells in the cochlea at birth. These cells can die off over time, leading to progressive hearing loss. Avraham's lab studied the functioning of microRNAs in the inner ears of mice and found that inactivating specific microRNAs led to loss of hair cells. This has implications for a therapeutic approach to prevent the loss of hair cells.

Currently, loss of hair cell function due to aging and environmental damage causes hearing loss in 10% of people worldwide. In humans and other mammals, the ability to grow new hair cells is lost before birth, so any damage after birth is irreversible (Deafness Research UK, 2006). A study by Douglas Cotanche in 1987 showing that chickens could regenerate hair cells after acoustic trauma gave hope for hair cell regeneration in humans.

The labs of D. Raible and E. Ruble at the University of Washington have collaborated on using the external lateral line hair cells of zebrafish as a model to identify both genetic mutations and drugs to confer protection against hair cell damage or stimulate hair cell regeneration (Owen, Coffin, Raible, & Rubel, 2009). Recent discovery of a line of deaf zebrafish has made possible the comparison of the genomes of hearing and deaf zebrafish strains, leading to the characterization of a specific gene coding for a protein (*Tmie*) that is involved in the mechanoelectrical transduction function of stereocilia (Gleason et al., 2009). The zebrafish model appears to be a promising approach for a better understanding of the genetic and physical components of hair cell function.

Two promising strategies for mammalian hair cell regeneration are transplantation or the induction of stem cells in the cochlea and the use of gene therapy to induce the remaining cells in the cochlea to differentiate into hair cells (Pauley et al., 2008). Such studies remain at the experimental stage and have not progressed to human clinical trials.

Brownstein and Avraham (2006) have reviewed approaches for future treatment of sensorineural hearing loss through vectors for gene therapy, manipulation of cell cycle regulation for hair cell regeneration, and stem cell treatment.

In 2008, J. V. Brigande's lab successfully transferred the hair cell gene *ATOH1* via viral transfection to the developing inner ears of embryonic mice (National Institute on Deafness and Other Communication Disorders, 2008). As a result, after birth the hair cell count was higher than normal in the treated mice. The next step will be gene transfer into deaf mice to determine whether hearing is restored.

Chen et al. (2009) were able to isolate human auditory stem cells from fetal cochleae. These cells retained the ability to differentiate into sensory hair cells and neurons. This new stem cell line gives researchers the ability to study the development of human cochlear neurons and hair cells and study therapeutic approaches to hair cell damage.

These studies are just a sampling of the avalanche of knowledge that is published and shared with researchers worldwide on the cellular mechanisms of hearing. Left unaddressed in this review is the work of researchers on untangling the gene-protein interactions in cell cycle regulation and cell-cell signaling systems that regulate the development of the functioning inner ear. Other researchers are studying the actual physical orientation of filaments and membranes in the inner ear through electron tomography. This rapidly accelerating wave of information not only is the beginning of a revolution in understanding the mechanism of human hearing but also has implications for the unintended consequences of controversial biotechnologies, which leads to our next topic.

Introduction to Bioethics

> Current developments in genomics challenge the established framework of biomedical ethics because the empirical facts of the genomic science change too fast for the reflections of ethics to keep pace. At the same time, as practical applications of new technologies are being developed, scientists call for pragmatic moral guidance. (Lunshof, Chadwick, Vorhaus, & Church, 2008, p. 406)

Callahan (2003) discusses the historical foundations of bioethics. Medical ethics had its origins in the Hippocratic oath and in the moral precepts of religion. In the late 1960s the field of bioethics developed in response to the inability of medical ethics to respond effectively to biomedical advances to protect the rights of medical patients and human research subjects. This early or traditional bioethics was based on four moral principles, which are self-explanatory:

1. Autonomy—freedom of informed choice and self-determination
2. Nonmaleficence, "cause no harm"
3. Beneficence—treatment or research should benefit the patient or subject
4. Justice—equal and fair treatment

However the continuing pace of change and the new issues arising, from biobanking to human gene patents to stem cell research and human cloning, go beyond traditional bioethics approaches and call for a more contemporary bioethics paradigm to guide society. Callahan (2003) raises three issues:

1. Future biomedical technology may be able to enhance people's physical and genetic characteristics. What should be the ethical standard for use of this technology?

2. What health standards should we establish as a result of this biomedical technology? What kind of biomedical research is acceptable to achieve these standards?
3. How will we define what is a human being? What ways of life are acceptable and how do we reconcile the individual's right to choose versus society's needs?

Although Callahan's questions are proposed to society as a whole, the Deaf community should consider these questions to be able to explain its point of view to hearing society. Possible questions to ask within Callahan's framework are the following:

1. Is restoration of hearing to deaf and hard of hearing people an enhancement or a compensation for hearing loss? Depending on the perspective, should the Deaf community oppose such restoration as an unethical enhancement of the human body or support it as an appropriate compensation?
2. What should the social standards be for diversity in health and physical condition? Can general support for disability as a category of diversity occur in society? There is some precedent for acceptance of disability as such a category by the American Psychological Association in its *Ethical principles of psychologists and code of conduct* (2002).
3. Does the Deaf community as a cultural group of human beings have the right to exist and lead lives as culturally Deaf people?

The leaders of the Human Genome Project understood that the discoveries of this project would have a significant impact on society in unanticipated ways and agreed that ethical studies would be as important as the actual discoveries themselves.

> The U.S. Department of Energy (DOE) and the National Institutes of Health (NIH) devoted 3% to 5% of their annual Human Genome Project (HGP) budgets toward studying the ethical, legal, and social issues (ELSI) surrounding availability of genetic information. This represents the world's largest bioethics program, which has become a model for ELSI programs around the world. (U.S. Department of Energy Office of Science, Human Genome Program, 2008, para.1)

The ethical, legal, and social issues Web page of the Human Genome Project identifies multiple social concerns that could and are developing based on the information being collected through genome studies, including but not limited to the issues of fair use of genetic information, privacy rights, the psychological impact of genetic differences, the use of genetic information in reproductive decision making, and the education of doctors and other health service providers, patients, and the general public in genetic capabilities and the potential implications for human life.

In response to increasing concerns about biotechnology worldwide, the United Nations Educational Scientific and Cultural Organization approved a Declaration of Bioethics and Human Rights in 2005 to set bioethical standards in support of human dignity and fundamental freedoms. This includes a recognition that health does not depend only on medical research but also on psychosocial and cultural factors that promote the welfare of individuals and communities. Since this has significant implications for the Deaf community, this declaration should be carefully considered as part of the discussion on how genetic research and cochlear implant technology might affect the Deaf community.

It is particularly urgent for the Deaf community to become educated about the implications of genome research since, as has been noted, about 50% to 60% of severe to profound congenital and early-onset deafness is due to genetic causes (Morton & Nance, 2006). As a case in point, recessive mutations in the *GJB2* gene for connexin 26 account for approximately 50% of deafness in some populations (Nance, 2003). Arnos et al. (2008) studied alumni of Gallaudet University to compare the number of deaf and hearing offspring of contemporary marriages of deaf individuals with data collected from marriages of deaf people from 100 to 200 years ago and found a fivefold increase in the number of deaf couples who only had deaf children in contemporary times. The *GJB2* gene is the cause of deafness in the vast majority of families of deaf parents who have only deaf children. This provides strong evidence for an increase in the frequency of *GJB2* deafness in the United States in the past 200 years. The study predicts that the future Deaf community will be increasingly composed of individuals with *GJB2* deafness.

DNA markers for the *GJB2* mutations have been identified and are being used for genetic screening for different purposes: diagnostic (to determine the genetic status of a person), carrier (to determine whether hearing people carry a recessive gene for deafness), and prenatal (to determine the genetic status of a fetus). In light of the increasing number of Deaf community members with *GJB2* deafness, the existence of genetic screening for their condition will have an impact on their lives. The purposes served by genetic screening for deafness can be either positive (for example, increase self-knowledge about personal hearing status, guide individuals in mate selection, and enable expectant parents to prepare for their infants' special needs) or negative (selective elimination of unwanted genetic characteristics). One thing is clear: with the accelerating pace of technological development, more than 900 tests for a wide range of genetic conditions are already available, with new tests announced regularly and sometimes made available directly to consumers (U.S. National Library of Medicine, 2010).

The Deaf community and its advocacy groups have not yet addressed the long-term ethical implications of potential applications of genome research and genetic technology to deafness. However the response to cochlear implants provides some thoughts on how to frame a response to these issues.

The Ethical Use of Cochlear Implants: Deaf Positions

Vigorous debate in the late 1990s about the ethical use of cochlear implants addressed issues such as the validity of the sociocultural model of deafness as a life to be lived versus the medical model of deafness as a condition to be cured; the implication of the lesser worth of Deaf people inherent in "fixing" their deafness; whether surgical intervention for a non–life-threatening condition is justifiable; balancing parental rights and informed consent for cochlear implantation of young deaf children; the question of decision making for the future of deaf children by parents, society, or the Deaf community; and, ultimately, the potential ethnocide of Deaf culture. Komesaroff (2007) provides an excellent review of these debates.

Bioethicists Hladek (2002) and Levy (2002) and scholars Hyde and Power (2006) continue to discuss this controversial issue. Hladek and Levy take the utilitarian position that cochlear implants are morally justifiable because they provide the potential for an open future for deaf children, enabling their access to hearing society. On the other hand, Hyde and Power argue that parents are not provided with complete information about all the options for their deaf children, including Deaf culture; thus they are denied truly informed consent.

The NAD Position Statement on Cochlear Implants

In 2000 the NAD posted a carefully thought-out position statement on cochlear implants that advocates the wellness model "preserving and promoting the psychosocial integrity of deaf" people rather than the medical model of deafness as an abnormal condition to be repaired. Within the framework of the wellness model, NAD

> recognizes the rights of parents to make informed choices for their deaf and hard of hearing children, respects their choice to use cochlear implants and all other assistive devices, and strongly supports the development of the whole child and of language and literacy. (NAD Position Paper on Cochlear Implants, 2000).

The NAD recommendations are thorough, balanced, and proactive:

- In-service training programs on the wellness model for medical professionals.
- Creation of cochlear implant teams of medical and rehabilitation staff and counselors for long-term support of implant recipients.

- Long-term commitment to habilitation strategies and psychological support by parents and support staff.
- Fair and equitable insurance coverage.
- Longitudinal research on the outcomes of childhood implants on communication and psychological development.
- Presentation of all options for deaf children, including Deaf culture and discussion of the benefits and risks of surgery to parents to ensure informed consent. (NAD, 2000)

However, one aspect of the NAD position paper should be revisited in the statement, "A pre-lingually deafened child . . . does not have the auditory foundation that makes learning a spoken language easy." This is not supported by more recent research. Neville and Bavelier (2002) have studied the effect of sensory deprivation on the brain's ability to organize itself (neuroplasticity) and found that in deaf people the auditory cortex reorganized to take on other functions, such as peripheral vision. These findings of brain plasticity are also supported by Moore and Shannon (2009), who state that implantation at an early age is important for successful auditory response and prevents loss of auditory function by cortex reorganization to support visual functions. We may conclude from this research that there are critical periods for brain development; therefore, it is reasonable to recommend early stimulation of the auditory cortex through cochlear implants for congenitally deaf children.

In addition, Schorr, Roth, and Fox (2008) studied 37 congenitally deaf children with cochlear implants and found that the children reported improved quality of life due to their cochlear implants. Earlier age of implantation was linked to better quality of life ratings. The authors concluded that the study reinforced the need for early detection and intervention for children with hearing loss to ensure the best possible outcomes.

PARALLELS TO DEAF CONCERNS—THE LITTLE PEOPLE OF AMERICA AND NEURODIVERSITY GROUPS

Founded in 1957, the Little People of America ([LPA] http://www.lpaonline.org/) is an organization equivalent to the NAD and advocates issues that affect people with dwarfism or, more formally, people of short stature. As does the NAD, the LPA provides social support and education for people with dwarfism and advocates its members' right to contribute to the diversity of our society. Medical advancements and genetics research have affected this group of people in ways similar to the Deaf community.

The LPA has developed several position statements to address these concerns, again similar to the NAD approach. In 2006 LPA posted a statement on extended limb lengthening (ELL), a surgical procedure that achieves symmetrical lengthening of arm and leg bones in people of short stature. This document has striking parallels to the NAD cochlear implant statement as it begins with a statement that LPA neither advocates nor condemns the surgical practice and recognizes that it has created controversy in the LPA community (LPA, 2006). It raises the similar concern of whether surgical intervention for a non–life-threatening condition is justifiable.

The LPA recommendations cover issues such as the following:

- Creation of ELL teams with medical and rehabilitation staff and counselors for long-term support of ELL patients.
- Long-term commitment to habilitation strategies and psychological support by support staff.
- Longitudinal research on the outcomes of ELL surgery.
- Consideration of the benefits and risks to ensure fully informed consent.
- Age of prospective patients so that they can participate in the decision making process. (Little People of America, 2006)

It is interesting that two groups with disabilities who identify themselves in cultural terms have a similar response to the impact of technology and similar language in their position statements.

However, in contrast to the NAD, the LPA has also addressed the implications of genetics research with position statements on both genetic research and preimplantation genetic diagnosis (PGD). The LPA's *Position statement on genetic discoveries in dwarfism* (2009) begins,

> The short statured community and society in general have become increasingly aware of eugenics movements (efforts to improve human qualities by selection of certain traits) in medical history in the U.S. and abroad and the traditional desire of parents to create perfect, healthy children. Along with other persons affected by genetic disorders, we are not only concerned as to how our health needs will be met under dramatically changing health care systems, but how the use of genetic technologies will affect our quality of life, medically, as well as socially. What will be the impact of the identification of the genes causing dwarfism, not only on our personal lives and our needs, but on how society views us as individuals? (LPA, 2009)

The LPA has also addressed the ethical implications of PGD (otherwise known as embryo screening), a procedure that allows prospective parents to screen embryos for a genetic condition and then carry to term children with an acceptable genotype (LPA, 2007). The most common forms of dwarfism are autosomal dominant genetic conditions. For couples with dwarfism with a dominant condition such as achondroplasia, there is a 25% chance that their child will have a homozygous dominant genotype, that is, will possess two copies of the dominant mutation that is lethal in the newborn. To avoid the heartbreak of carrying a child to term and then discover that the child will die, couples with this type of dwarfism welcome PGD to prevent pregnancies in which the child will not survive after birth. However, PGD also identifies embryos that have one copy of the genetic condition for dwarfism as well as unaffected embryos. LPA's position is that parents with dwarfism have the right to choose to implant the dwarf embryo; that the decision should be between the parents and their physician; and that parents should not be forced to have only children without dwarfism.

In 2008 the British Parliament enacted the Human Fertilisation and Embryology Bill with multiple amendments of their similar Act of 1990. One of the amendments specified that persons or embryos with known genetic abnormalities leading to the possibility of developing a physical or mental disability "must not be preferred" as donors or for use in implantation of an embryo into a host mother (U.K. Parliament, 2008). In other words, actively choosing to have a dwarf baby, or in the case of deaf parents, a deaf baby, is illegal under British law. This, in turn, implies that the British government's position is that children with physical or mental disabilities have lesser value or are not worthy of life. Burke (2007) points out that the language of the bill encompasses people with more than 1,300 known genetic conditions, a steadily expanding category due to current genetics research, who presumably will not be permitted to donate gametes for reproductive purposes or have access to reproductive services in the United Kingdom.

In light of this action by the British Parliament, which appears to devalue disability as part of human diversity, the LPA position statement ends movingly:

> For the vast majority of people with dwarfism, having a dwarfing condition creates physical and social challenges, but does not diminish the value of our lives and the diversity and perspective we add to our society. While we rejoice in the new prenatal medical technologies that have recently become available, we are committed to their being employed judiciously—ensuring that all ethical implications are thoughtfully and carefully considered. History has all too many accounts of earlier societies in which disastrous decisions were made about which individuals were to be deemed "worthy of life." (LPA, 2007)

There are obvious parallels for the rights of deaf parents to have deaf children. Genetic testing is increasingly available for families with a history of deafness. Genetic screening can currently test a limited number of genes, and that means that physicians and genetic counselors can provide diagnosis, identification of carriers, and reproductive counseling (Smith & Hone, 2003). It is reasonable to anticipate that an increasing number of genes will be tested in clients as genome research moves from the lab to clinical applications. It will be important for physicians and counselors to understand the limitations of genetic testing and explain those limitations to their patients/clients (Smith & Robin, 2002).

An interesting new development is the concept of neurodiversity, which arose from the disability rights movement in the past few years (Solomon, 2008) and argues that variations in neurodevelopment such as autism and other neurological conditions (dyslexia, attention deficit/hyperactivity disorder, and bipolar conditions, to cite a few) are part of the range of human diversity and should be valued as alternative ways of being. Researchers are engaged in tracking down gene variants related to the autism spectrum (Kalb, 2009). One example of the application of genetic screening technology readily available in medical centers is that approximately 90% of fetuses identified as carrying Down syndrome are terminated each year. Organizations such as the Autistic Self-Advocacy Network logically infer that this will apply to their conditions as well, thus depriving society of their unique talents. It would serve the Deaf community well to observe the ethical arguments and the fates of these neurodiversity groups.

Clearly the LPA has taken the lead in considering the implications of biomedical applications that other disability groups are beginning to address. As Nance (2003) states, both genomic research and cochlear implants present an ethical dilemma for society and the Deaf community, particularly in light of the fact that most deaf children are born to hearing parents. On a more positive note, advances in genetic knowledge have the potential to empower deaf couples to make informed reproductive decisions by allowing them to know whether their children will be hearing or deaf. On the other hand, the British Human Fertilisation and Embryology Bill of 2008 may prove to be the forerunner of a paternalistic hearing culture that regulates reproductive decisions for deaf individuals.

As Leigh (2009) comments, a careful social balancing act is required between valuing diverse kinds of human lives and the empowerment inherent in genetic technology for making decisions never before possible about human characteristics. "The increasing prevalence and acceptability of genetic testing, together with the real possibility of institutional eradication of genes of deafness based on political decisions" (p. 164) forces us to consider the impact of decisions made by the majority hearing culture in using this technology and the consequences for the long-term survival of the Deaf community.

Other Relevant Ethical Concerns for Cochlear Implants

An estimated 120,000 deaf people have had cochlear implants in the past decade (Moore & Shannon, 2009). In considering the millions of deaf people worldwide, this is barely scratching the surface. Access to cochlear implantation surgery and rehabilitation services is heavily dependent on adequate health insurance or government commitment to providing this service. Clearly, for people who do not have health insurance or who live in developing countries, cochlear implantation is unattainable. Hyde and Power (2006) have done research that shows that there are significant inequities in medical access to cochlear implantation surgery in First World countries. Gross inequities in medical access in the developing world mean that these countries have large populations of deaf people with limited or no access to cochlear implantation surgery (Tarabichi et al., 2008). One responsibility that the American Deaf community should consider is how to assist deaf Americans without health insurance and deaf people in developing countries to improve the quality of their lives.

Current surgical techniques "include direct electrical stimulation of the brain, bilateral implants and implantation in children less than 1 year old" (Moore & Shannon, 2009). Concerns of the Deaf community about implantation in infants must be balanced with increasing understanding of neuroplasticity in the infant brain, the importance of stimulating the auditory cortex (Neville & Bavelier, 2002), and studies that show quality of life is directly linked to age at first use of cochlear implants (Schorr et al., 2008).

Additionally, Moore and Shannon (2009) note that brain stimulation with an implant may be more critical to successful use of cochlear implants than improving the implant technology itself. Little is known about cochlear implant users' ability to perceive environmental sounds, but effective perception of those sounds has been shown to be a reliable predictor of success in using cochlear implants (Shafiro, Gygi, Cheng, Vachhani, & Mulvey, 2009). Therefore effective rehabilitation strategies are an increasingly important but little addressed area of cochlear implantation in which the needs of cochlear implant users have not been adequately met. To ensure a satisfactory auditory quality of life for a cochlear implant user, the implantation surgery is a necessary but insufficient step to guarantee user satisfaction. An intensive program of rehabilitation therapy and guided brain stimulation to teach the cochlear implant user how to make sense of auditory stimuli are critical components for successful adaptation to the cochlear implant.

Conclusion

It is not possible to address every possible issue in this chapter because the intersection of genome research and medical development of cochlear implants with the concept of human rights inherent in bioethics and the immediate personal concerns of deaf and hearing people creates a complex tangle of conflicting moral, cultural, social, and personal rights and responsibilities on a foundation of rapidly accelerating discoveries in biomedical research. This is not reason for despair but cause for hope that in our plural and diverse society there is recognition of and respect for people with disabilities.

Caulfield and Brownsword (2006) point out, "In a pluralistic society there needs to be room to discuss and debate all perspectives that inform the content of human dignity. . . . [with the caveat that] not all perspectives should serve as a justification for science policy" (p. 76). Reindahl (2000) notes that "the right to define has been an instrument of power. . . . in the oppression of, and discrimination against, people" (p. 95). Nondisabled researchers persist in placing deafness within a medical model of disability and insist on the right to define who is disabled and what disability is. If the bioethical discussions of genome research and cochlear implantation do not include the full participation and viewpoints of deaf people, who have a vested interest in these areas, then these advances will be seen as discrimination against deaf people. The Deaf community has participated in an ongoing discussion to define the ethical use of cochlear implants (Komesaroff, 2007; NAD, 2000).

Similarly, the Deaf community must become involved in the bioethical discussion of genome research or risk having decisions made for them. The Deaf community should also recognize that it does not stand alone. The Human Genome Project, the United Nations Educational Scientific and Cultural Organization Declaration of Bioethics and Human Rights, the work of bioethicists, scholars, and genetics researchers (for example, Arnos, 2008; Burke, 2007; Hyde & Power, 2006; Komesaroff, 2007; Leigh, 2009; Nance, 2003), and the activism of other disability groups all reaffirm the value of every human life.

> *Never doubt that a small group of thoughtful committed people can change the world. Indeed it is the only thing that ever has.*
>
> —*Margaret Mead*

Acknowledgment

The author appreciates the invaluable assistance of Dr. Kathleen Arnos and Dr. Larry Dillehay in reviewing the manuscript.

References

Agrawal, Y., Platz, E. A., & Niparko, J. K. (2008). Prevalence of hearing loss and differences by demographic characteristics among US adults: Data from the National Health and Nutrition Examination Survey, 1999–2004. *Archives of Internal Medicine, 168*(14), 1522–1530.

American Psychological Association. (2002). *Ethical principles of psychologists and code of conduct. 2010 Amendments.* Retrieved January 5, 2010, from http://www.apa.org/ethics/code/index.aspx

Arnos, K. S. (2002). Genetics and deafness: Impacts on the Deaf community. *Sign Language Studies, 2*(2), 150–168.

Arnos, K. S. (2008). Ethical and social implications of genetic testing for communication disorders. *Journal of Communication Disorders, 41*(5), 444–457.

Arnos, K. S., Welch, K. O., Tekin, M., Norris, V. W., Blanton, S. H., Pandya, A., et al. (2008). A comparative analysis of the genetic epidemiology of deafness in the United States in two sets of pedigrees collected more than a century apart. *The American Journal of Human Genetics, 83*(2), 200–207.

Brownstein, Z., & Avraham, K. B. (2006). Future trends and potential for treatment of sensorineural hearing loss. *Seminars in Hearing, 27*(3), 193–204.

Burke, T. B. (2007). British bioethics and the human fertilisation and embryology bill. Retrieved January 10, 2010, from http://deafecho.com/2007/12/british-bioethics-and-the-human-fertilisation-and-embryology-bill

Callahan, D. (2003). Individual good and common good: A communitarian approach to bioethics. *Perspectives in Biology and Medicine, 46*(4), 496–504.

Caulfield, T., & Brownsword, R. (2006). Human dignity: A guide to policy making in the biotechnology era? *Nature Reviews Genetics, 7*(1), 72–76.

Chen, W., Johnson, S. L., Marcotti, W., Andrews, P. W., Moore, H. D., & Rivolta, M. N. (2009). Human fetal auditory stem cells (hFASCs) can be expanded in vitro and differentiate into functional auditory neurons and hair cell-like cells. *Stem Cells, 27*(5), 1196–1204.

Cotanche, D. A. (2008). Genetic and pharmacological intervention for treatment/prevention of hearing loss. *Journal of Communication Disorders, 41*(5), 421–443.

Davis, R. L. (2003). Gradients of neurotrophins, ion channels, and tuning in the cochlea. *The Neuroscientist, 9*(5), 311–316.

Deafness Gene Mutation Database. (2010). Retrieved February 11, 2010, from http://hearing.harvard.edu/db/genelist.htm

Deafness Research UK. (2006). *Hair cell research.* Retrieved January 9, 2010, from http://www.deafnessresearch.org.uk/factsheets/hair-cell-research.pdf

Lilach, M., Friedman, L. M., Dror, A. A., Mor, E., Tenne, T., Toren, G., et al. (2009). MicroRNAs are essential for development and function of inner ear hair cells in vertebrates. *Proceedings of the National Academy of Sciences, 106*(19), 7915–7920.

Gleason, M. R., Nagiel, A., Jamet, S., Vologodskaia, M., López-Schier, H., & Hudspeth, A. J. (2009). The transmembrane inner ear (*Tmie*) protein is essential for normal hearing and balance in the zebrafish. *Proceedings of the National Academy of Sciences USA, 106*(50), 21347–21352.

Grillet, N., Schwander, M., Hillebrand, M., Sczaniecka, A., Kolatkar, A., Velasco, J., et al. (2009). Mutations in *LOXHD1*, an evolutionarily conserved stereociliary protein, disrupt hair cell function in mice and cause progressive hearing loss in humans. *American Journal of Human Genetics, 85*(3), 328–337.

Grillet, N., Xiong, W., Reynolds, A., Kazmierczak, P., Sato, T., Lillo, C., et al. (2009). Harmonin mutations cause mechanotransduction defects in cochlear hair cells. *Neuron, 62*(3), 375–387.

hear-it.org. (2009, July). Gene research advancing. *hear-it.org quarterly newsletter*. Retrieved July 10, 2009, from http://www.hear-it.org/page.dsp?page=6413

Hereditary Hearing Loss Homepage. (2008). Retrieved January 4, 2010, from http://hereditaryhearingloss.org

Hladek, G. A. (2002). Cochlear implants, the Deaf culture, and ethics: A study of disability, informed surrogate consent, and ethnocide. *Monash Bioethical Reviews, 21*(1), 29–44.

Hyde, M., & Power, D. (2006). Some ethical dimensions of cochlear implantation for deaf children and their families. *Journal of Deaf Studies and Deaf Education, 11*(1), 102–111.

Kalb, C. (2009, May). Erasing autism. *Newsweek*. Retrieved July 29, 2009, from http://www.newsweek.com/id/197813

Komesaroff, L. (Ed.). (2007). *Surgical consent: Bioethics and cochlear implantation*. Washington, DC: Gallaudet University Press.

Konings, A., Van Laer, L., Michel, S., Pawelczyk, M., Carlsson, P. I., Bondeson, M. L., et al. (2009). Variations in *HSP70* genes associated with noise-induced hearing loss in two independent populations. *European Journal of Human Genetics, 17*(3), 329–335.

Leigh, I. W. (2009). The influences of technology. In I. W. Leigh (Ed.), *A lens on Deaf identities* (pp. 146–165). New York: Oxford University Press.

Levy, N. (2002). Reconsidering cochlear implants: The lessons of Martha's Vineyard. *Bioethics, 16*(2), 134–153.

Little People of America. (2006). *Extended limb lengthening*. Retrieved July 11, 2009, from http://www.lpaonline.org/mc/page.do?sitePageId=56366&orgId=lpa

Little People of America. (2007). *Preimplantation genetic diagnosis position statement*. Retrieved July 11, 2009, from http://data.memberclicks.com/site/lpa/LPA_PGD_Position_Statement_2007.doc

Little People of America. (2009). *Position statement on genetic discoveries in dwarfism*. Retrieved July 29, 2009, from http://www.lpaonline.org/mc/page.do?sitePageId=84634&orgId=lpa#LPAPosition

Lunshof, J. E., Chadwick, R., Vorhaus, D. B., & Church, G. M. (2008). From genetic privacy to open consent. *Nature, 9*(5), 406–411.

Moore, D. R., & Shannon, R. V. (2009). Beyond cochlear implants: Awakening the deafened brain. *Nature Neuroscience, 12*(6), 686–691.

Morton, C. C., & Nance, W. E. (2006). Newborn hearing screening—a silent revolution. *New England Journal of Medicine, 354*(20), 2151–2164.

Nance, W. E. (2003). The genetics of deafness. *Mental Retardation and Developmental Disabilities Research Reviews, 9*(2), 109–119.

National Association of the Deaf. (2000). *Cochlear implants*. Retrieved July 10, 2009, from http://www.nad.org/issues/technology/assistive-listening/cochlear-implants

National Institute on Deafness and Other Communication Disorders. (2008). *Gene transfer in mice produces functional hair cells crucial to hearing.* Retrieved July 25, 2009, from http://www.nidcd.nih.gov/news/releases/08/09_24_08.htm

Neville, H., & Bavelier, D. (2002). Human brain plasticity: Evidence from sensory deprivation and altered language experience. *Progress in Brain Research, 138,* 177–188. Retrieved July 25, 2009, from http://www.bcs.rochester.edu/people/daphne/articles/Amsterdam_chapter.pdf

Owen, K., Coffin, A., Raible, D., & Rubel, E. (2009). *Zebrafish: A serendipitous solution.* Retrieved January 9, 2010, from http://www.ifrahl.org/articles/Zebrafish%20in%20Hearing%20Health.pdf

Pauley, S., Kopecky, B., Beisel, K., Soukup, G., & Fritsch, B. (2008). Stem cells and molecular strategies to restore hearing. *Panminerva Medicine, 50*(1), 41–53.

Reindahl, S. M. (2000). Disability, gene therapy and eugenics—a challenge to John Harris. *Journal of Medical Ethics, 26*(2), 89–75.

Ruel, J., Emery, S., Nouvian, R., Bersot, T., Amilhon, B., Van Rybroek, J., et al. (2008). Impairment of *SLC17A8* encoding vesicular glutamate transporter-3, *VGLUT3,* underlies nonsyndromic deafness *DFNA25* and inner hair cell dysfunction in null mice. *American Journal of Human Genetics, 83*(2), 278–292.

Schorr, E. A., Roth, F. P., & Fox, N. A. (2008). Quality of life for children with cochlear implants: Perceived benefits and problems and the perception of single words and emotional sounds. *Journal of Speech, Language, and Hearing Research, 52,* 141–152. Retrieved July 20, 2009, from http://jslhr.asha.org/cgi/content/abstract/1092-4388_2008_07-0213v1

Shafiro, V., Gygi, B., Cheng, M., Vachhani, J., & Mulvey, M. (2009, July). Factors in the perception of environmental sounds by patients with cochlear implants. *AudiologyOnline.* Retrieved July 13, 2009, from http://www.audiologyonline.com/articles/article_detail.asp?article_id=2260

Solomon, A. (2008, May). The autism rights movement. *New York Magazine.* Retrieved July 29, 2009, from http://nymag.com/news/features/47225

Smith, R. J., & Hone, S. (2003). Genetic screening for deafness. *Pediatric Clinics of North America, 50*(2), 315–329.

Smith, R. J., & Robin, N. H. (2002). Genetic testing for deafness—*GJB2* and *SLC26A4* as causes of deafness. *Journal of Communication Disorders, 35*(4), 367–377.

Tarabichi, M. B., Todd, C., Khan, Z., Yang, X., Shehzad, B., & Tarabichi, M. M. (2008). Deafness in the developing world: The place of cochlear implantation. *Journal of Laryngology and Otology, 122*(9), 877–880.

Thys, M., Van Den Bogaert, K., Iliadou, V., Vanderstraeten, K., Dieltjens, N., Schrauwen, et al. (2007). A seventh locus for otosclerosis, *OTSC7,* maps to chromosome *6q13–16.1. European Journal of Human Genetics, 15*(3), 362–368.

U.K. Parliament. (2008). *Human Fertilisation and Embryology Bill 2007–08.* Retrieved January 10, 2010, from http://services.parliament.uk/bills/2007-08/humanfertilisationandembryologyhl.html

United Nations Educational, Scientific, and Cultural Organization. (2005). *Universal declaration on bioethics and human rights*. Retrieved July 27, 2009, from http://unesdoc.unesco.org/images/0014/001461/146180E.pdf

U.S. Department of Energy Office of Science, Human Genome Program. (2008). *Ethical, legal, and social issues*. Retrieved July 27, 2009, from http://www.ornl.gov/sci/techresources/Human_Genome/elsi/elsi.shtm

U.S. Department of Energy Office of Science, Human Genome Program. (2009). *Human genome project information*. Retrieved January 4, 2010, from http://www.ornl.gov/sci/techresources/Human_Genome/home.shtml

U.S. National Library of Medicine. (2010). *Genetic testing*. Retrieved January 10, 2010, from http://www.nlm.nih.gov/medlineplus/genetictesting.html

Van Eyken, E., Van Laer, L., Fransen, E., Topsakal, V., Lemkens, N., Laureys, W., et al. (2006). *KCNQ4*: A gene for age-related hearing impairment? *Human Mutation, 27*(10), 1007–1016.

3

COCHLEAR IMPLANTS AND DEAF COMMUNITY PERCEPTIONS

John B. Christiansen and Irene W. Leigh

During the past quarter century, there has been significant opposition to cochlear implantation, especially the implantation of children, among many people who consider themselves part of the culturally Deaf community. Beginning in the 1980s, national organizations of deaf people throughout the world, as well as the World Federation of the Deaf, have frequently gone on record against pediatric cochlear implantation (Andersson, 1994; Bloch, 1999; Christiansen & Leigh, 2002/2005; Lane, Hoffmeister, & Bahan, 1996). Although this opposition has been tempered somewhat during the past decade, especially in the United States where the National Association of the Deaf (NAD) now formally supports cochlear implantation as one of a "multitude of options" that parents are encouraged to consider for their deaf child (National Association of the Deaf, 2000), it remains to be seen how widespread this transformation might actually be. It is one thing for the NAD to issue a position paper that purportedly ushers in a new era and quite another to ascertain the extent to which Deaf people themselves actually share these revised sentiments. This is particularly true now that the number of cochlear implant users has increased dramatically since the appearance of the NAD position paper.

At the beginning of the new millennium, there were approximately 35,000 cochlear implant users around the world, almost all in wealthy nations, about evenly divided between children and adults (Christiansen & Leigh, 2002/2005). During the past decade this number has increased substantially. Information available on the Web site of the National Institute on Deafness and Other Communication Disorders (2011) indicates that as of December 2010, the Food and Drug Administration estimated that 219,000 people around the world had received a cochlear implant (including approximately 42,600 adults and 28,400 children in the United States). There is also an increasingly important distinction between the number of implantees and the number of cochlear implants. This is because of the increasing number of bilateral cochlear implants, a trend that has grown substantially since the mid-2000s (Valente, Hosford-Dunn, & Roeser, 2007). It is likely that at least 7,000 people used, or at least had, two cochlear implants as of early 2009 (Nussbaum, 2009), and by the end of 2010 this number was most likely well over 10,000 and increasing rapidly (Christiansen, 2010). It is not known how many implantees are still using the device, but it is likely that most are.

One attempt to measure some of the attitudes related to cochlear implants, both for adults and for children, among a subset of the Deaf population was a survey that we conducted among Gallaudet University faculty, students, staff, and alumni in 2000. Some of the results of this survey, which included responses to closed-ended questions as well as extensive written comments to open-ended queries, are reported in our book *Cochlear implants in children: Ethics and choices* (Christiansen & Leigh, 2002/2005). In an effort to see if any of these attitudes have changed since then, we conducted a "semireplication" of this study in 2008 using the same statements for participants to respond to. Among other things, we were interested in trying to determine if the protest related to the selection of Jane Fernandes as the ninth president of Gallaudet University, which occurred on campus in 2006, might have led some people to become less tolerant of cochlear implants and cochlear implant users. As will be discussed in greater detail below, one of the consequences of this protest was a heightened awareness of the importance of Deaf culture and American Sign Language (ASL) on campus, and we wondered if this might have led some people to become less tolerant of cochlear implants and cochlear implant users.

Before describing the results of the new study and comparing them with our initial investigation, it is important to note that the samples for these two studies were not selected in exactly the same way, nor was the study itself conducted the same way both times. For one thing, in 2000, we included a small random sample of alumni in our survey along with faculty, staff, and students. In 2008, alumni were not included, although there is little doubt that a good number of the faculty and staff members who replied are in fact former Gallaudet students. In addition, except for a nonrandom sample of 20 Gallaudet summer school students in 2000, the respondents in the earlier study were selected randomly. Respondents to the 2008 survey were not selected randomly.[1]

---

1. The 2008 survey was nonrandom primarily because we decided, both for logistical and budgetary reasons, to make the questionnaire available online for those who had access to Gallaudet University's Web-based "Blackboard" system. Several notices were sent to the campus community via a daily public service announcement that is routinely distributed each morning to those who have access to the university's e-mail system. Potential respondents were asked to complete the Institutional Review Board approved questionnaire on Blackboard and submit it online when they were done. The researchers had no access to these responses until the survey was over, and Shannon Augustine, a professional staff person with the Office of Academic Technology on campus, made the completely anonymous results available to us. We are grateful to Ms. Augustine for assisting in the design of the online questionnaire and for compiling and sharing the collective responses with us.

Table 1. Composition of the Gallaudet University Samples, 2000 and 2008 (%)

	Year of Survey	
	2000	2008
Hearing status		
Deaf	63%	62%
Hard of hearing	12%	11%
Hearing	23%	27%
Gallaudet University affiliation		
Faculty/Staff	38%	19%
Students	33%	80%
Alumni	29%	N/A
Gender		
Female	64%	78%
Male	35%	22%
Race/Ethnicity		
White	80%	75%
African American	9%	7%
Other/Unknown	11%	17%
Deaf community affiliation		
Yes	75%	77%
No	16%	14%
Not sure	8%	8%
Number of respondents	138	238

Table 1 summarizes the composition of the two samples on several important background variables. In 2000, there were 138 responses to the mailed questionnaire; in 2008, 238 people responded to the online version.

Clearly, most of the respondents in both samples are White and most consider themselves part of the Deaf community. The distribution of deaf, hard of hearing, and hearing respondents in the two surveys is very similar, with a slightly higher proportion of female responses in 2008. The most obvious difference between the two samples is in terms of the respondents' affiliation with Gallaudet University. As noted, no alumni were included, at least formally, in the 2008 survey. In 2000, students accounted for one third of the respondents; in 2008, students made up 4 out of every 5 respondents. In fact, of the 238 responses to the 2008 survey, 59% were actually undergraduate students (not shown in Table 1).

To make it easier for the reader to compare the responses from the two studies, we have listed seven statements to which participants were asked to respond that will be discussed in this chapter. Response choices ranged from Strongly Disagree to Strongly Agree, with a No Opinion or Don't Know option in the middle of the five-point scale.[2]

1. It is possible for a person to use a cochlear implant and still have an identity as a Deaf person.
2. Hearing parents should be permitted to get a cochlear implant for their child under the age of 5 if they study the issue carefully and believe this to be the best decision for the child and the family.
3. Gallaudet University should do more to encourage students with cochlear implants to come to Gallaudet.
4. It would be a good idea to have a "cochlear implant center" at Gallaudet to help meet the needs of students (including MSSD and Kendall school students [that is, precollege programs on campus]) with cochlear implants.
5. Faculty and staff should be encouraged to sign with voice whenever possible to make the university more "user-friendly" for students who use voice communication more than sign, as many cochlear implant users do.
6. The Deaf community in America will eventually disappear because so many children are getting cochlear implants.
7. A cochlear implant may be an appropriate choice for a hearing person who becomes deaf later in life and does not want to be part of the Deaf community.

Results

Table 2 reports the percentage of respondents in each survey who either Strongly Agree or Agree with each of the above statements.

As is readily apparent from Table 2, there are some interesting similarities as well as differences between the two surveys. It should be noted that these results include all of the respondents, deaf, hard of hearing, and hearing, to the two surveys; we will discuss some of the differences among these three subpopulations below.

---

2. Two statements from the 2000 survey, specifically "When using his/her cochlear implant, an implanted person can usually hear as well as a hearing person" and "The cochlear implant center should provide information for people interested in learning more about cochlear implants," were not included in the 2008 survey.

Table 2. Respondents Who Strongly Agree or Agree with the Statements (%)

Statement	Year of Survey 2000	Year of Survey 2008
1. It is possible for a person to use a cochlear implant and still have an identity as a Deaf person.	51%	61%
2. Hearing parents should be permitted to get a cochlear implant for their child under the age of 5 if they study the issue carefully and believe this to be the best decision for the child and the family.	35%	37%
3. Gallaudet University should do more to encourage students with cochlear implants to come to Gallaudet.	59%	54%
4. It would be a good idea to have a "cochlear implant center" at Gallaudet to help meet the needs of students (including MSSD and Kendall school students [i.e., pre-college programs on campus]) with cochlear implants.	53%	80%
5. Faculty and staff should be encouraged to sign with voice whenever possible to make the University more "user-friendly" for students who use voice communication more than sign, as many cochlear implant users do.	34%	18%
6. The Deaf community in America will eventually disappear because so many children are getting cochlear implants.	25%	26%
7. A cochlear implant may be an appropriate choice for a hearing person who becomes deaf later in life and does not want to be part of the Deaf community.	69%	65%

Note. MSSD = Model Secondary School for the Deaf.

Respondents in 2008 were clearly more likely to support the idea that it is possible for someone to have a cochlear implant and, at the same time, have an identity as a Deaf person than was the case in 2000 (statement 1). In addition, there was considerably more support for a cochlear implant center on campus in 2008 than there was in 2000 (statement 4). Finally, there was much less support for the proposition that faculty should be encouraged to sign with voice in 2008 than there was 8 years earlier (statement 5). Among the other statements, there are few differences between the two periods.

Table 3 reports the percentage of respondents in each survey that either Strongly Agree or Agree with each of the above statements separated by their hearing status. As was the case in 2000, there are some important differences among deaf, hearing, and hard of hearing respondents on several of the statements. For statement 2, for example, which focuses on support for pediatric implantation, a much larger

Table 3. Respondents Who Strongly Agree or Agree with the Statements by Hearing Status (%)

	Year of Survey					
	2000			2008		
Statement Number	D	HoH	H	D	HoH	H
1	37%	71%	81%	70%	85%	86%
2	16%	53%	78%	30%	35%	77%
3	54%	65%	71%	64%	65%	61%
4	41%	71%	78%	90%	96%	100%
5	24%	59%	47%	21%	27%	21%
6	34%	6%	9%	40%	27%	11%
7	66%	41%	91%	70%	65%	94%

proportion of hearing respondents compared to those who are deaf or hard of hearing agreed with this statement in both surveys. In addition, the proportion of deaf people in agreement with the statement increased, whereas the proportion of hard of hearing people who agreed decreased from 2000 to 2008. For statement 1 (which asks whether it is possible to have a cochlear implant and still retain one's identity as a culturally Deaf person), there continues to be a difference between deaf respondents on the one hand and hearing and hard of hearing respondents on the other. Whereas deaf respondents were clearly more likely to agree with statement 1 in 2008 than they were in 2000, they were not as likely to agree as those who are hearing or hard of hearing.

There also continues to be some differences in the responses to the last two statements: Deaf respondents are considerably more likely to have concerns about the future of the Deaf community (statement 6) compared with their hearing and hard of hearing counterparts, and are somewhat less supportive of implantation for those who lose their hearing later in life compared to hearing respondents (although not compared to hard of hearing respondents) (statement 7). Still, a large majority of all responses to the last statement was affirmative in 2008, and this particular result does not appear to us to be a surprise. This represents an implicit recognition of the diversity of deaf people in general, not all of whom can be referred to as culturally Deaf.

Although there are some differences, there are similarities among the respondents as well. For example, for statements 3 and 4, there was considerable agreement among all three subgroups in 2008. Perhaps the most interesting finding here is the large increase from 2000 to 2008 in the percentage of respondents agreeing with statement 4, that it would be a good idea to have a cochlear implant center at the university. As far as encouraging students with implants to come to Gallaudet is concerned (statement 3), it is clear that in 2008 over 60% of all respondents agreed with this statement. Deaf respondents who, as noted, included a large number of undergraduate students, expressed considerably more agreement with this statement in 2008 than did deaf respondents (which included a much smaller proportion of undergraduate students) in 2000. Taken together, the level of agreement to these two statements indicates a somewhat greater acceptance of students with cochlear implants on campus in 2008 compared to 2000, an issue that will be discussed in more detail below.

The responses to statement 5 in Table 3 show that the support for signing with voice has declined across-the-board on campus. Although what was called the "simultaneous method," that is, signing and speaking at the same time, was more or less the standard form of communication on campus during the 1970s and 1980s, this is clearly no longer the case. Today, signing in ASL, which does not support simultaneous signing and speaking, is preferred. Thus, although there may be a more welcoming environment for students with cochlear implants at Gallaudet, this welcome mat does not appear to include a general willingness to use one's voice to make the university more "user-friendly" for students who use voice communication.

In addition to these quantitative results from the 2008 Gallaudet campus survey, we also asked a couple of open-ended questions to give respondents an opportunity to comment on some of the issues raised in the questionnaire. One of the questions was: Have you ever considered a cochlear implant for yourself? Why or why not? Hearing respondents, of course, did not comment on this question, but many deaf and hard of hearing people did. Survey respondents were also given an opportunity to comment on any aspect of the survey, and some of the comments, noted below, focus on other issues, particularly the question of whether pediatric implantation is appropriate. First, some of the comments about whether implantation might be considered for oneself:

- I am satisfied with myself. I can't hear at all, my cochlea hair is dead, and there is no way the cochlea implant can work. I am fifth deaf generation in my family. I have almost 100% accessibility with communication. I am able to write in English very well. I am a native user of ASL.
- I don't see the need to—why cut my brain open?
- 50 staples on a shaved head just to "be fixed?" No, thank you.
- I do not want to hear somebody fart right next to me.

Not surprisingly, some respondents already had a cochlear implant, and their experiences with the device varied greatly. Some comments:

- I already had a cochlear implant when I was 6 years old and never liked it. It always gave me headaches when the battery was dying. I never wanted it in the first place and it was my parents' decision.

- I am sick of people telling me what I should be or should not be. I am a proud deaf individual who happens to have a cochlear implant.
- Since getting my implant 6 years ago, I have experienced zero negative reactions or comments from other members of the Deaf community. I think the message has sunk in that the decision to get a CI is a strictly private one, and a person should not be criticized for it.
- I am still part of the Deaf community and function much better in the hearing world with the CI than with the hearing aid.

As noted above (see Table 3, statement 2), deaf and hard of hearing respondents are less likely than those who are hearing to support pediatric cochlear implantation. What follows is a sample of some of the comments made regarding this issue:

- I completely disagree with cochlear implanting when deaf babies are only 6 months because surgeons could make a mistake that messes up babies' very tiny heads and brains.
- It ruins Deaf culture and doctors recommend them to parents of deaf children just to make money and never mention ASL and Deaf culture. It's suitable for hearing people who lose their hearing later in life.
- I respect the use of cochlear implants for specific individuals. However, I believe that parents should wait until their daughter/son reaches a specific age where they are able to make a life-altering decision whether they should get a cochlear implant or not.
- Parents don't have the right to force cochlear implants upon their children when they just want to do the "easy" way and assume that having cochlear implants automatically makes one person hearing.
- There is a lot of negativity [regarding implantation before age 5]. However, my standard answer . . . is that parents will always make decisions they believe will be beneficial to their child.

Comments about the Deaf Community and Gallaudet University also frequently appeared in the survey. For example:

- I think the saddest part of CI is that many who have them are never exposed to ASL or the Deaf community. It's not the CI itself that threatens the Deaf community but the thought that it's a fix for deafness. Or even the thought that deafness is bad. That's what is truly the problem.
- Gallaudet must recruit more students with CIs and market the fact that we have a world-class audiology and speech center that offers mapping services right on campus. It appears that CIs are more and more accepted at Gallaudet.

- It amazes me that at Gallaudet we are more accepting of sexual orientation and sexual identity choices including transsexual surgery than we are of CI surgery. . . . We say celebrate diversity. Let's walk the talk.
- Many people have hearing aids, CIs, etc., but will not use them for fear of not fitting in with other students.
- It is completely acceptable for people with CIs to identify as Deaf and participate in the Deaf community.

Discussion

In our book *Cochlear Implants and Children: Ethics and Choices* (Christiansen & Leigh, 2002/2005), we wrote that in

> the last few decades of the 20th century, the topic of cochlear implants emerged as perhaps the single most divisive issue among deaf and hard-of-hearing people, educators, parents of deaf children . . . and others concerned about the welfare and future of deaf people and the Deaf community. (p. vii)

Given the results of our on-campus survey, it appears that many of the issues that were important at that time are still with us, although there have been some important changes as well. In this section we will examine some of these issues.

The events of 2006 at Gallaudet University do not appear to have had much impact on the trend toward greater acceptance of cochlear implants in the Deaf community. This general conclusion is supported by the results of our 2008 on-campus survey, especially the overall increase from 2000 to 2008 in the percentage of respondents agreeing with the statement that it is possible for a person to use a cochlear implant and still have an identity as a Deaf person. Although agreement with this statement increased for deaf respondents in 2008 compared to 2000, comparatively more hard of hearing and hearing respondents affirmed this statement. We suggest the possibility that hearing and hard of hearing individuals who have had to adjust to the Gallaudet University environment recognize the importance of flexibility in comparison to some Deaf respondents, who may take a more essentialist or strict perspective on what it means to have a Deaf identity that does not involve audition per se.

In addition, although opposition to pediatric implantation among certain members of the Deaf community continues unabated, there continues to be much less opposition to cochlear implantation among those who are old enough to decide for themselves if they want this technology. This trend is also apparent from the NAD's various pronouncements over the years, the growing number of culturally Deaf people who have decided to get an implant, and the general absence of criticism directed at older people who have a cochlear implant. As an example, one of the authors of this chapter got a cochlear implant in 2001 and has never been criticized for doing so (Christiansen, 2011). Many other people in the Deaf community, known to one or both of the authors, have chosen to get an implant and, in general, they have successfully maintained strong social and familial ties with their nonimplanted Deaf peers.

As far as Gallaudet University is concerned, based on the 2008 survey result indicating that almost two-thirds of deaf respondents agree or strongly agree that Gallaudet should do more to encourage students with cochlear implants to enroll at the university, we expect that Gallaudet is increasingly likely to be a welcoming place for students with implants. However, this openness is likely to occur only if these students endeavor to become fluent in ASL and only if they are interested in affirming at least part of their identity as a culturally Deaf person (as many cochlear implant adolescents are; see Leigh & Maxwell-McCaw, this volume). This in fact was demonstrated by a panel of students with cochlear implants held at Gallaudet in the spring of 2008 (Leigh, 2009). Those students who could use ASL comfortably reported feeling very accepted by the Gallaudet University community. In contrast, those who struggled with ASL tended to feel less comfortable. The dramatic increase in the number of 2008 respondents who affirm the need for a cochlear implant center on the Gallaudet University campus (statement 4) is also a case in point. In fact, there has actually been a cochlear implant education center at the Laurent Clerc National Deaf Education Center on campus since 2000. Additionally, the Hearing and Speech Center at Gallaudet University now offers cochlear implant services.

This leads us to examine the responses to statement 5: Faculty and staff should be encouraged to sign with voice whenever possible to make the university more "user-friendly" for students who use voice communication more than sign, as many cochlear implant users do. Tables 2 and 3 reveal a significant drop in the percentage of those agreeing with this statement from 2000 to 2008. This could be a direct response to the 2006 protest at Gallaudet University, during which one of the critical issues was the support of ASL in and of itself and the need to separate a signed language from any accompanying spoken language. Even though the 2006 protest regarding the appointment of Jane Fernandes as the ninth president of Gallaudet was not specifically about cochlear implants, one of the issues that emerged during the protest was whether or not Dr. Fernandes was "Deaf enough" (Davis, 2007; Humphries & Humphries, 2011). That is, was she sufficiently committed to ASL and other attributes of Deaf culture to lead the university? Although a number of protest leaders, particularly some members of the Gallaudet faculty, strongly objected to the characterization of the protest in this manner, the fact remains that many protesters did articulate their concerns by using this rationale (this was especially evident on some of the blogs that emerged during the protest).

The new Gallaudet University mission statement (2009), which was developed in the aftermath of the protest, states that Gallaudet University is, among other things, a bilingual institution of higher education that ensures the use of ASL and English. This mission emphasizes the centrality of ASL alongside English as part of the university curriculum. Although it may appear to contravene the acceptability of cochlear implantation, in fact a bicultural identity is an attractive option for many young deaf people with a cochlear implant (see Leigh, 2009 for a brief review). If Gallaudet University itself continues to accommodate the needs of implanted students (mapping—that is, software programming—services, speech therapy as needed, and so on), in tandem with a bicultural identity reflecting comfort with ASL, Deaf cultural values, and English, this may be a positive outcome for all concerned.

In this context, the recent activities of several organizations, including the Deaf Bilingual Coalition (DBC), Audism Free America (AFA), and the NAD are important to mention. The mission statement of DBC is as follows: "The Deaf Bilingual Coalition promotes the basic human right of all Deaf infants and young children to have access to language and cognitive development through American Sign Language (ASL)" (Deaf Bilingual Coalition, 2007). AFA describes itself as "a grassroots Deaf activist organization . . . which advocates for Deaf American rights, cultural resurgence, and seeks primarily to challenge the ideological foundations of audism in America" (Audism Free America, 2009). Since their conception, both organizations have employed a number of confrontational tactics, especially with respect to the Alexander Graham Bell Association of the Deaf and Hard of Hearing, (AG Bell) an organization whose mission is that of advocating independence through listening and talking, in an effort to promote their messages. One example of these confrontational tactics was a 1-day protest and rally in April 2009 that was held in front of the Volta Bureau in Washington, DC. According to an unsigned posting on the bionic ear blog, "The purpose of the rally is to call attention to the denial of linguistic and human rights of Deaf citizens and to highlight how the Volta Bureau/AG Bell Association has worked to perpetuate the denial of these rights" (Bionic Ear Blog, 2009). Another example occurred in the summer of 2008 in Milwaukee, Wisconsin. Several hundred people attended the first convention of the DBC in Milwaukee at the same time that AG Bell was holding its 48th biennial convention, and DBC rallies were held outside the convention center (Johnson, 2008).

Although the DBC efforts have not focused primarily on pediatric cochlear implantation, DBC advocates do stress the importance of a strong, visually oriented Deaf community that stands in opposition to those who would focus on remediation of hearing loss and emphasize various forms of spoken language. Explicit in their message is that there is no need for pediatric implants as long as deaf children are exposed to a vibrant Deaf community and a vibrant, visual language such as ASL. This latter message has also been strongly espoused by AFA. They see much of the current research related to the physical, psychological, social, and cultural impact of cochlear implants on deaf infants, children, and youth as not truly legitimate without significant participation of culturally Deaf researchers (see a sampling of current psychosocial research in Leigh & Maxwell-McCaw, this volume).

In addition to the efforts of the DBC and AFA, the more formal, 130-year-old NAD has also been active, especially by focusing on traditional advocacy efforts related to captioning, ASL, access to court proceedings, infant screening, and so on. Information about cochlear implants on the NAD's Web site is somewhat limited but does include the organization's 2000 position paper as well as a few links to other resources. In general, it appears that, in contrast to the year 2000, issues related to cochlear implantation are currently not very high on the NAD's list of priorities. Whether this simply represents a growing acceptance of a form of technology that a rapidly increasing number of deaf children and adults are using, or whether it simply means that the NAD has formally or informally chosen to more or less allow the issue to evolve on its own is difficult to determine.

In sum, what seems to be occurring is that, in contrast to the situation at the beginning of the 21st century, cochlear implantation has moved away from the forefront of attention among many people in the Deaf community, although the AFA is attempting to resurrect strong opposition to the procedure in the framework of audism, presumed denigration of ASL, and concern about the actual benefits of cochlear implantation. It is worth reemphasizing that there is clearly still a good amount of opposition to pediatric implants, especially among some of those who identify strongly with the Deaf community as well as those individuals who are generally opposed to surgery on an otherwise healthy person for ethical reasons. As noted in Table 3, less than one third of the deaf respondents in 2008 agreed with statement 2, which states that parents should be permitted to get a cochlear implant for their child under the age of 5 if they study the issue carefully and believe this to be the best decision for the child and the family. However, what is particularly striking here is that the percentage of deaf respondents who currently agree with this statement is about twice what it was in 2000. Moreover, as noted earlier, the majority of 2008 deaf respondents are, in fact, Gallaudet undergraduate students, a population one might expect to be most likely opposed to the idea of pediatric implantation, in part because of the campuswide focus on the use of ASL and visual stimuli.

In any event, although there is still significant opposition, we expect that this opposition will continue to gradually diminish over the years, paralleling the 2000 and 2008 survey results, as increasing numbers of cochlear implant users arrive at Gallaudet. Additionally, the results of research in the past decade demonstrate the impressive speech and listening performance of many young implantees, although variability in results continues to be an issue (Belzner & Seal, 2009; Marschark, 2007). It is still true that cochlear implants do not turn a deaf person into a hearing person, and children with cochlear implants still typically need support services (Christiansen & Leigh, 2002/2005).

One major issue that has developed in recent years is the trend toward bilateral implantation, especially among children. Preliminary research here suggests that children who receive two cochlear implants relatively early in life do even better, at least in terms of speech perception and localization acuity (identifying the location of sound), than do children who receive one implant (Litovsky et al., 2006; Peters, Litovsky, Parkinson, & Lake, 2007). If this trend continues, it could conceivably become somewhat less likely that future bilateral implant users will need the type of support services that many young implant users frequently require today. If this happens, this may serve to reinforce the current pattern of decreasing opposition to pediatric cochlear implantation.

The prevalence of cochlear implantation has led some to consider whether the Deaf community's very existence will be affected, at least in those countries where implantation is widespread. This may be one reason for some of the ambiguous responses to cochlear implantation evidenced by a number of Deaf people and scholars. The relative size (and perhaps the absolute size as well) of the Deaf community is probably decreasing, most clearly in Australia (Hyde, Ohna, & Hjulstadt, 2006; Johnston, 2004), even taking into consideration the fact that there are ongoing new entrants into the Deaf community among those curious about this community (Carty, 2006; see discussion below). In the United States, in the early 1970s Schein and Delk (1974) estimated the Deaf population—really "prevocationally deaf"—to be about 400,000. Recent very rough estimates on the Gallaudet Research Institute's Web site (2008) put the number at no more than this. Of course, the U.S. population has increased by approximately 100 million people since the mid-1970s, so the relative size of the Deaf population has most likely decreased. In a related estimate, Mitchell, Young, Bachleda, and Karchmer (2006) extrapolated a possibly larger number of individuals who use ASL from population estimates of increasing numbers of people identified with hearing loss. However, this estimate may be tempered by the increasing number of children with cochlear implants, especially bilateral implants, who may be relying more on spoken language than children who received only one implant. In addition, as Mitchell et al. point out, estimates of ASL users must take into account the fact that many of these users (including hearing siblings and interpreters) are not deaf people.

Certainly, there is a desire on the part of a large number of people for more "members" in the Deaf community. Some go as far as to opine that the Deaf community is being maintained by later entries, more specifically late signers, oral deaf adults, and hard of hearing individuals (Carty, 2006; Hyde, Power, & Lloyd, 2006). At the same time, there is an apparent "circling the wagons" mentality, in which people are expected to adhere to the essentialist definition of what it means to be Deaf and strongly identify with those characteristics that constitute the core of the community, especially valuing and using ASL. Suffice it to say that at the present time, there is an ongoing core of ASL users. Consequently, our expectation is that the core will be maintained at least for the near future. The long-term prognosis for the Deaf community is that it will continue to exist, perhaps less in countries where pediatric cochlear implantation is increasingly the standard, but most definitely in countries where cochlear implantation is not the standard for economic and societal reasons.

In this regard, it is worth noting that a recent article in the *Los Angeles Times* (Roan, 2009) estimates that approximately 40% of deaf children under the age of 3 in the United States now get either one or two cochlear implants (compared to 25% in 2004, when almost all implantees got only one). How many children is this? Based on information from the Population Reference Bureau's (2009) World Population Data Sheet, we estimate that approximately 380 deaf babies are born in the world each day (based on the generally accepted assumption that 1 child in every 1,000 live births will be born deaf). Moreover, of the approximately 380,000 births worldwide each day, the Population Reference Bureau estimates that approximately 10% are in what the United Nations classifies as "more developed nations." The 38 or so deaf children born each day in these nations are clearly the ones most likely to receive a cochlear implant; few of the approximately 342 deaf children born each day in "less developed nations" are likely to have access to this technology.

The population of the United States represents approximately 4.5% of the world's total and approximately 25% of the total population of world's more developed nations. Extrapolating from this, we would estimate that, on average, about 9 or 10 deaf babies are born in the United States each day. Assuming the figure in the *Los Angeles Times* is reasonably accurate (it is based on information from the three cochlear implant companies), it is likely that in the near future about half of these children will receive an implant.[3]

Regarding the last statement of the survey, which focuses on the cochlear implant being an appropriate choice for a hearing person who becomes deaf later in life and does not want to be a part of the Deaf community, the trend toward agreement with this statement is relatively strong. The typical assumption is that such individuals remain culturally hearing, but in fact there is variability in terms of becoming accommodated to the new hearing status (Leigh, 2009). Although some would prefer to remain fully within their respective hearing communities, a good number will gravitate toward associations with other late deafened peers like themselves (Goulder, 1997).

---

3. Of course, deaf infants and toddlers (under the age of 3) are not the only children who get a cochlear implant. Many older deaf children are implanted as well. However, the clear trend is to implant younger children, often those younger than 12 months, so it seems reasonable to estimate that at least half of all severely to profoundly deaf children in the United States will be implanted in the not-too-distant future (compared to an estimated 80% of deaf children implanted in Australia [Marschark, 2007]).

A study done by Maxwell-McCaw (2001) that focused on deaf identity categorization reported that an equal number of participants who self-identified as late deafened were categorized as having hearing, Deaf, or bicultural identities. This is a group of individuals who appear to have positively internalized who they are and to be comfortable participating in a study advertised as a deaf-acculturation research project.

Conclusion

This chapter emphasizes that a wholesale rejection of cochlear implants, or cochlear implant users, does not appear to be imminent. Although there are pockets of resistance, especially in terms of pediatric implantation, there is nonetheless increasing acceptance that cochlear implant technology is now part of the range of possibilities for the child or adult who is deaf. Moreover, and in contrast to the tensions of the past, it is likely that culturally Deaf people will increasingly be comfortable with cochlear implant users who embrace ASL and the Deaf community. For the Deaf community to continue to thrive, old perceptions need to be cast aside as the community reconstitutes itself by meeting these technological challenges and by putting its unique interpretation on them. The implications for the future, both at Gallaudet University and in the wider Deaf community, remain to be seen.

References

Alexander Graham Bell Association for the Deaf and Hard of Hearing. (2009). *Who we are*. Retrieved August 2, 2009, from http://agbell.org/NetCommunity/Page.aspx?pid=550

Andersson, Y. (1994). Do we want cochlear implants? *WFD News*, 1, 3–4.

Archibold, S., & Wheeler, A. (2010). Cochlear implants: Family and young people's perspectives. In M. Marschark & P. Spencer (Eds.), *Oxford handbook of deaf studies, language, and education* (pp. 226–240). New York: Oxford University Press.

Audism Free America. (2009). *Audism Free America: To promote and protect the civil liberties of Deaf people and their linguistic birthrights*. Retrieved August 2, 2009, from http://audismfreeamerica.blogspot.com

Belzner, K., & Seal, B. (2009). Children with cochlear implants: A review of demographics and communication outcomes. *American Annals of the Deaf, 154*(3), 311–333.

Bionic Ear Blog. (2009). Retrieved December 6, 2009, from http://www.meryl.net/ci/2009/03/audism_free_ame.html

Bloch, N. (1999). Update: The NAD and childhood cochlear implants. *The NAD Broadcaster, 21*(5), 5.

Carty, B. (2006). Comments on "W(h)ither the Deaf Community." *Sign Language Studies, 6*(2), 181–189.

Christiansen, J. B. (2010). *Reflections: My life in the Deaf and hearing worlds.* Washington, DC: Gallaudet University Press.

Christiansen, J. B., & Leigh, I. W. (2002/2005). *Cochlear implants in children: Ethics and choices.* Washington, DC: Gallaudet University Press.

Davis, L. J. (2007). Deafness and the riddle of identity. *The Chronicle Review, 53*(19), B6.

Deaf Bilingual Coalition. (2007). *DBC's mission.* Retrieved May 26, 2009, from http://deafbilingual.blogspot.com/2007/08/welcome-to-our-temporary-deaf-bilingual.html

Gallaudet Research Institute. (2008). *Current estimates (2004): How many deaf people are there in the United States?* Retrieved May 16, 2009, from http://research.gallaudet.edu/Demographics/deaf-US.php

Gallaudet University. (2009). Retrieved June 28, 2009, from http://www.gallaudet.edu/x20518.xml

Goulder, T. (1997). *Journey through late deafness: Results of a focus group study.* San Diego, CA: California School of Professional Psychology Rehabilitation Research and Training Center on Mental Health for Persons Who Are Hard of Hearing or Late Deafened.

Humphries, T., & Humphries, J. (2011). Deaf in the time of the cochlea. *Journal of Deaf Studies and Deaf Education, 16*(2), 153–163.

Hyde, M., Ohna, E., & Hjulstadt, O. (2006). Education of the deaf in Australia and Norway: A comparative study of the interpretations and applications of inclusion. *American Annals of the Deaf, 150*(5), 415–426.

Hyde, M., Power, D., & Lloyd, K. (2006). Comments on "W(h)ither the Deaf Community." *Sign Language Studies, 6*(2), 190–201.

Johnson, M. (2008, June 30). Deaf groups clash at meeting: Advocates of hearing aids, signing disagree. *Journal Sentinel.* Retrieved December 10, 2009, from http://www.jsonline.com/news/milwaukee/29571839.html

Johnston, T. (2004). W(h)ither the Deaf community? Population, genetics, and the future of Australian Sign Language. *American Annals of the Deaf, 148*(5), 358–375.

Lane, H., Hoffmeister, R., & Bahan, B. (1996). *A journey into the Deaf-World.* San Diego, CA: DawnSignPress.

Leigh, I. W. (2009). *A lens on Deaf identities.* New York: Oxford University Press.

Litovsky, R. Y., Johnstone, P. M., Godar, S., Agrawal, S., Parkinson, A., Peters, R., Lake, J., et al. (2006). Bilateral cochlear implants in children: Localization acuity measured with minimum audible angle. *Ear and Hearing, 27*(1), 43–59.

Marschark, M. (2007). *Raising and educating a deaf child* (2nd ed.). New York: Oxford University Press.

Maxwell-McCaw, D. (2001). Acculturation and psychological well-being in deaf and hard-of-hearing people (Doctoral dissertation, The George Washington University). *Dissertation Abstracts International, 61*(11–B), 6141.

Mitchell, R., Young, T., Bachleda, B., & Karchmer, M. (2006). How many people use ASL in the United States? *Sign Language Studies, 6*(3), 306–335.

Mukari, S. Z., Ling, L. N., & Ghani, H. A. (2007). Educational performance of pediatric cochlear implants recipients in mainstream classes. *International Journal of Pediatric Otorhinolaryngology, 71*(2), 231–240.

National Association of the Deaf. (2000, October). *NAD position statement on cochlear implants (2000).* Retrieved May 20, 2009, from http://www.nad.org/issues/technology/assistive-listening/cochlear-implants

National Institute on Deafness and Other Communication Disorders. (2011). *Who gets cochlear implants?* Retrieved March 21, 2011, from http://www.nidcd.nih.gov/health/hearing/coch.asp

Nussbaum, D. (2009, April). *Evolving trends and practices.* Paper presented at the Cochlear Implants and Sign Language Conference, Washington, DC.

Peters, B. R., Litovsky, R., Parkinson, A., & Lake, J. (2007). Importance of age and postimplantation experience on speech perception measures in children with sequential bilateral cochlear implants. *Otology & Neurotology, 28*(5), 649–657, S1–S2.

Population Reference Bureau. (2009). *2009 world population data sheet.* Retrieved August 31, 2009, from http://www.prb.org/pdf09/09wpds_eng.pdf

Roan, Shari. (2009, August 3). Cochlear implants open deaf kids' ears to the world. *Los Angeles Times.* Retrieved August 5, 2009, from http://articles.latimes.com/2009/aug/03/health/he-deaf-children3

Schein, J. D., & Delk, M. T., Jr. (1974). *The Deaf population of the United States.* Silver Spring, MD: National Association of the Deaf.

Valente, M., Hosford-Dunn, H., & Roeser, R. (2007). *Audiology: treatment* (2nd ed.). New York: Thieme.

4

HOW DEAF ADULT SIGNERS EXPERIENCE IMPLANTS: SOME PRELIMINARY CONCLUSIONS

Khadijat Rashid, Poorna Kushalnagar, and Raja Kushalnagar

We define "Deaf adult signers" as adults who use sign language as a primary mode of communication some or all of the time and who have a large number of Deaf friends, family members, or colleagues with whom they regularly socialize. In recent decades, legal, social, and technological changes have significantly reshaped Deaf communities. One of the more recent changes was the development of cochlear implants (CIs).

We define "signing deaf adults" broadly, since not all deaf adults who sign employ the same communication mode consistently, and people can switch modes depending on circumstances. For example, deaf adults who are employed in a primarily hearing workplace but have deaf spouses might employ speech at work but sign at home or during leisure hours. Other deaf adults who have hearing partners but work in primarily deaf workspaces might sign mostly during work hours and then use speech communication at home or with friends. Yet others might sign all the time or only rarely. This special population of Deaf adult signers is the focus of this chapter.

When CIs were first introduced in the late 1980s and early 1990s, the Deaf community's reaction was overwhelmingly negative. The National Association for the Deaf released a position document that considered the implants "highly experimental . . . experimentation with children" (National Association of the Deaf, 1991) especially since doctors advocated implanting children earlier for maximum efficacy. Implant technology appeared to provide yet another avenue by which those with a medical perspective of deafness sought to determine the direction and future prospects of the Deaf community. Yet less than 2 decades later, anecdotal evidence suggests that with heightened understanding of what implants can and cannot do, CIs are becoming increasingly acceptable within the Deaf community.

Although the history of CIs in medical research goes back to the 1960s, it was only after they were approved for commercial use in 1984 that CIs started to be considered an alternative to hearing aids. By April 2009, approximately 188,000 people worldwide had received CIs (National Institute on Deafness and Other Communication Disorders, 2009). Although not all deaf adults have embraced the technology wholeheartedly, a striking number of deaf adults now sport implants or have implanted their minor deaf children. In this chapter, we seek to examine the trend in the number of deaf signers who underwent cochlear implantation as well as what their reported experiences and attitudes toward those implants have generally been. More broadly, we are interested in identifying trends in the attitudes of Deaf adult signers toward CIs.

Unfortunately, there has been relatively little of a scholarly nature written about the genesis and effects of this movement within the Deaf community and the concomitant changes in attitude that accompanied and accelerated this trend. What research there has been on the impact of CIs on deaf people has tended to focus on the generic, mostly nonsigning population rather than the Deaf signers who were the first, most ferocious opponents of the implants and who are now moving to a space where implants are accepted as just one in a range of options available to deaf people. It is important here to clarify what we mean by "deaf" and "Deaf." We define "deaf" people as these with hearing loss who do not employ sign language as a primary mode of communication in any sphere of their lives and who do not interact much, if at all, with other deaf people as colleagues or friends. In this context, "Deaf" people reflect the group we call "Deaf adult signers."

Review of the Literature

Hallberg and Ringdahl (2004) were among the first to study how implants affected deaf adults. Their study's stated aim was to "gain a deeper insight into the subjective experiences of the effects of CIs on the quality of life" (p. 116). The results of that study illustrated a profound difference between how deaf and Deaf people viewed their deafness and the impact of CIs on them. The authors asserted that the primary emotion expressed by their 16 interviewees was one of "coming back to life" and again becoming part of the living world, with the unstated corollary that being deaf was akin to being dead to the rest of the world. However, Padden and Humphries noted in their seminal book *Deaf in America* (1990) that culturally Deaf people already have a rich language and ample access to social opportunities. They also noted that although culturally Deaf individuals are aware that they miss much audiological information that the hearing world takes for granted, they also generally consider their lives as being on a par with everyone else situated in a minority culture within a dominant majority.

Wolff (2007) studied a small group of prelingually deaf adults and found that, in general, they considered their CIs to have brought about positive quality of life changes after implantation. However, even his small sample of 6 was considerably diverse, with half of them involved with the Deaf community and half primarily users of spoken language. Wolff's interviewees had fewer negative feelings about their deafness and considered the CI a tool that better facilitated communication with their hearing family members and colleagues.

Other studies of CI use by deaf adults have focused on postlingually deafened adults who are often not members of the Deaf community. These studies have tended to emphasize the economic and audiological benefits rather than the social and psychological outcomes that this study is interested in. Thus, Cheng and Niparko (1999) and Zeng (2004) looked at the costs and benefits of CIs in dollar terms, whereas Waltzmann and Cohen (1999) and Manrique et al. (1995) looked at audiological and speech processing aspects of CIs.

Chee et al. (2004) looked at the benefits that the CI conferred on its subjects' quality of life. However, the 30 adults surveyed were all deaf from birth or an early age, and there was no indication of the deaf individuals' primary mode of communication. Although signing was one of the options included on the multiple-choice questions, it was not cross-referenced with responses, so we could not ascertain which data referred specifically to Deaf adults. Other research studies have been conducted primarily at the behest of the CI companies, and the results focus on specific CI models and brands. Waltzmann and Cohen (1999) researched the Clarion CI; Castro, Lassaletta, Bastarrica, and Alfonso (2005) focused on the Med-El brand; and other research that focused on the advantages and disadvantages of CIs is considerably older and likely outdated, since these studies were carried out before the current generation of multichannel CIs were developed. An example of this is Tyler (1994) and Tyler and Kelsay (1990), who conducted surveys on deaf adults considering CI surgery and then again surveyed these individuals a few months after the surgery was concluded. Again, these studies did not specify how many of the recipients were primarily signers. Consequently, we cannot conclude if any or even a minority of those in the study was Deaf or simply deaf individuals with CIs.

In early 2009, almost 62% of an estimated 67,000 American CI recipients were adults (National Institute on Deafness and Other Communication Disorders, 2009). The number of signers and the onset of their deafness within this group are unknown. There is plenty of information about the cost and postimplant rehabilitation appropriate for the CI adult patients, but little coherent summary information is available on how well deaf American adult signers are living with CIs and how satisfied they are with the implant-related outcome.

In this chapter, we highlight a few themes that appear to be intrinsic to the experience of all those who underwent cochlear implantation as adults and use sign language in their daily lives. This chapter addresses the following questions:

- What aspects of CI-related experiences appear to affect the overall quality of life of those who use sign language in their daily lives?
- Are there varying levels of attitudes toward CI usage?
- Do CI adult signers report satisfaction with their implant use in situations where listening and/or speaking are necessary?

- Did they perceive family and/or friends' support to be important for their decision to get an implant?
- Do the CI signers perceive their health professionals to be working effectively as partners in delivering state-of-the-art care and empowerment?
- Are there barriers to considering implantation that Deaf adult signers should be aware of and be prepared to overcome?

Survey Development and Procedure

We explored the above questions by applying survey techniques in Web-based data collection. Qualitative interviews with 10 adult CI recipients were first conducted to obtain reports of their pre- and postimplant experiences. Broad interview questions related to CI experiences and outcomes were developed based on relevant literature. CI recipients were asked to elaborate on the factors that they felt were important to their decision making prior to implantation. They were also asked about their experiences and satisfaction following CI surgery and rehabilitation. Their qualitative responses were analyzed for common themes and used to generate items. Item reduction and selection of similar items that were the most clearly worded were achieved by input from 3 other CI recipients.

The anonymous online survey was a 30-item self-administered questionnaire using a 10-point Likert scale with responses ranging from "not at all" to "very much." All items were worded as statements. The respondents were asked to rate how strongly the statements applied to their CI experience. This CI experience survey was sent to electronic mailing lists and posted on Web sites targeted at CI users. The study was approved by the Gallaudet University institutional review board, and all participants provided informed consent. Confidentiality was ensured because participants were not asked to provide identifying information such as name, location, and workplace.

Response data were downloaded and entered into SPSS statistical software (SPSS Inc., Chicago, IL). We conducted reliability testing to ensure consistency across survey responses. Cronbach's alpha for all items ranged between .90 and .93, which is considered "very good" by convention. We kept items that showed an acceptable range of responses. Three items had high agreement response (ceiling effect) from more than 75% of respondents, and these were removed from the scale. The final questionnaire had 27 items that were included in the analysis for this study (see Appendix A).

Participants

The CI experience online survey was viewed by 290 people. Of these, 105 proceeded to answer the common core set of demographic questions about age, education, onset of deafness, and age of language acquisition for American Sign Language (ASL) and English. Within this group, 51 respondents continued to answer questions specific to the CI experience. Two respondents reported that they had not acquired ASL nor did they use it at home, work, or in the community. These 2 nonsigners were excluded from the sample group. The age range in the final sample (N = 49) is 19 to 62 years old.

Within the total sample of 49 adult respondents, 12 respondents received their first implantation as children (between ages 4 and 17) and 6 of these child recipients elected a second implantation in the other ear when they were adults. Their survey responses were compared to 37 deaf signers who were implanted for the first time when they were adults. Only one item ("I felt I fully understood what the CI process involved before I made my decision") yielded significant group difference. This is expected, as the parents made the decision for those who were implanted as children. For all other items, no significant group differences were found for the child-implanted adult group and adult-implanted group. These two groups were merged into one group for all analyses, including or excluding the one item mentioned above.

The following table presents the statistics on our 49 valid respondents. Table 1 provides a demographic summary of the survey sample, consisting of primarily Caucasian females with postsecondary education. Adult CI signers in our study were likely to have had some experience with hearing aids prior to implantation ($r = .61$; $p < .001$). Among participants who wore hearing aids prior to cochlear implantation, only 28% perceived their functional hearing ability to be average or above average. The other 72% of participants rated their functional hearing ability (with hearing aids) prior to implantation to be below average or poor. At the time of survey completion, 9 unilateral CI participants reported using hearing aids on the non-CI side. Fifteen other participants are bilateral CI users.

Approximately 65% of the respondents came from an all-hearing family background, and most learned English before acquiring ASL as a second language. All participants reported using ASL in the community. When asked about frequency of ASL usage at home, 59% of participants reported using ASL frequently or at all times. This figure dropped to 49% for high frequency of ASL usage in the workplace. This includes using ASL directly or through interpreters to communicate with coworkers.

Results

- What aspects of CI-related experiences appear to effect the overall quality of life of those who utilize sign language in their daily lives?
- Are there varying levels of attitudes toward CI usage?

Table 1. Characteristics of CI Signer Survey Participants (N=49)

Characteristics	Percentage	Characteristics	Mean (SD)
Gender			
Male	35	Age	41 (12.69)
Female	65		
Ethnicity			
Caucasian	85	Years of hearing aid usage	21 (14.87)
Hispanic	6	Age implanted as an adult	37 (10.81)
African American	4		
Asian	4		
Highest education level			
High school	2	Age first learned ASL	15 (9.96)
Some college	14	Age first learned English	3 (3.09)
College graduate	22		
Graduate degree	61		
Hearing level in better ear			
Moderate-severe	2		
Severe	10		
Profound	80		
Progressive loss	4		
Did not report	4		
Deaf family members			
Most or all	8		
Sibling(s) or extended only	18		
Mixed	8		
None	65		

In a multivariate statistical analysis, "ASL usage" was used as a predictor variable to evaluate its influence on all items in the survey. Separate analyses were conducted for ASL usage at home, work, and in the community. For example, the researchers wanted to know if the frequency of ASL usage at home predicted the deaf signer's perception of their CI experience in the survey, First, the deaf signer participants were divided into three groups: frequently use ASL at home, sometimes use ASL at home, and rarely use ASL at home. Second, all survey items were entered as dependent variables. Finally, multivariate analyses were run to compare these three groups on all survey items. This same procedure was used again in separate analyses for "ASL usage at work" and "ASL usage in the community."

For ASL usage at home, a significant between-group effect ($p < .05$) was found on 4 of 25 items.

1. Compared to high ASL users at home, participants who do not use or use little ASL at home were more likely to report that their CI devices are not user-friendly. This suggests that these participants are likely to be heavy CI users who communicate in spoken language at home and will expect more out of their CI usability.
2. A significant group difference was found between high ASL usage and low ASL usage at home on an item that asked about the respondents' belief that their understanding of speech perception will improve with more practice and speech therapy. Participants who do not use or use little ASL at home rated higher on an item that asked about their belief that their understanding of speech perception will improve with more practice and speech therapy (mean score = 9 out of 10 on a Likert scale) than high ASL usage at home participants (mean score = 7 out of 10 on a Likert scale).
3. Adults with CIs who reported that they sometimes use ASL at home rated significantly higher on an item that asked about their perceived ability to participate in groups than other groups of participants who never or always use ASL at home. This likely suggests that participants who use ASL sometimes at home are more affected in their communication than other participants. For example, participants who never use ASL at home are likely to have established better spoken communication with their family members. Similarly, other participants who always use ASL at home do not have a reason to expect that the CI will help improve their group participation at home.
4. The group who never used ASL at home was reportedly least satisfied with overall CI usage compared to the other two groups. One possible interpretation of this finding is the level of expectation among CI users who do not sign at home. These participants use spoken language to communicate with other members at home and therefore may have greater expectations from CI functionality and usage.

For reported ASL usage at work, significant between-group effect was found on several items that asked about perceived impact of CI on group participation. Participants who use ASL less frequently at work were more likely to perceive increased CI benefit for group participation and sense of inclusion in the workplace, increased speech understanding and communication, and greater satisfaction with CI-related outcomes.

For reported ASL usage in the community, there were no significant group differences on any survey items.

- Do CI adult signers report satisfaction with their implant use in situations where listening and/or speaking are necessary?

A regression analysis was conducted on the full model consisting of all CI-related experiences in the survey as predictor variables with overall satisfaction as a dependent variable. The adjusted R^2 for this model was .97. R^2 provides an idea of how much CI-related survey items (predictor variables) as one group contributes to an overall satisfaction item (dependent variable). The survey items explain 97% of the overall satisfaction item, which is very good. The other 3% could be other factors or issues that we did not ask about in the survey. Within the full model, three predictors made the highest contribution to overall satisfaction among adult signers who have CI(s). The predictors that have a larger contribution to overall postimplant satisfaction are (1) unexpected benefits of CI, (2) usefulness of the CI in monitoring their own voice quality and loudness, and (3) the positive influence of the CI on becoming comfortable with oneself as a deaf or hard of hearing person.

- Do the CI signers perceive their health professionals to be working effectively as partners in delivering state-of-the-art care and empowerment?

Among those who received a CI for the first time as adults, 51% reported that they underwent psychological evaluation as part of the pre-CI candidacy procedure although correlation analysis showed that psychological evaluation was not associated with informed decision about CI surgery. However, among deaf signers who were implanted as an adult for the first time, there is a moderate correlation between having had a psychological evaluation and perceived satisfaction with the CI ($r = .30$; $p < .02$).

There is a significant correlation between opting for a second CI and perceived valuation of medical providers in empowering the respondents' total communicative quality of life ($r = .71$; $p < .003$). Having a positive relationship with medical providers appears to contribute to a person's decision to get a second CI. Deaf signers' perception of medical provider's role in empowering or supporting their total communicative quality of life is associated with CI satisfaction ($r = .579$; $p < .001$).

- Did they perceive family and/or friends' support to be important to their decision to get an implant?

There was a ceiling effect for an item that asked if the family was supportive of the Deaf adult signer's decision to get an implant. A large percentage of participants in this study reported that their families were supportive of their decision to get an implant.

On other items that asked the respondents to rate how important their family's or friends' support was in making a decision to get an implant as an adult, only the friends' support item emerged as having a significant correlation with age. This means that as one ages, friends' support becomes more important in the deaf signer's decision to get an implant as an adult.

Interestingly, on another item that asked about the deaf signer's perception of the difficulty involved in dealing with family expectations at the time of cochlear implantation, age of acquisition for ASL was associated with greater difficulty in dealing with family expectations. In other words, the later the deaf signer learns ASL, the more likely the deaf signer will report some difficulty in dealing with family expectations associated with getting an implant. The family may view the CI as capable of providing greater functionality to the deaf signer who has been using spoken language all of his or her life; however, the deaf person may hold a different opinion about how much functionality the CI will provide.

Regression analyses were conducted on "age of ASL acquisition" as the predictor and three attitude-related items as dependent variables. The attitude-related items were worded as follows: (1) My getting a CI created tensions between deaf friends and me, (2) I feel that Deaf communities react differently to my CI, and (3) I would implant my child. Age of ASL acquisition did not have a significant effect on any of those items.

Regression analyses were also conducted using "age of English acquisition" as the predictor with the same attitude-related items. Age of English acquisition was a significant predictor for the item, "My getting a CI created tension between deaf friends and me" ($t = 4.00$; $p < .001$). On this item, signers who learned English later were more likely to rate higher tension between themselves and deaf friends.

On the item, "My getting a CI created tensions between deaf friends and me," deaf signer participants who always/frequently use ASL in the community or the workplace rated this item significantly higher than other deaf signer participants who sometimes use ASL in the community ($t = 2.7$; $p < .05$) or occasionally use ASL in the workplace ($t = 3.58$; $p < .008$).

There is a gender effect (t-value range: 4.09–7.56; $p < .05$), with female signers rating significantly higher on the following items than male signers:

1. I feel that Deaf communities react differently to my CI.
2. If better CI technology came along, I would get it.
3. I am satisfied with my implant.
4. My CI helps monitor my own voice loudness and quality.
5. My implant helps me make myself understood with fewer clarifications.
6. I feel my implant is not user-friendly.

We interpret all of the above issues to be due to one of two possible factors. One is increased sensitivity and expectations for their implant among females, and the second is the desire to be "inclusive" in the society if females perceive themselves to be at greater disadvantages compared to deaf male signers.

In addition to the Likert-scaled questions, survey respondents filled out qualitative questions about their experiences with implants. These responses provided a richer level of detail to the answers we obtained through the scaled questions.

The first question was "How have hearing people (i.e., family and friends) around you responded to your being implanted?" As might be expected, the reaction of survey respondents' hearing family and friends was overwhelmingly positive. The majority of respondents mentioned that their family and friends supported them and saw the implantation as "a positive step" toward improving communication. Of the 47 people who answered this question, only 1 responded "unknown." All the others had varying degrees of positive responses, although these were intermixed with what the respondents considered unrealistic expectations. Following is a typical response from this category:

> Family unfortunately continues to have high expectations and still "expect" me to wear it at all times, and insist that I "perform better" with it on, and I don't really think that's true. Sometimes I leave it off while wearing it, and they think I'm "performing better!" I think the CI process has reversed in some way the grieving process that hearing parents have for deaf children, so it causes more stress for everybody involved, I think. Ugh! My mother still looks around my head to see if I'm wearing it (especially if she's trying to get my attention) and I'm 27 years old! I think the CI has made them more "lazy" and dependent on the CI to get my attention, as if they've forgotten how to be parents of a deaf child.

Hearing family members and friends of people in this category (about 25% of the sample) tend to believe that the CI is a cure-all and will lead to better hearing almost overnight, not realizing the amount of work and therapy that is required for most CI implantees to obtain the most benefit from their CI. This can lead to an increased element of frustration for the implanted deaf individual, since, as one eloquently described it,

> They act like I'm hearing and get frustrated when I ask them not to all talk at the same time or to get my attention before talking to me—"frustrated" as in "pissed off," like they think that I'm faking deafness.

However, for the majority of the sample, hearing friends and family members have proved to be encouraging and accepting of the implant and supportive of the deaf person's decisions in getting it.

Surprisingly enough, the response to the question "How have deaf people (i.e., family and friends) around you responded to your being implanted?" is not very different from those of the implantees' hearing family members and friends. We found it surprising because of the dramatic nature of the Deaf community's reaction to implantation only 2 decades ago. Perhaps time—or greater familiarity with the devices and knowledge of their limitations and benefits—has muted this reaction. Respondents reported that most of their Deaf friends were cautiously supportive, although a few voiced misgivings or opposition to the implantation. Typical is the reaction this person outlined:

> The majority have been accepting, and several Deaf people have asked me lots of questions about it. I know some Deaf people who are opposed to CIs for deaf babies, but seem OK with me as an adult having one.

Less than half report receiving negative reactions from deaf friends regarding their getting an implant, surely a 180° change from even just a decade ago. These whose deaf friends and family were not as positive about the implants were actually more lukewarm in their attitude than negative, and this was primarily because of concern about the negative side effects of implants on the recipient rather than identity-related concerns. Respondents stated that their friends still considered them as primarily Deaf, even with the implant, and as one person said, "They realize I am the same person as I was before, I'm still Deaf the same way I was before." According to our respondents, they still had some Deaf friends who rejected the implants and expressed their negative attitudes to these friends, but in general most people keep their opinions to themselves if these opinions are negative.

Finally, we asked our survey respondents to tell us about the unexpected disadvantages of implants they have experienced. Approximately 21% of this group reported no disadvantages or no "unexpected" disadvantages. Of the rest, there was a variety of responses with no single recurring negative mentioned more than 3 times. These included the following:

- Inability to get magnetic resonance imaging.
- Weight of the implant and battery, resulting in headaches or sore ears.
- Length of time it takes to get used to the implant and to develop speech/listening skills and the lack of resources to accomplish these goals.
- Dizziness/headaches/not being able to hear as well when sick.
- Problems with batteries (short life, weight, difficulty replacing/ordering, etc.)
- Taunting from Deaf community members.
- Heightened expectations on the part of those who do not really understand how implants work and having to explain over and over.
- Low quality materials and design.
- Being unused to an extremely noisy world.
- Inability to immediately understand speech and other sounds.

In conclusion, it seems from this research that there has been a slow but very perceptible shift on the part of Deaf community members toward implants. Although not all members have wholeheartedly embraced cochlear implantation, the signing Deaf community seems to have come to terms with it for deaf adults at least, and more members as reflected in our study results are finding it acceptable not only to get implants for themselves but also to implant their children. Consequently, the attitudes of Deaf community members are no longer viewed as an insurmountable barrier to these signing deaf adults who want to obtain implants or implant their deaf children. Perhaps this is a result of culturally Deaf individuals leading the way, but whatever the cause, it seems that an increasing number of signing deaf adults have declared a truce in the war against cochlear implantation.

Appendix A

COCHLEAR IMPLANT EXPERIENCE SURVEY: 27 ITEMS

EVALUATING YOUR EXPERIENCE WITH COCHLEAR IMPLANT(S)

- You will read questions that ask how you feel about yourself.
- Please circle *ONE* number on each scale that *BEST* describes how the statement applies to you.

1. **My feelings about cochlear implants were the same after implantation as before . . .** *(please circle one number)*

   NOT AT ALL 0 1 2 3 4 5 6 7 8 9 10 VERY MUCH

2. **When I first started using it, I had a difficult time with my implant . . .** *(please circle one number)*

   NOT AT ALL 0 1 2 3 4 5 6 7 8 9 10 VERY MUCH

3. **I am satisfied with my implant . . .** *(please circle one number)*

   NOT AT ALL 0 1 2 3 4 5 6 7 8 9 10 VERY MUCH

4. **My CI helps monitor my own voice loudness and quality, as well as improve speechreading ability . . .** *(please circle one number)*

   NOT AT ALL 0 1 2 3 4 5 6 7 8 9 10 VERY MUCH

5. **My decision making process was quick and easy . . .** *(please circle one number)*

   NOT AT ALL 0 1 2 3 4 5 6 7 8 9 10 VERY MUCH

6. **My CI experience allowed me to be more comfortable with myself as a deaf or hard of hearing person . . .** *(please circle one number)*

   NOT AT ALL 0 1 2 3 4 5 6 7 8 9 10 VERY MUCH

7. **I felt I fully understood what the CI process involved before I made my decision . . .** *(please circle one number)*

   NOT AT ALL 0 1 2 3 4 5 6 7 8 9 10 VERY MUCH

8. **My implant helps me speechread better . . .** *(please circle one number)*

   NOT AT ALL 0 1 2 3 4 5 6 7 8 9 10 VERY MUCH

9. **I believe that with time, practice, and speech therapy, I will understand speech and sounds more . . .** *(please circle one number)*

   NOT AT ALL 0 1 2 3 4 5 6 7 8 9 10 VERY MUCH

10. **I rely on reading CI materials and listening to other people's experiences to help with CI-related decision making . . .** *(please circle one number)*

    NOT AT ALL 0 1 2 3 4 5 6 7 8 9 10 VERY MUCH

11. **I can distinguish among different kinds of sound . . .** *(please circle one number)*

    NOT AT ALL 0 1 2 3 4 5 6 7 8 9 10 VERY MUCH

12. **I feel my medical providers have empowered me or showed me how to improve my total communicative quality of life . . .** *(please circle one number)*

    NOT AT ALL 0 1 2 3 4 5 6 7 8 9 10 VERY MUCH

13. **Different deaf communities react differently to my CI . . .** *(please circle one number)*

    NOT AT ALL 0 1 2 3 4 5 6 7 8 9 10 VERY MUCH

14. **I would implant my child . . .** *(please circle one number)*

    NOT AT ALL 0 1 2 3 4 5 6 7 8 9 10 VERY MUCH

15. **My friends' support was important to me in deciding to get the implant . . .** *(please circle one number)*

    NOT AT ALL 0 1 2 3 4 5 6 7 8 9 10 VERY MUCH

16. **It was difficult to deal with my family's expectations for my CI . . .** *(please circle one number)*

    NOT AT ALL 0 1 2 3 4 5 6 7 8 9 10 VERY MUCH

17. **With my implant, I feel more inclusive in hearing groups . . .** *(please circle one number)*

    NOT AT ALL 0 1 2 3 4 5 6 7 8 9 10 VERY MUCH

18. **My family's support was important to me in deciding to get the implant . . .** *(please circle one number)*

    NOT AT ALL 0 1 2 3 4 5 6 7 8 9 10 VERY MUCH

19. **My implant helps me in the workplace . . .** *(please circle one number)*

    NOT AT ALL 0 1 2 3 4 5 6 7 8 9 10 VERY MUCH

20. **My getting a CI created tensions between deaf friends and I . . .** *(please circle one number)*

    Not At All 0 1 2 3 4 5 6 7 8 9 10 Very Much

21. **The implant gave me other benefits that I did not expect . . .** *(please circle one number)*

    Not At All 0 1 2 3 4 5 6 7 8 9 10 Very Much

22. **My sources of information were helpful . . .** *(please circle one number)*

    Not At All 0 1 2 3 4 5 6 7 8 9 10 Very Much

23. **My implant helps me make myself understood with less clarifications . . .** *(please circle one number)*

    Not At All 0 1 2 3 4 5 6 7 8 9 10 Very Much

24. **If better CI technology came along, I would get it . . .** *(please circle one number)*

    Not At All 0 1 2 3 4 5 6 7 8 9 10 Very Much

25. **I sometimes forget to wear my implant . . .** *(please circle one number)*

    Not At All 0 1 2 3 4 5 6 7 8 9 10 Very Much

26. **I have the resources to find and maintain cochlear implant rehabilitation . . .** *(please circle one number)*

    Not At All 0 1 2 3 4 5 6 7 8 9 10 Very Much

27. **I feel that my implant is not user-friendly . . .** *(please circle one number)*

    Not At All 0 1 2 3 4 5 6 7 8 9 10 Very Much

NOTE: The following items were removed due to ceiling effect:

a. **My family was supportive of my decision to get an implant . . .**

b. **My implant provides me with more advantages than a hearing aid . . .**

c. **My implant helps alert me to environmental cues . . .**

References

Castro, A., Lassaletta, L., Bastarrica, M., & Alfonso, C. (2005). Quality of life in cochlear implant patients. *Acta Otorrinolaringologica Espanola, 56*, 192–197.

Chee, G. H., Goldring, J. E., Shipp, D. B., Ng, A. H. C., Chen, J. M., & Nedzelski, J. M. (2004). Benefits of cochlear implantation in early-deafened adults: The Toronto experience. *Journal of Otolaryngology, 33*(1), 26–31.

Cheng, A. K., & Niparko, J. K. (1999). Cost-utility of the cochlear implant in adults. *Archives of Otolaryngology—Head & Neck Surgery, 125*(11), 1214–1218.

Hallberg, R. M., & Ringdahl, A. (2004). Living with cochlear implants: Experiences of 17 adult patients in Sweden. *International Journal of Audiology, 43*(2), 115–121.

Manrique, N., Huarte, A., Molina, M., Perez, N., Espinosa, J. M., Cervera-Paz, F. J., et al. (1995). Are cochlear implants indicated in prelingually deaf adults? *Annals of Otology, Rhinology & Laryngology. Supplement, 166*, 192–194.

National Association of the Deaf (2000). *Position statement on cochlear implants.* Retrieved April 8, 2011, from http://www.nad.org/issues/technology/assistive-listening/cochlear-implants

National Institute on Deafness and Other Communication Disorders. (2009). *Cochlear implants.* Retrieved April 8, 2011, from http://www.nidcd.nih.gov/health/hearing/coch.asp

Padden, C., & Humphries, T. (1990). *Deaf in America: Voices from a culture.* Cambridge, MA: Harvard University Press.

Tyler, R. S. (1994). Advantages and disadvantages expected and reported by cochlear implant patients. *American Journal of Otology, 15*(4), 523–531.

Tyler, R. S., & Kelsay, D. (1990). Advantages and disadvantages reported by some of the better cochlear-implant patients. *American Journal of Otology, 11*(4), 282–289.

Waltzmann, S. B., & Cohen, N. L. (1999). Implantation of patients with prelingual long-term deafness. *Annals of Otology, Rhinology, & Laryngology. Supplement, 177*, 84–87.

Wolff, R. (2007). *The effect of self-efficacy on prelingually deaf adults' decision to have cochlear implants and subsequent life changes.* Unpublished doctoral dissertation, Walden University.

Zeng, F. G. (2004). Trends in cochlear implants. *Trends in amplification, 8*(1), 1–34.

5

MY CHILD CAN HAVE MORE CHOICES: REFLECTIONS OF DEAF MOTHERS ON COCHLEAR IMPLANTS FOR THEIR CHILDREN

Julie Mitchiner and Marilyn Sass-Lehrer

Deaf children have more opportunities in the 21st century than ever before. Many of these opportunities are accompanied by a host of choices thrust upon parents/caregivers in the first few months of their child's life. Although the literature focuses almost exclusively on the decisions and opportunities that hearing families face, few researchers have investigated deaf families' experiences (Meadow-Orlans, Mertens, & Sass-Lehrer, 2003; Meadow-Orlans, Spencer, & Koester, 2004). The proliferation of cochlear implants has added a level of complexity to the decisions confronting both hearing and deaf families. The issues, concerns, and, ultimately, decisions these families make may be different. This chapter describes the insights of three deaf families who chose cochlear implants for their children and their views on language, literacy, and Deaf culture.

Background

Although the strong negative reaction to cochlear implantation within the Deaf community in the early 1990s has lessened, there continues to be considerable controversy about the potential harmful versus beneficial consequences of this technology for young children (Lane, 2005; Marschark, 2007; Wever, 2002). It is still uncommon for culturally Deaf parents to elect to have their children implanted. Wever (2002) suggested that parental decisions regarding cochlear implantation may be influenced by their beliefs about what it means to be deaf. That is, those who perceive that being deaf is a "disability" are more apt to consider technologies that will remediate what they consider a deficit. Skepticism about the effectiveness of cochlear implants led Julie, the first author of this chapter, to take a closer look at her own feelings about cochlear implants and her identity as a culturally Deaf person. She wondered why deaf parents would elect this procedure for their children.

> My attitudes and perspectives about young deaf children getting cochlear implants have gradually evolved since the first time I heard about deaf people getting cochlear implants. Growing up with deaf parents and attending deaf schools, I have a strong sense of pride of being deaf and being part of the Deaf community. I do not look at myself as disabled. I often say if I were given a choice to hear or stay deaf, I'd choose to stay deaf. It is who I am. My family, my friends, and my community have taught me that being deaf is part of our culture and is a way of life. Many deaf people have succeeded in life without having the ability to hear. They've become lawyers, doctors, scientists, and teachers. It has nothing to do with the ability to hear. It has to do with many other factors such as the person's attitude, values, beliefs, and motivation.
>
> I used to oppose strongly the idea of deaf people getting cochlear implants. It indicates the need to "fix" the problem. I felt betrayed and angry that doctors implanted deaf children. What does this say about me? It tells me that there is something wrong with me. Being deaf is natural to me, and putting "machines" inside children's heads frightened me. I believed that it would destroy deaf children's sense of pride and they'd end up viewing themselves as disabled. I had heard stories that many deaf children ended up throwing away their cochlear implants when they got older. One of my friends had her cochlear implant surgically removed. She was ashamed to have a cochlear implant. She was stuck with a huge scar on her head. In the past, mostly hearing parents chose to have their deaf children implanted and it was almost nonexistent in deaf children with deaf parents. Most deaf parents shared the same beliefs as me. It seemed to me that the deaf community did not want to interact with families who chose to have their deaf children implanted. Many of us criticized these parents and blamed doctors for "brainwashing" the parents. We believed that doctors didn't share all of the options with the families, and they often offered only one solution, which was to get a cochlear implant. It was frequently recommended by health care providers that deaf children with cochlear implants attend oral programs rather than schools for deaf children using sign language so that these implanted deaf children would have maximum exposure to spoken language.

The numbers of deaf children with deaf parents/caregivers receiving implants appear to be growing due to advances in technology and the explosion of available information. A rising number of families with deaf parents/caregivers, like hearing parents, have decided to have their young deaf children implanted (D. Nussbaum, personal communication, February 2008). The rapid increase in cochlear implantation is due to several factors, including enhanced technologies, improved surgical procedures, and an escalation in the literature on the outcomes for young children.

Julie explains her changing views about implants this way:

My attitude about cochlear implants began to change slightly as I increased my knowledge about cochlear implants. I began to accept the idea of having adults receive cochlear implants, especially those who became deaf later in life. I was still completely against the idea of having parents make decisions about their children getting cochlear implants. I believed that the children should wait until they were old enough to make decisions themselves. . . . However, an increasing number of researchers have suggested that the earlier the children got their implants, the better they were able to access sound and develop speech skills.

In 2000 when I first started working in a deaf program with preschoolers, my school boldly initiated a Cochlear Implant Education Center to share resources and information with families about cochlear implants. They also implemented a pilot class with preschoolers. They had a separate class only for children with cochlear implants in a small room next to my classroom. They had a hearing teacher with a hearing teacher aide. They used sign-supported spoken language as the communication approach. I had the opportunity to interact with the children from the pilot class. The more I interacted with them, the more I realized the role I need to play to support these children. My attitude began to change, and I realized I had many misconceptions about cochlear implants. The biggest misconception was that cochlear implants would change deaf children, and they would not maintain a sense of deaf pride. I began to realize that cochlear implants are simply tools. At the same time, I began to take courses in bilingual education in American Sign Language (ASL) and English and learned about the positive benefits of bilingualism. My hearing co-teacher and I began to discuss how we could better educate children with cochlear implants. We came up with several ideas and met with the administrators at the school about a new class. We wanted to teach children with cochlear implants. Since my co-teacher was hearing, she could provide spoken English language support, and I as a deaf teacher could provide sign language support. This way all children would get the best of both languages. My co-teacher and I taught a range of children, children with cochlear implants, children who were hard of hearing, and children who were profoundly deaf. The outcomes were positive. Children with cochlear implants could easily code-switch between spoken language and sign language. I remember one time when one of my students signed to me about something and then the next minute she used spoken language to tell my co-teacher the same thing she had just signed to me. This is what we wanted to accomplish. Deaf children were able to have deaf role models and maintain a sense of deaf pride with deaf teachers. We began to publicize our approach to other programs. My attitudes about children getting cochlear implants changed completely and I began to be open to it.

Several researchers have shown improvement in spoken language skills for children who received implants prior to 3 years of age and an increase in the number of children who use spoken language as their preferred mode of communication up to 5 years after implantation (e.g., McConkey Robbins, Burton Koch, Osberger, Zimmerman-Phillips, & Kishon-Rabin, 2004; Sharma, Dorman, & Spohr, 2002; Watson, Archbold, & Nikolopoulous, 2006; Yoshinaga-Itano, 2006). Although researchers have primarily focused on improvements in spoken language, a few have examined improvements in specific areas of language (Geers, Moog, Biedenstein, Brenner, & Hayes, 2009).

WHY A COCHLEAR IMPLANT FOR DEAF CHILDREN IN DEAF FAMILIES?

Researchers have suggested that deaf children who are highly fluent in American Sign Language (ASL) are superior in academic achievement, reading and writing, and social development to deaf children who are not fluent signers (Singleton, Supalla, Litchfield, & Schley, 1998; Snoddon, 2008; Strong & Prinz, 1997, 2000). Deaf children consistently perform at higher levels on tests of both ASL and English in large part due to the early and consistent visual access to language (Israelite & Ewoldt, 1992). Early accessible and natural communication between parents and their deaf children results in a strong language foundation that is equal in all aspects to the language foundation that hearing children acquire from their hearing parents (Volterra & Iverson, 1995; Volterra, Iverson, & Castrataro, 2006). Family values and cultural traditions likewise are easily passed on when families and their children share the same language and communication modality.

Deaf children with deaf parents in general have demonstrated better outcomes than their peers with hearing nonsigning parents although many of these children have chosen not to use hearing technologies of any kind (Gallaudet Research Institute, 2006; Newport & Meier, 1985). Some deaf parents are now expressing a desire for more. That is, not only do they want their children to be academically successful and linguistically fluent in ASL and written English, but they also want their children to be competent users of spoken English. Many parents believe that by providing access to spoken English their children will have the same opportunities as their hearing peers. Deaf parents interviewed for the National Parent Project (Meadow-Orlans et al., 2003) emphasized high expectations for their children and the opportunity for their children to have the same choices and opportunities as all children.

Professionals and families alike have misconceptions about cochlear implants. Medical and other health care professionals tend to be leery about the use of sign language with children who have cochlear implants. Although research and practice are slowly dismantling the myth that sign language interferes with the development of spoken language, additional misinformation about cochlear implants persists. Cochlear implants are not a cure for being deaf and do not make deaf children into hearing children. Hearing technologies, such as hearing aids and cochlear implants, provide access to information from sound but do not fully restore hearing (Blamey, 2003). Although hearing technologies are extremely beneficial to some, others find these technologies unhelpful or choose not to use them. Families, both deaf and hearing, often find it difficult to obtain current, accurate, and nonbiased information about the outcomes for children who have cochlear implants (Johnson, 2006; Li, Bain, & Steinberg, 2003). For families who are deaf, these obstacles may be complicated by the lack of clear communication with professionals (Meadow-Orlans et al., 2003). On the other hand, professionals may make assumptions that families who are deaf have already decided against cochlear implantation and therefore do not provide them with the same information that they provide hearing families.

Purpose and Research Questions

There is a plethora of resources and information about cochlear implants that are readily accessible to hearing parents, however, there is virtually no research to date and little information or resources available that specifically address deaf parents who have children with cochlear implants. This chapter presents an effort to ascertain how deaf parents obtained information about cochlear implants and what resources were most helpful to them.

Deaf families have unique strengths and challenges. Through the use of ASL, Deaf families are able to provide full access to language for their children from birth. Deaf children with fluently signing parents acquire language at the same rate as hearing children through spoken language (Meier, 1991; Petitto, 2000; Volterra & Iverson, 1995; Volterra et al., 2006). ASL provides a foundation for the acquisition of other languages (including English) and appears to provide an advantage for acquiring spoken English for children who have cochlear implants (Preisler, Tvingstedt, & Ahlström, 2002; Yoshinaga-Itano & Sedey, 2000; Yoshinaga-Itano, 2006).

Deaf families considering cochlear implants for their children have unique challenges. For example, hearing parents can easily provide spoken English support at home, whereas deaf parents may need to rely on other resources. A pilot study was conducted in 2008 to learn more about the perspectives of deaf parents who had decided on cochlear implants for their children and to discover how they were supporting literacy and language development in ASL and English. The results of this investigation may provide professionals working with deaf families with suggestions for how to provide better information and support.

An interview protocol was designed to answer the following questions:

1. What do deaf families hope their children will be able to accomplish with cochlear implants?
2. How do deaf families support their children's language development in ASL and English?
3. What educational choices and decisions do they make?
4. What advantages as well as challenges do they face in supporting their children's language, literacy, and cultural development?

Interviews with these families provided a glimpse into their personal goals and beliefs as well as their successes and challenges for supporting their children's development.

Participants and Research Setting

Participants interviewed for this investigation were mothers who are deaf and have young children with cochlear implants. All parents used both ASL and written English with their children. The population of deaf parents with deaf children who have cochlear implants is quite small compared to the population of hearing parents with deaf children who have cochlear implants, making it difficult to find a large number of participants. A "snowball" approach was used to locate families to participate. Julie contacted Cochlear Implant Children of Deaf Adults, a support group for deaf parents with deaf children who have cochlear implants. This group has connections with deaf families with children with cochlear implants across the country. The support group was formed to provide support for deaf parents seeking advice and to share experiences about their journey. An invitation to participate in this investigation was posted on the support group's listserv site. Only four families expressed interest. One of the families was eliminated from participation in the study because the child had not yet undergone cochlear implantation. The fact that only three families agreed to participate may have been an indication of some reluctance among these nonparticipating families to trust that the researcher, who was herself deaf, would be accepting of their decisions, be nonjudgmental, and maintain confidentiality.

Description of Participants

Sierra comes from a multigeneration deaf family. She has a son who was born deaf and received a cochlear implant when he was around 18 months old. Her husband is hard of hearing.

---

* All identifying information has been changed to protect confidentiality.

Jasmine was the only deaf member of her birth family. She and her deaf husband have several young children. Their daughter received her cochlear implant when she was 20 months old. Her daughter was exposed to ASL from the time she was born. After receiving her cochlear implant, spoken language developed rapidly.

The third mother interviewed for the study, Lauren, also is from a multigeneration deaf family. She grew up in mainstream settings and was part of both hearing and Deaf communities. She and her late deafened husband have several children. Their daughter received her cochlear implant at age 7.

Each participant was asked where and how they would be most comfortable doing the interview. All three interviews were conducted in different parts of the United States.

Data Collection

The data for this study were derived from interviews with the above three participants. Each interview was slightly different depending on the comfort level of the interviewee and her individual experiences. From time to time, questions needed to be restated to ensure that the participants understood the terminology used. For example, not all of the participants shared the same understanding of the term "literacy." Consequently, the interviewer needed to explain that she was interested in learning about the family's experiences with reading, writing, and book sharing. Whereas one participant wanted to talk more about her decision making process and the Deaf community's reaction, others shared more about how they supported their child's language development in ASL and English.

Table 1. Descriptions of the Participants

Mothers who were interviewed in the study	Sierra	Jasmine	Lauren
Mother's family background	Comes from multigenerations of deaf families	Hearing parents	Comes from multigenerations of deaf families
Hearing status of the participants and their spouses	Mother is deaf and spouse is hard of hearing	Both parents are deaf	Mother is deaf and spouse is late deafened
Time of child's hearing loss	From birth	From birth	From birth
Age of child's implantation	18 months old	20 months old	7 years old
Age of child at the time of the study	2 years old	3 years old	10 years old

All of the videotaped interviews were translated from ASL to English. ELAN, an electronic transcribing tool, was used to create annotations of the videos. Each interview required close to 30 hours to transcribe. Each participant was sent a copy of the transcription of their interview with the goal of ensuring that they felt the transcriptions reflected what they said and meant. Feedback was requested for this purpose. Some of the feedback was related to word choices used to translate from ASL to English. Other feedback from the mothers pertained to clarity or additional information based on their answers.

Data Analysis

The transcriptions of each of the interviews were reviewed several times to identify themes that emerged from the data. Highlighting pens with different colors were used to differentiate these themes. During the first level of coding, all comments that had significance and relevance to the main questions and purpose of the interview or appeared to provide additional insight into the participants' decisions or feelings were identified. The next level of coding involved identifying statements describing their reasons for deciding to have their children implanted, the support the participants received for their decisions, and comments about their children's language use and beliefs.

Because of the large number of comments related to language, these comments were differentiated into three categories: languages used at home, school, and with friends. These comments also reflected the participants' beliefs about using both ASL and English. An additional category was created to identify participants' beliefs about language use and practice in general. Other themes that emerged included the impact of the cochlear implant on the child, the family, their decision about educational placements, and their thoughts about the Deaf and hearing communities' support for children and families with cochlear implants.

The next step in the thematic analysis included a more in-depth exploration of each of the themes identified. Using the software program Excel, insights and other observational notes as well as specific comments that reflected each theme were recorded. This process provided a useful way to connect the participant's own words and the themes with the research questions.

Findings

The following discussion highlights the main themes that emerged from the interviews with quotations from the parents that support their perspectives and beliefs related to the central research questions:

1. What did these families hope to accomplish with cochlear implants?
2. How did these families support their children's language development in ASL and English?
3. What educational choices and decisions did they make?
4. What advantages and challenges do they face in supporting their children's language, literacy, and cultural development?

"I Want to Give Her Wings, Put Wings on Her."

During the first part of the interviews, all of the mothers shared their reasons for their decisions to have their children implanted. Before they made the decision, each family questioned whether cochlear implants actually worked. They relied on different sources of information. All of the mothers mentioned that they had observed other children with cochlear implants and noted that these children were able to speak clearly. They depended on hard of hearing and hearing people they trusted to assure them that the cochlear implant was beneficial in developing spoken language. Sierra relied on people who had access to spoken English to inform her that a child with a cochlear implant could speak clearly. Sierra had doubts about the effectiveness of cochlear implants based on what she had heard from various sources. In addition, she did not trust the audiologists and speech therapists who claimed the cochlear implants worked. Some people in the Deaf community felt audiologists and speech therapists patronize them by saying their speech was good or that their cochlear implants worked, when they really did not.

> At the party, he (a little boy with a cochlear implant) spoke a lot. I observed him and asked my husband, who is hard of hearing, if he could hear him speaking. He listened to him and said he spoke clearly. In the past, I've heard that CIs were lousy and didn't work. This time, it was successful for real. It was the first time that I really understood. Oh, it really works! (Sierra)

Lauren also had doubts and wanted to see the evidence for herself.

> I wanted to see how these children who have CIs functioned in an oral environment. I wanted to see and observe. I went to a second place (spells place), another oral program in (town). I went there and observed with my daughter. I observed and observed. I was impressed with these kids (pause), their ability to listen and talk fluently.

In an e-mail following the interview, Lauren added,

> I am obviously not able to know if they're talking fluently. I had a hearing parent who was a close friend of mine who had a deaf 4-year-old come with me. She was considering implanting her child at that time. She was the one who said she could understand almost everything that the kids were saying.

Jasmine also did some investigations on her own.

> I've seen children at (names school) who had CIs; they were signing and speaking. I noticed that. I became curious about what's up with CIs. (Jasmine)

The mothers' reasons for choosing a cochlear implant were strongly related to their desires to provide their children with more communication and language choices. Even though they had a range of different reasons, they repeatedly emphasized giving their children more choices in life and the ability to communicate with more people. All three of the mothers emphasized this point:

> Really, he could learn not only spoken English but learn other spoken languages and have the opportunity to interact with anyone and not limit himself only to those who can only sign. He can have more choices. (Sierra)
>
> We thought why not give our daughter the opportunity to have the ability to hear and develop spoken language. It'll become easier for her to participate in both communities. She can switch back and forth between the two, including our hearing families. (Jasmine)
>
> I wanted to see her have more opportunities in the world, because it's a hearing world and I don't want to limit her choices only to having to find jobs within the deaf world such as in deaf education or whatever related to sign language (shakes head). For her, she can go for it. Nowadays and in the future, it will be different compared to my time and my parents' time a long time ago. It was in the heydays for deaf people back then. The Deaf communities are getting smaller and smaller and spread all over and becoming thinner. It means it's becoming limited in different places. I don't want that. I want her to have more choices; I encourage it. Go, go, go. (Lauren)

"I'm a Part of Both Worlds—Hearing and Deaf Community"

The three participants indicated that their beliefs and perspectives on language development strongly influenced their reasons for choosing to implant their children. These mothers wanted their children to maintain both ASL and

English so that they would be able to shift back and forth between both language communities.

Their own experiences of being deaf also had an impact on their decision. They all expressed the wish that their children would have more opportunities than they had. All of them talked about needing to depend on interpreters and the challenges in communicating directly with hearing people. They indicated that their ability to engage in meaningful relationships with hearing people who do not sign is limited. They wanted their children to have the abilities to have direct and meaningful communication with both deaf and hearing people.

> I am fully deaf and I can't talk, nothing. I've worked in the hearing world for a few years. It was very tough, mostly dealing with communication. A little request required a lot of work. I had to bring my writing pad so I could communicate with them. It wasn't easy. (Sierra)
>
> We acknowledged that we've had a hard time fitting in with our hearing families. It is hard to communicate with them. There is no communication between our families and it has caused separation between our hearing families and us. The Deaf community and the hearing community are separated because of that. (Jasmine)
>
> I'm part of both worlds—hearing and Deaf community. I go back and forth between both communities, but I (grimaces) still have frustrations, because my speech is limited. I know it. My hard of hearing friends are more involved. I was envious because I wanted to be able to be involved more. Anyway, I grew up in a mainstreamed setting until I was almost in the eighth grade. I was in a hearing school. I had hearing interpreters. Throughout college, university, and my master's years, I was in hearing settings. Except, I was in a deaf school for a short period of time. I was comfortable in both settings, and I wanted my daughter to have similar opportunities that I had, but MORE, similar or more than that. (Lauren)

All of the mothers interviewed for this study said that their children showed little benefit from hearing aids and that this was one of the primary reasons they chose cochlear implants.

Sierra and Jasmine thought about waiting until their children were older so that they could make their own decision. However, doctors, audiologists, and others stressed the importance of implanting children before they were 18 months old. The mothers were told that their children would require less speech therapy and have an easier time acquiring spoken language if their children were implanted early. Both mothers felt they had to make the decision as quickly as possible. Sierra's son was 15 months old when she decided to proceed with a cochlear implant and was able to rush the procedure so that her son could be implanted by the time he was 18 months old. Watching a video about the surgery facilitated her decision to speed up the process of getting her son a cochlear implant:

> It wasn't easy watching the video of the surgery. However, along the video, it included text of descriptions about the surgery on the side. I was reading it also. One of the descriptions said, "Best results for CI happens before the child is 18 months old." I saw that. At that time, my son was 15 to 16 months old. I was surprised. 18 months old! I did not realize that. I thought I could take my time and wait until later. 18 months old! At that moment, it struck me. I began to realize if I want to consider it, I must decide soon. It's not like I can wait too long, then it'll be too late. That window of opportunity would be closed shut. I told myself, "Do it!" (Sierra)

Jasmine's daughter, on the other hand, received her CI when she was around 20 months old.

It was different for Lauren. Her daughter was 3 years old when Lauren first considered a cochlear implant. At that time, the Food and Drug Administration did not recommend an implant for children under the age of 3. Lauren set a surgery date, but as the date approached, she changed her mind because of the lack of support from the Deaf community where she lived. Lauren's daughter's teachers were surprised with the family's decision to get a cochlear implant and did not encourage their decision. She later moved to another part of the country where her daughter received a cochlear implant when she was 7 years old. Lauren expressed regret that her daughter had been implanted late. She felt that her daughter's spoken language skills would be more similar to her oral deaf peers if she had been implanted at a younger age.

"She Already Has a Strong Language Foundation in ASL"

Throughout the interview, the mothers shared examples about how families, teachers, and friends supported their children's language development in ASL and English. Their children acquired ASL from birth naturally through daily interactions and did not have access to spoken language until they received their cochlear implants.

> I signed to him all the way. I read books to him and talked with him through signing. (Sierra)
>
> ASL is our language and I sign to her through natural ways of exposing her to ASL. I don't teach her directly but through natural interactions. She also receives exposure to ASL from her teachers of the deaf who come here for home visits. She has been acquiring ASL fine from me and her father and including her teachers and several friends. (Jasmine)

According to their mothers, all of the children's ASL skills were on age level and communication within the family was very effective.

> There is an age range of language development; my son is more on the later side of the range. Some children acquire language earlier. He is in the age range, but at the end of the range. He seems to be very physical. (Sierra)

The mothers believed they had a dominant role in supporting their children in acquiring ASL. The mothers mostly taught their children ASL through natural interactions and play.

> Yes, he will play with toy cars and bridges. I'll tell him that the car is going over the bridge or the car fell off the bridge. A lot of talk about dramatic events like the car falling off the bridge or crashing with another car. It's his thing. We'll also play kickball, and I'll use signs to talk about that. (Sierra)
>
> I don't really teach her directly on academic topics. It tends to be through natural interactions. The teacher of the deaf will expose new signs and teach these new signs to her. She/he gave me a few suggestions on how to expand my child's vocabulary by describing things. She/he will share different ideas. I'm not a teacher myself. I'm a parent. I focus on being a parent and I don't teach her one-to-one directly, but through exposing her to ASL naturally. Sometimes I will use what I learned from the teachers and expose her to new words. (Jasmine)
>
> Now, for example, we have family time at home during the evening. We sit together. Whatever the topic is, we do activities together. During that time, we always must use ASL. During dinnertime when we sit together, we use ASL, because of access, ACCESS, for all. It's our priority. It's important. We use ASL. (Lauren)

"The Problem Was, Who Will Teach My Child Spoken Language?"

The mothers expressed that they were unable to provide their children with support for spoken language development themselves. They relied on other sources such as hard of hearing or hearing family members, many speech therapists, hearing teachers, and peers.

> We have a system at home. My husband will speak all of the time. I sign to him all of the time. We've split our roles, so he will know to respond to his dad by speaking and to me by signing. (Sierra)
>
> I mostly signed with her, but exposing her to speech, there was no one, because I couldn't do it. But, I taught her ASL and CASE [Conceptually Accurate Signed English]. Her language development was typical for her age level for sign language. (Lauren)

> Since both my husband and I use ASL, it's my daughter's first language. However, the problem was who will teach her spoken language? What do we do?, we thought. I noticed with my son, he's hearing, but he was able to acquire spoken language outside of our home by attending regular school; he was able to acquire spoken language there. So, I thought why couldn't my daughter do the same thing? She could be placed in a spoken language environment, and she would be exposed to the language. At home, my daughter would still sign just like my son. He is hearing. I thought, why not? (Jasmine)

The mothers noticed dramatic changes with their children's spoken language after their children received their cochlear implants. They strongly believed that their children were able to acquire spoken language quickly because they already had a first language as a foundation for learning a second language. Jasmine's daughter began recognizing her own name and sounds about 2 to 3 months after the surgery. She was able to respond to sounds from another room.

> About 1 year after my daughter received her CI, she began picking up spoken language rapidly. They (teachers) said my daughter made the 2-year-progress of acquiring spoken language in 1 year. Because of ASL. (Jasmine)
>
> After she got her CI, there was a BIG difference! I encouraged her to develop speech skills. With her hearing aids, she developed a little bit and then it plateaued; (looks disappointed) she was at the same level as me when I grew up. I was aware of that. I went ahead with a CI and her language developed rapidly, and now it's still developing more and more and more. I was surprised, Wow! That was the reason why I wished it happened earlier. (Lauren)
>
> So, sometimes signs will be used to reinforce his spoken language; that's nice. The teachers do that, too. They support his language development by making connections to spoken words through sign. He was able to pick up spoken language quickly, then separating both languages and focusing only on spoken language. It's harder for him to acquire spoken language without support from ASL. Oh, most definitely! If it wasn't for signing, he would be very delayed big time. That's for sure. (Sierra)
>
> Through sign, he has full access to a language. He has a language. Plus, it provides him with a strong language foundation. He is able to develop spoken language on top of that foundation. He is "riding" on it. (Sierra)

"He Code-switches Between Both Languages All the Time."

All three children began acquiring spoken language soon after they received cochlear implants. The mothers commented that when their children had access to both languages, they began to code-switch between both languages. They sometimes mixed languages. The language used depended on with whom they were interacting, e.g., a deaf person, a hard of hearing person, or a hearing person.

> When my son is with me, he'll talk less. He will sign more and be more visual focused. With my husband, he'll talk more. He code-switches between both languages all the time. . . . Really, more like every 5 seconds. (Sierra)
>
> Sometimes he will mix both languages. With me, he'll use his voice to speak, "open," "more," and other words. When he signs, "cow," he will say, "Moo, moo." (Sierra)
>
> On weekends, she signs all day, really. She'll speak with her brother a little bit. When she is with other KODAs [Hearing Kids of Deaf Adults], she will speak with them. With my husband and me, she will sign with us. (Jasmine)
>
> She is purely bilingual. Yes, in the mornings, if it's today, for example, she signs with me all of the time, all the time. When her sister and her brother speak with each other, she will listen to them, and then turn to them to speak to them. When she is done speaking to them, she'll turn back to me and sign to me, and turn back to talk with her siblings. Her sister and brother will sign and talk to her because sometimes she does not understand them, unless they are talking face-to-face, in a context they are familiar with, and about other specific things. They must be in a "perfect" environment too, you know? Or, it will be distorted (shakes head), they mostly speak to each other and will sign a little bit. They'll fill in signs in between their conversations. With me, she signs more in ASL. With them, she uses Signed English and speaking (nods). (Lauren)

The mothers reported that their children's rate of development with spoken language varied. Jasmine felt her daughter had made great progress, but she had not yet caught up with her peers. Based on a spoken language evaluation, Jasmine's daughter was a couple of months delayed for her age, but Jasmine believed her daughter would eventually catch up. Sierra's son had just received his cochlear implant about 6 months prior to the interview, and Sierra thought he was making good progress. Lauren was concerned about gaps in her daughter's spoken language that she attributed to late implantation.

> When reading a book, if one person reads aloud, the book has to be at second grade level with some context exposure and without showing the lip movement. The lips are covered. As the person reads aloud, she can listen and understand in a quiet environment at the second grade level. Not third grade or fourth grade. She is in the fourth grade level in school. She is unable to follow fourth grade level texts. She misses a lot, so there is a gap. (Lauren)

Lauren reported that her daughter was able to speak almost fluently. In school, she speaks most of the time and also has interpreters as a backup. She orders meals at restaurants by herself and does not depend on interpreters or writing on paper to communicate. Lauren is content with her daughter's development and considers her hard of hearing.

> My daughter participates in extracurricular activities and church activities totally on her own. If she wasn't implanted and hadn't had the ASL foundation preimplantation and intensive AVT [auditory-verbal therapy] after implantation (5 days a week!), she wouldn't be this independent. Tell me, how many deaf ASL nonspeaking children would be comfortable totally alone (without an interpreter) during achievement night (a weekly church thing for young women age 10–12 focusing on teamwork and leadership), dance sessions, primary classes in church every Sunday? The CI gives her SO MUCH access in the hearing world! She is still deaf, Deaf, and labels herself HOH [Hard of Hearing], and she does have so many opportunities now than if she was never implanted and gotten intensive habilitation. I have no regrets whatsoever; except that I wish I hadn't listened to the Deaf community when my girl was 3 years old. (Lauren via e-mail)

"I Want for Her to Be Fluent in Both Languages."

The interviewer explored the issue of bilingualism, ASL, and spoken English in depth. All of the mothers believed strongly in the importance of maintaining bilingualism. They all supported and advocated their children's language development in both ASL and English. All of the mothers valued ASL and their children's membership in and relationships with the Deaf community. Being deaf connects the children to their families. Sierra stated very clearly that her son is deaf and must have ASL. This issue, according to Sierra, was nonnegotiable and therefore not open for further discussion. Jasmine said that ASL can be beneficial for all children including hearing children.

> I think the value is having access. Having access is most important because ASL can be used anytime and anywhere. In a noisy environment, if the CI is broken or whatever, he will always have ASL. It's all set. He won't have to worry about that. He is not hearing. He will have some challenges. Spoken language is nice and he has access to it, yes, but not fully. He will always face barriers with spoken language. That is what I value about signing. Among other bonuses like culture, community, and so forth, but number one, he is still deaf. He must have access to language all the time, that's what is nice about ASL. (Sierra)
>
> I believe that ASL supports both hearing and deaf children. Most of the children do not learn how to speak until they are 2 years old. Why not give them an opportunity to be exposed to ASL to develop early communication

> skills. Also, sometimes, CIs get lost or broken and are unused during bath time or swimming. Children can use ASL to communicate as a backup. That's one of the reasons why my husband and I prefer to include ASL. (Jasmine)
>
> ASL is to me . . . a family's heritage. I have many old signs that I learned from my mother. I feel moved, wow. It is important for me to share that with my offspring. I want to pass on that to my children. I want them to have that same feeling, of family passing on the language. In the Deaf community, we share the same language. I feel at HOME, "HOME." (Lauren)

The mothers also highly valued their children learning English, because it is the majority language in this country. They believed that it is essential to develop skills in English to be able to function in the larger hearing society and believed that their children's English skills would make it easier for them to communicate with hearing people.

> English is a majority language. It's important to be skilled, so we can compete in the hearing world. We have to. It's important to be an expert in English to be able to COMPETE. (Lauren)
>
> Yes, I value English, reading and spoken, too. Learning English helps her to fit in the majority of the world and fit in with our society. I don't want her to be separated from the hearing world. I don't have many hearing friends, but just a few. Most of my friends are deaf. At work, I don't hang out with my hearing coworkers. It's hard to fit in with them. (Jasmine)
>
> [Spoken English provides him with] the ability to communicate with anyone he wants. Spoken language is mostly used here [in our society]. That's what I value about learning that. He can communicate and learn from different people. The language itself . . . it's nice. I'm not in awe of it. It's not special to me, no. It just happens that it's out there to use, so let's take advantage of this opportunity. (Sierra)

Even though the mothers had strong beliefs in bilingualism, they stressed the need to provide additional support for their children's spoken language development. Lauren admitted that she had been giving more value to her daughter's spoken language than to her ASL skills. She felt content with her daughter's ASL abilities and thought that learning ASL at home was sufficient. All of the mothers sought programs and services that provided abundant spoken language support. Sierra's son received multiple speech therapy services and attended a mainstream school to develop spoken language skills. He also attended a deaf school that practiced a bilingual approach in ASL and spoken English.

Jasmine's daughter attended a childcare program with hearing peers and an auditory-verbal program daily. She also received speech therapy on a regular basis. Lauren had chosen to place her daughter in a mainstream setting with an interpreter to reinforce her spoken language. Both Jasmine and Lauren expressed the importance of having hearing students around as spoken language models.

> It's funny. I . . . I just realize just now that I'm not a good ASL advocate. Oh. I'm more focused on her getting speech therapy. In class, I made sure she has opportunities to speak for herself. I did not want interpreters to take over like a crutch. She can do it. I encourage her. I'm more focused on her spoken language. Why? It's because she already has ASL in her life. It's her first language. When I sign to her in ASL, she understands me fully. It's fine. She signs fluently. Actually it's odd, she does not sign in ASL. Mostly, she signs in CASE. Why? It's because of her personality, first of all. She is quiet and polite. (Lauren)
>
> I urged my husband to use spoken language with our son. When our son finally showed interest in speaking with his dad, his dad became more motivated to speak with our son more. My challenge is to monitor him and make sure he is ok and has access to both languages to communicate effectively. It's a lot of work; it's not a fun thing. Having a CI is a lot of work. (Sierra)
>
> The reason why she is going there [oral/auditory program] is because she can receive spoken language exposure. Her parents are deaf, and we can't train her at home. She needs spoken language exposure as much as possible. We hope that the oral/auditory program will help her acquire spoken language more because the classroom is small and the FM (Frequency Modulated) system is available there. They also provide a lot of support in scaffolding my daughter's spoken language. (Jasmine)

The mothers demonstrated a desire to maintain a balanced bilingual approach in ASL and English to support their children's development in both languages. However, Lauren and Jasmine commented on the limited resources that were available. They believed that the programs available focused only on ASL or spoken language. Sierra, on the other hand, was able to find a relatively new program that practices a bimodal and bilingual approach. The mothers described an ideal setting for their children's education:

> With that, I prefer deaf schools. I expect in the classrooms, spoken language will be used. At a deaf school, in the first-grade class, spoken language is being used all day. Except during art, PE, and in the cafeteria, sign language is used. Children have both; they develop spoken language in classes and ASL skills in social settings. They miss nothing. To me, that's an ideal environment. It's nice. They have both and they'll be comfortable there with their identity, culture, community, and everything else in one place. That's an ideal place. In a mainstream setting, can they have that? While playing sports, it'll be a challenge to listen to what is being said on the field. My son is still deaf. (Sierra)

My perfect idea is for deaf schools to have an oral-only program and a sign-only program and students can attend both programs alternatively. That's beautiful and perfect. I would place my daughter there and she can have more options with an understanding that the schools have hearing kids, too. (Lauren)

The most important thing is following where my daughter feels comfortable. We could place her at the deaf school and I hope by then the spoken language program will be expanded. Also, if she has good peers and has good models to be around. (Jasmine)

Overall, the mothers recognized that each individual is different, and there is no single right way to best support children with cochlear implants. Each child has unique needs and different experiences that may affect their language development. The mothers felt that there were more opportunities for the children to grow when they had two languages to rely on. They could use their knowledge of ASL if spoken language alone was insufficient. They would have options.

"I Always See Myself as a 'Colossus'"

The last section of the interview focused on the mothers' hopes for the Deaf community and the hearing community related to children having cochlear implants. The mothers expressed hope that a relationship between Deaf and hearing communities would be better formed.

There is still some resistance within the Deaf community in terms of supporting children with cochlear implants and their families. The mothers shared their experiences about how they have dealt with myths and misunderstandings that some Deaf people have about cochlear implants. Sierra shared a negative experience with the Deaf community. An acquaintance approached her in a tactful way asking why she wanted to "kill" and "destroy" the Deaf community. Sierra responded,

> I want to talk about it. I want to analyze it. We can't stop CIs from happening. People think we can stop it completely. It is not possible. It won't happen. Let's put it aside. We should shift our focus more to how we keep ASL alive. I think the key is to make everyone understand that the child with a CI is still deaf. These children still will miss out in a spoken language environment. ASL still provides full access to a language. If technology gets better and better in the future, I . . . I can't stop what's happening. We can't dwell on that, we have to focus on the now. What can we do about it? Later on, we'll adjust to meet the challenges. We'll make the changes. I think it is important that we continue this dialogue. (Sierra)

The mothers strongly believed that the hearing community needed to understand that the child with a CI is still deaf. Deaf children still need ASL in their lives. The mothers expressed a desire for the hearing community to become more supportive about maintaining bilingualism in ASL and English. They believed that this is a way for both communities to be connected.

> In the hearing communities, many people perceive that children don't need sign language. I still think children should be encouraged to use sign language because the CI equipment may break down among other things. More deaf children are having two CIs now. Most hearing parents argue that if one breaks down, the child still can use the second one and learning sign isn't necessary. But still. . . . That's their perspective. In the hearing community, they are supportive toward CIs. I understand that because English is their native language. The families don't want their children to be left out or isolated. Many deaf children who use ASL with hearing families are often left out. So, it's hard for them. (Jasmine)
>
> I hope to see a strong bridge formed between both communities and see more deaf people being supportive of both rather than being against each other. That's not a good idea. I always see myself as a "colossus," a giant standing between both communities. I'm trying to get both communities to work together by sharing ideas. I want to see more colossuses in the Deaf community for the sake of preserving the Deaf community. People need to change and be more open and accepting. At the same time, we need to show why ASL is very important for literacy. And also have more deaf people become accepting of CIs, by saying, "Sure. It's a great tool. It gives us more opportunities. Go for it." (Lauren)

Conclusion

The three families interviewed for this study provided unique insights into the reasons they decided on cochlear implants for their children and what they have chosen to do to support their children's bilingual development. Even though there was some initial reluctance to discuss their experiences, the mothers gradually warmed up to the interviewer and shared their children's successes, frustrations, and hopes for the future.

All of the mothers interviewed were clear that the main reason they chose a cochlear implant for their child was their hope that this assistive device or tool would provide their child with greater opportunities, independence, and access than they themselves had. These deaf mothers, like many hearing mothers who have decided to have their children implanted, reported that they wanted the best for their children and believed that it was important to provide them with choices that would potentially enhance their access to hearing people.

All of the mothers were proud of their Deaf heritage and language and felt strongly about the value of a strong foundation in ASL and the importance of preserving ASL and their child's connection with the Deaf community. On the other hand, their concerns about providing their children with sufficient exposure and opportunities to use spoken English caused at least one of the mothers to reflect on the fact that she might have been putting more value on her daughter's spoken language progress than she realized.

Being deaf and fluent ASL users seemed to provide these mothers with a degree of confidence in their children's ability to succeed regardless of their ability to acquire spoken language. They attributed their child's rapid acquisition of English to a strong ASL foundation. They also, however, expressed frustrations with the lack of understanding on the part of both the Deaf and hearing communities.

Some deaf people, although their attitudes toward cochlear implants may have changed, are still not supportive and are often critical of deaf parents who have chosen this technology for their children. Some hearing people, on the other hand, do not understand the importance of acquiring both ASL and English and promoting a bilingual and bimodal approach for deaf children (Christiansen & Leigh, 2002). Another challenge faced by these parents was finding appropriate services and programs for their children that provide sufficient support for developing spoken language, as well as opportunities to use ASL and interact with deaf peers and adults. For many deaf parents, the educational and social aspirations for their deaf children are of equal importance and often create conflict when it comes to making decisions regarding the best educational placement for their child (Meadow-Orlans et al., 2003). Wilkens and Hehir (2008) raised concerns about the paucity of program options where deaf children can get both strong academic preparation and speech and language services while also having opportunities to develop social relationships with deaf peers and adults.

These in-depth interviews with deaf parents suggest several hypotheses that warrant further investigation. The small number of participants cannot be interpreted as representing the views of all deaf parents who have chosen cochlear implants for their children. A larger and more extensive investigation is needed to get a full picture of the reasons deaf parents choose cochlear implants for their children, how their children are progressing, and their challenges and successes. Further, it would be helpful to know what professionals could do to provide more support to these families. The importance of parent-to-parent support and involvement to the overall academic and well-being of deaf children is well documented (Hintermair, 2000, 2004; Lederberg & Golbach, 2001; Luckner & Velaski, 2004; Meadow-Orlans et al., 2003). And yet, deaf parents considering cochlear implantation for their children find limited opportunities to network with other deaf parents with whom they can discuss their unique issues and concerns. The experiences of these families may be very helpful to other deaf families who are considering a cochlear implant for their children. Additionally, hearing families and professionals can benefit from learning from the experiences of deaf adults and gaining understanding of the value of ASL and Deaf community connections for all children who are deaf.

ACKNOWLEDGMENTS

The authors would like to thank the mothers for their participation in this study. Their contributions are critical in gaining a deeper understanding to provide the best possible support for all deaf children. This pilot study was in partial fulfillment of the first author's requirement for her doctoral program at George Mason University. Julie Mitchiner wishes to thank her professor Dr. Joe Maxwell and her classmates for their guidance in this study.

REFERENCES

Blamey, P. (2003). Development of spoken language by deaf children. In M. Marschark & P. E. Spencer (Eds.), *Oxford handbook of deaf studies, language, and education* (pp. 232–246). New York: Oxford University Press.

Christiansen, J. B., & Leigh, I. W. (2002). *Cochlear implants in children: Ethics and choices*. Washington, DC: Gallaudet University Press.

Gallaudet Research Institute. (2006). *Regional and national summary report of data from the 2005–2006 Annual Survey of Deaf and Hard of Hearing Children and Youth*. Washington, DC: Author.

Geers, A., Moog, J., Biedenstien, J., Brenner, C., & Hayes, H. (2009). Spoken language scores of children using cochlear implant compared to hearing age-mates at school entry. *Journal of Deaf Studies, 14*(3), 371–385.

Hintermair, M. (2000). Hearing impairment, social networks, and coping: The need for families with hearing-impaired children to relate to other parents and to hearing-impaired adults. *American Annals of the Deaf, 145*, 41–51.

Hintermair, M. (2004). The sense of coherence—A relevant resource in the coping process of mothers with hearing impaired children? *Journal of Deaf Studies and Deaf Education, 9*, 15–26.

Israelite, N., & Ewoldt, C. (1992). *Bilingual/bicultural education for deaf and hard-of-hearing students: A review of the literature on the effects of native sign language on majority language acquisition*. Toronto: Queen's printer for Ontario.

Johnson, R. E. (2006). Cultural constructs that impede discussions about variability in speech-based educational models for deaf children with cochlear implants. *Perspectiva Florianópolis, 24*, 29–80.

Lane, H. (2005). Ethnicity, ethics and the Deaf-World. *Journal of Deaf Studies, 10*(3), 291–310.

Lederberg, A. R., & Goldbach, T. (2002). Parenting stress and social support in hearing mothers of deaf and hearing children: A longitudinal study. *Journal of Deaf Education and Deaf Studies, 7*(4), 330–345.

Li, Y., Bain, L., & Steinberg, A. G. (2003). Parental decision making and the choice of communication modality for the child who is deaf. *Archives of Pediatric Adolescent Medicine, 157*, 162–168.

Luckner, J. L., & Velaski, A. (2004). Healthy families of children who are deaf. *American Annals of the Deaf, 149*(4), 324–335.

Marschark, M. (2007). *Raising and educating a deaf child* (2nd ed.). New York: Oxford University Press.

McConkey Robbins, A., Burton Koch, D., Osberger, M. J., Zimmerman-Phillips, S., & Kishon-Rabin, L. (2004). Effect of age at cochlear implantation on auditory skill development in infants and toddlers. *Archives of Otolaryngology—Head & Neck Surgery, 130*, 570–574.

Meadow-Orlans, K., Mertens, D., & Sass-Lehrer, M. (2003). *Parents and their deaf children: The early years.* Washington, DC: Gallaudet University Press.

Meadow-Orlans, K., Spencer, P., & Koester, L. (2004). *The world of deaf infants: A longitudinal study.* New York: Oxford University Press.

Meier, R. (1991). The acquisition of language by deaf children. *American Scientist, 79*(2), 60–70.

Newport, E., & Meier, R. (1985). The acquisition of American Sign Language. In D. Slobin (Ed.), *The crosslinguistic study of language acquisition* (Vol. 1, pp. 881–938). Hillsdale, NJ: Erlbaum.

Petitto, L. A. (2000). On the biological foundations of human language. In K. Emmorey & H. Lane (Eds.), *The signs of language revisited: An anthology in honor of Ursula Bellugi and Edward Klima* (pp. 449–471). Mahwah, NJ: Erlbaum.

Preisler, G., Tvingstedt, A., & Ahlström, M. (2002). A psychosocial follow-up study of deaf preschool children using cochlear implants. *Child: Care, Health and Development, 28*(5), 403–418.

Sharma, A., Dorman, M., & Spohr, A. (2002). Early cochlear implantation in children allows normal development of central auditory pathways. *Annals of Otology, Rhinology & Laryngology, 111*, 38–41.

Singleton, J., Supalla, S., Litchfield, S., & Schley, S. (1998). From sign to word: Considering modality constraints in ASL/English bilingual education. *Topics in Language Disorders, 18*(4), 16–30.

Snoddon, K. (2008). American sign language and early intervention. *The Canadian Modern Language Review/La Revue Canadienne des Langues Vivantes, 64*(4), 581–604.

Strong, M., & Prinz, P. (1997). A study of the relationship between American Sign Language and English literacy. *Journal of Deaf Studies and Deaf Education, 2*(1), 37–46.

Strong, M., & Prinz, P. (2000). Is American Sign Language skill related to English literacy? In C. Chamberlain, J. Morford, & R. Mayberry (Eds.), *Language acquisition by eye* (pp. 131–141). Mahwah, NJ: Erlbaum.

Volterra, V., & Iverson, J. (1995). When do modality factors affect the course of language acquisition? In K. Emmorey & J. Reilly (Eds.), *Language, gesture and space* (pp. 371–390). Hillsdale, NJ: Erlbaum.

Volterra, V., Iverson, L., & Castrataro, M. (2006). The development of gesture in hearing and deaf children. In B. Schick, M. Marschark, & P. Spencer (Eds.), *Advances in the sign language development of deaf children* (pp. 46–70). New York: Oxford University Press.

Watson, L. M., Archbold, S. M., & Nikolopoulous, T. P. (2006). Changing communication mode after implantation by age at implant. *Cochlear Implants International, 7*, 77–91.

Wever, C. C. (2002). *Parenting deaf children in the era of cochlear implantation. A narrative-ethical analysis.* Unpublished doctoral dissertation, Radboud University, Nijmegen, The Netherlands.

Wilkens, C. P., & Hehir, T. P. (2008). Deaf education and bridging social capital: A theoretical approach. *American Annals of the Deaf, 153*(3), 275–284.

Yoshinaga-Itano, C., & Sedey, A. (2000). Speech development of deaf and hard of hearing children in early childhood: Interrelationships with language and hearing. *The Volta Review, 100*(5), 181–211.

Yoshinaga-Itano, C. (2006). Early identification, communication modality, and the development of speech and spoken language skills: Patterns and considerations. In P. Spencer & M. Marschark (Eds.), *Advances in the spoken language development of deaf and hard-of-hearing children* (pp. 298–327). Oxford: Oxford University Press.

6

COCHLEAR IMPLANTS: IMPLICATIONS FOR DEAF IDENTITIES

Irene W. Leigh and Deborah Maxwell-McCaw

How can a certain piece of technology influence one's identity? In the case of cochlear implants, what is the relationship between having a cochlear implant and one's identity development? This chapter will attempt to address this by exploring the concept of identity, how it evolves, what deaf-related identities are all about, the various perceptions of cochlear implants, and their role in psychosocial/identity development.

First of all, what is identity? When people are asked that question, they tend to answer: "Identity is who I am." When we explore further, we discover that identity is a construction that reflects multiple aspects that define who a person is. Specifically, identity reflects a composite of the biological (including race, gender, age, physical characteristics), psychological (cognition, competencies, motivations, self-awareness), social (cultural influences, social roles, relationships), and religious/spiritual aspects (Tatum, 1997). Not only that, identity changes throughout the life span. It is easy to recognize that each of the aspects just mentioned will evolve in terms of one's awareness of his or her race or ethnicity, emerging cognitive development, changing social roles ranging from childhood to adulthood, and expression of religion, for example. Even further, identity aspects can change from situation to situation as individuals modify their self-perceptions to fit specific situations. In this case, interactions with different types of people can influence psychological motivations, and perceptions of the self may be reshaped depending on the situation (Kegan, 1982). In this chapter, however, we will focus specifically on identities that may be affected by whether one has a cochlear implant or not.

For many who are uninitiated, it may be baffling to consider that a piece of equipment, specifically a cochlear implant, has the power to convey an identity or influence one's identity. An understanding of what the cochlear implant represents and how it can influence one's interaction with his or her social environment will serve to address this baffling relationship. But first, we will explore the concept of D/deaf identities and how these reflect different ways of living with hearing differences.

Authors' Note: A significant portion of this chapter represents a condensation of information presented in Leigh, I. W. (2009). A lens on deaf identities. *New York: Oxford University Press.*

Deaf Identities

D/deaf identities have a long history, starting with reports of people in ancient Egypt, Greece, and Rome, as well as during the Old and New Testament periods who could not hear and who communicated differently (Abrams, 1998; Baumann, 2008; Eriksson, 1993; Miles, 2000; Moores, 2001; Rée, 1999; Van Cleve & Crouch, 1989). Whether these individuals were accepted or rejected depended in great part on how their respective societies framed the meaning of disability and the inability to hear. How these individuals themselves defined their identities is lost to history.

Descriptions of approaches to educating children who were deaf began appearing in the 1500s and beyond (see Moores, 2001; Rée, 1999; Van Cleve & Crouch, 1989 for reviews). To read about the "Paris banquets" of post-Revolutionary France is to recognize the presence of a proud Deaf group capable of independent and intellectual thinking who held forth in expressing their perceptions of what it meant to be part of a Deaf constituency (Mottez, 1993; Quartararo, 2008). Not only was this discourse aimed at contradicting hearing authority figures who focused on deficiency and disability (Branson & Miller, 2002), but it also presaged the emergence of formal study related to what it meant to espouse a Deaf identity, an identity forged through centralized education of deaf children in residential schools for the deaf. In these schools, deaf children developed and reinforced social relationships with deaf peers. These relationships led to socialization parameters as these children transitioned away from the educational sphere; these parameters emerged as Deaf cultural ways of being (Burch, 2002; Rée, 1999; Van Cleve & Crouch, 1989).

So, exactly what is a culturally Deaf identity? This identity actually has been around for the past 2 centuries at the very least but has been subsumed within the terms of "Deaf community" or "Deaf-World" (Burch, 2002; Lane, Hoffmeister, & Bahan, 1996; Miles, 2000; Rée, 1999; Van Cleve & Crouch, 1989; Woll & Ladd, 2003). Essentially, as deaf people found each other, they created a Deaf center that relies on language and thought expressed through visual relationships incorporating body movements, eye contact, facial expressions, and other markers of signed languages. In short, as Bahan (2008) conceptualizes it, they became a "visual variety of the human race." With increased focus on academic study of deaf lives, authors such as Carol Padden and Tom Humphries (1988) led the way to the popularization of the term "Deaf culture" as a way of describing who Deaf people were, based on a Deaf form of normality and a common understanding of how Deaf people live, relate with others, love, and work. The key component is the use of the eye in daily interactions. Auditory components of daily living, including the use of spoken language, were not seen as important, relatively speaking, since Deaf people felt that they have deciphered visual equivalents to auditory events surrounding their environment.

But not all deaf people claim Deaf culture identities and not all necessarily organize their world around their use of vision. There are some who gravitate toward spending a significant amount of time in the hearing society surrounding them. They feel at home using spoken language and in interconnections with hearing peers. They are comfortable relying on whatever auditory skills they can develop and depend on technology to enhance their ability to interpret sound and linguistic inputs. They feel "culturally hearing" (Leigh, 1999, 2009) and attempt to conform to norms for spoken language. Those who experienced a loss of hearing after having internalized spoken language and become "late deafened" are more likely to be culturally hearing. Others who fall into this category include those who grew up with severe to profound hearing levels but were not exposed to sign language, and, as a result, developed spoken language. For the culturally hearing, their sense of belonging, however, can be tenuous, depending on communication ease, background noise, and the patience of those hearing people who are interacting with them. At times they still may desire to be "with their own kind" (deaf people like themselves—other "oral" deaf people; Bain, Scott, & Steinberg, 2004; Leigh, 1999, 2009; Oliva, 2004).

These different perceptions of deaf lives have given rise to various theories of deaf identities and how these are internalized. The description of the culturally hearing as described in the preceding paragraph falls into the first of Neil Glickman's (1996) four categories of deaf identities. His categorization has become the standard in the field, much used by researchers (e.g., Bat-Chava, 2000; Maxwell-McCaw, 2001) to try to understand how deaf people categorize themselves and at times transition from one identity category to another. His theory, based on racial identity development theories, is primarily a psychological theory in terms of how oppressed minority groups can evolve to develop a positive identity based on their interactions both in their own group and with the majority group. Thus, identities in this case are shaped by the psychological impact of social interactions.

The second category covers cultural marginality. Glickman (1996) describes individuals falling into this category as not fully identifying with or having a sense of belonging with either Deaf or hearing groups. These individuals fall into two types. The first type is the individual with inadequate access to spoken or signed languages, which exacerbates social marginality and heightens psychological marginality in terms of confusion regarding identity, poorly differentiated understanding of self and other, and difficulties with self-regulation of emotions and behavior (Glickman, 1996). The other type reflects linguistically competent individuals who are in the process of actively exploring their sense of identity as culturally hearing or culturally Deaf.

The third category is that of identification as culturally Deaf. Glickman (1996) refers to this category as that of immersion. Deaf identity and Deaf culture are uncritically embraced. These individuals often fit the prototypical type of deaf person: they are fluent in American Sign Language (ASL) or their native signed language, typically marry a deaf spouse, work in the Deaf world, and socialize primarily only with other Deaf people. Lastly, the fourth category represents an integrative awareness that one can be bicultural. In this category, the individual can integrate the values of both Deaf and hearing cultures and comfortably navigate either one as the situation demands. Multiple studies have indicated that individuals who fall into the bicultural category appear to be the most optimally adjusted psychosocially (Cornell & Lyness, 2004; Hintermair, 2008; Jambor & Elliott, 2005), although Maxwell-McCaw (2001) found both deaf immersed and biculturals were optimally adjusted.

How do people gravitate toward these identity categories and internalize who they are? And how does this affect one's identity? Social connections and exposure to specific groups are clearly one factor that figures prominently in how deaf individuals configure their identity descriptions. Shared and effective ways of communicating with peers, whether via spoken or signed languages, will facilitate the strengthening of social relationships and of social identities with specific groups for which they have affinity. This has been demonstrated by a variety of studies investigating social relationships (e.g., Bat-Chava, 2000; Kluwin & Stinson, 1993). Generally, individuals who prefer signed languages will identify with those who also use their language, whereas those preferring spoken language will identify with like-minded peers. Today, more and more deaf and hard of hearing individuals are identifying themselves as bicultural, preferring to gravitate between various social environments and shifting language use as needed.

According to Maxwell-McCaw and Zea (2011), the concept of acculturation provides an additional pathway to understanding how deaf identities evolve. They suggest that, similar to groups immigrating to America and navigating between their home culture and the new American culture, Deaf people must navigate their membership between two very different cultures, Deaf and hearing cultures. As a result, they suggest that there are several factors in addition to social influences that can ultimately shape the acculturation process to both Deaf and hearing cultures. These factors include the level of psychological identification to Deaf and hearing cultures, the degree of cultural involvement, preferences for one culture or the other, competence in the language used, and knowledge of the cultures. By assessing one's process of acculturation to each group, we can examine how one adjusts to these groups according to the situation. Assumptions about the psychological impact of different identities are removed from the measure. For example, Hintermair (2008), using the Deaf Acculturation Scale, which was translated into German, found that those participants who actually preferred to be marginal and not defined by a cultural status quo (via Deaf or hearing cultures) actually demonstrated positive psychological resources, facilitating their adjustment. So, in this case, marginalization does not necessarily assume maladjustment as many racial identity theories suggest. Nevertheless, if a deaf spoken language user is new to Deaf culture and its relevant signed language, that person could still be marginal if she or he does not identify fully with hearing peers. But with increased exposure to Deaf cultural ways of being and mastery of the signed language, that person is said to be acculturating to Deaf culture. For individuals with a cochlear implant, a complex constellation of issues come into play, particularly since Deaf and hearing cultures often have contradicting attitudes toward the implants, with hearing cultures most typically seeing the implant as a great technology intervention to restore the lost sense of hearing.

In addition to the impact of socialization on identity, one factor not accounted for in the above theories is the simple impact of biology—the degree of hearing loss—on identity. In other words, what is it that ultimately determines whether the deaf person becomes primarily a visually oriented person or primarily auditorily oriented? One author (Maxwell-McCaw), progressively deafened since early childhood and implanted with a cochlear implant in adulthood, makes an interesting observation on how one's primary orientation to the world may affect and shape identity. Ironically, as a child, Maxwell-McCaw always needed to use her eyes to help make sense of her auditory world. As a result, learning ASL came easily and intuitively because it just "made sense" to her visually. She was already very used to "organizing" her world through her eyes. Thus, her transition into Deaf culture was eased by the sense that even as an oral deaf person, the ultimate tie that bound her with other deaf signing people was that she, too, used her eyes to navigate the world. Now, as an implanted adult, and a "high-end" user at that, able to talk on the phone and interact more easily with hearing individuals often without lipreading, she slowly feels her "orientation" shifting. The technology actually makes it possible, for the first time in her life, to really "navigate" the world more auditorily. Her primary reminder that she is deaf comes at moments when her battery dies unexpectedly or in large group settings. Yet socially, she prefers her deaf friends because she is still most at ease and relaxed when she is in signing environments. Perhaps this is partly due to a long history with them, in addition to the fact that understanding speech in groups, particularly in noisy environments, is still difficult with a cochlear implant. Still, she asks herself: What if this technology had been available to her as a child? Would she have organized her world primarily visually or auditorily? Who would have been her "reference" group? Would she be seeking out other implanted peers? Signing deaf peers? Or hearing peers who have similar interests as herself? She is not sure. So, what about today's children who are being implanted at such an early stage in their development, especially at an age when their brains are at an early stage of plasticity? One possible answer is the use of a bimodal approach (see Morere, this volume, for example).

Although many factors influence how variations in deaf identities may be shaped and formed, cochlear implants—as a technology that is capable of altering one's very way of being in the world, whether that person is a person of the "eye" or the "ear"—lend additional complications in this process. Indeed, cochlear implants have ideologically come to represent two very different and often contradictory constructs in Deaf and hearing cultures.

The Passion Surrounding Cochlear Implants

Cochlear implants were developed with the goal of restoring hearing where none existed or where hearing was lost. The medical profession saw the issue of hearing restoration as a critical one for research and development (Christiansen & Leigh, 2002/2005). The first to undergo cochlear implantations in the 1960s and 1970s were individuals who desperately wanted to hear and were willing to undergo experimental surgery. Many in the scientific community were skeptical about the potential effectiveness of cochlear implants, viewing efforts to develop this technology as misguided efforts to stimulate already dead nerves (Christiansen & Leigh, 2002/2005; House, 1995; Schindler, 1999). As time went on and research proceeded against all odds, including difficulty in obtaining financial support, not only the scientific community but also the Deaf community began to take note.

Deaf people in France and Australia were among the first to protest this new development, with those in the United States chiming in somewhat later (Blume, 1999; Christiansen & Leigh, 2002/2005; Lane et al., 1996). The focus of their protest was centered on their claim that they were happy with their identities as Deaf people. They viewed themselves as functioning satisfactorily in society, and saw no reason to be "fixed." Implantation was viewed as a process of invading a healthy body and creating an artificial modification when one could easily be happy following a culturally Deaf way of life. Their fundamental principle was that having grown up deaf, they are the experts on how deaf people can maneuver through life. Yet, hearing society has tended to view deaf people in general as less intelligent, as less capable or competent, and with limitations that bar them from full participation in society rather than assessing how existing barriers make it difficult for deaf people to achieve. This has led to frustration, the fermenting of a visceral reaction to what a number of deaf people perceive as the imposition of a technology on their people, or another potential threat of cultural genocide, and a battlefield mentality. The tenor of this opposition started off strong and has continued to this day among various segments of the community, as indicated in some of the chapters in this book. This opposition has also made a critical number of parents leery of reaching out to Deaf informants to get answers to questions about life for their deaf child, fearing that they will be denigrated for even considering the cochlear implant (Christiansen & Leigh, 2002/2005).

Despite the protests of notable members in the Deaf community, cochlear implant research proceeded to clinical trials in the 1980s, with the result that increasing numbers of individuals were implanted, particularly deaf children (Christiansen & Leigh, 2002/2005). Because it involved surgery, parents typically struggled with the decision to implant their child and in most cases decided to proceed, feeling that the potential for spoken language was worth the procedure. It is important to note that 95% of these parents are hearing with little knowledge or contact with Deaf culture. Initially, pediatric candidates for the procedure had previously lost their hearing or had no benefit from existing auditory amplification. Whether they were viable candidates was subject to question, but as time went on, data supporting their improvement in open set tests of speech recognition began to appear. As technology has continued to improve, data continue to reveal improvement, in not only speech recognition but also speech production and spoken language development, particularly in comparison with deaf children who use hearing aids. However, it must be kept in mind that variability in improvement was present early on and continues to be present to this day. The specific factors contributing to this variability are multiple and probably interactive, which makes it difficult to pinpoint the reasons for the variability.

The increasing number of cochlear implantees has led the Deaf community to recognize that vehement opposition and highlighting Deaf culture success stories have not resulted in any significant dent in the inexorable increase of people getting the cochlear implant, including those who are culturally Deaf, and the trend toward bilateral implantation is beginning to gain momentum (see Christiansen & Leigh, this volume). As indicated in the results of the Christiansen and Leigh survey reported in this book, there is an increasing, albeit for some, grudging, acceptance of this technology, coupled with ongoing concern about the increased use of pediatric implantation without the consent of the children involved. This has generated a shift in focus toward evaluating the attitudes of the cochlear implantees regarding Deaf culture and Deaf identities. Additionally, how to combine the focus on audition with the focus on vision has become the linchpin of attention at this time, as can be seen throughout this book. Such a focus is particularly critical as educational systems grounded in residential and day schools for deaf children that incorporate the use of ASL in the curriculum grapple with increasing numbers of children with cochlear implants and with parents, both hearing and deaf, asking for comparatively more focus on the use of spoken language alongside the signed language component. These are culturally Deaf parents who *are* comfortable with the use of a signed language but do not want to minimize any opportunity for exposure to and internalization of spoken language (see Mitchiner & Sass-Lehrer, this volume). Nevertheless, results from the Christiansen and Leigh (this volume) study do show increasing levels of endorsement by Deaf respondents of the idea that deaf people can have both cochlear implants and a Deaf identity compared with the results of the 2000 study reported by Christiansen and Leigh (2002/2005).

Implications for Identity

In the 1980s and 1990s, deaf adults who decided to get the cochlear implant faced the fury of Deaf protesters who considered them beyond the pale and ostracized them from the community as people who wanted to be "hearing" and who therefore rejected Deaf culture values (Christiansen & Leigh, 2002/2005). These Deaf protesters railed against the perception that theirs was a spoiled, defective identity rather than a normal variety of the human race (Cherney, 1999; Crouch, 1997; Lane, Hoffmeister, & Bahan, 1996; Tellings, 1996). They felt that inserting a piece of technology into a human being created a so-called cyborg that hearing people deemed to be better than a Deaf person relying on vision to accommodate to the world. This creation of an apparent artificial hearing identity appeared to run the danger of creating "outsider" status for some cochlear implantees, who can never fully be a part of hearing culture due to the technical limitations of implants in replicating normal sound, nor of Deaf culture due to the focus on auditory sounds and spoken language that typically accompanies implantation (Ladd, 2007; Leigh, 2009).

The cochlear implant issue even divided Deaf families, as exemplified by a set of Deaf parents going as far as to disown their culturally Deaf adult daughter after she opted to get a cochlear implant because she wanted access to environmental sounds (Leigh, 2002). Eventually, the parents recognized that their daughter was still their beloved culturally Deaf daughter and reconciled with her. Closure in situations such as this create an atmosphere for the increased acceptability of cochlear implantation, but this is interposed with Deaf individuals accusing Deaf parents of betraying their culture when they decide on cochlear implantation for their deaf child. Clearly, all these perceptions suggested the need for research to examine claims of harm and rejection, psychological adjustment and identity, particularly since Deaf people mentioned their worry about potential long-term educational and mental health implications such as language delays, confusing identity issues (am I Deaf or hearing?), social difficulties, and possible psychological trauma related to denying one's true self as a Deaf person.

STUDIES OF PSYCHOSOCIAL FUNCTIONING

There is a small but growing corpus of research on the psychosocial functioning of children, youth, and adults with cochlear implants in addition to the rapidly expanding database on receptive and expressive spoken language outcomes. A group of studies covering information on psychosocial functioning was gathered from parents who provided their perceptions on how their cochlear-implanted children functioned. In general, these studies indicate that parents perceive their children as demonstrating improved quality of life, greater self-esteem, confidence, and outgoing behavior compared with the time before implantation. Nonetheless, even though they generally felt that social well-being was positive, age appropriate socialization experiences with hearing peers was not guaranteed because of issues with spoken communication skills, limited access to communication in groups due to noise and difficulties in following the course of conversations, and hearing peer attitudes (Bat-Chava & Deignan, 2001; Bat-Chava, Martin, & Kosciw,

2005; Chmiel, Sutton, & Jenkins, 2000; Christiansen & Leigh, 2002/2005; Kluwin & Stewart, 2000; Nicholas & Geers, 2003).

Very satisfactory perceptions of social well-being were reported by parents of 62 Danish cochlear-implanted children (Percy-Smith et al., 2006). In a follow-up study investigating factors that affect the social well-being of 167 children with cochlear implants based on information derived from structured interviews with their parents, similar positive results were obtained (Percy-Smith et al., 2008a). There was stronger evidence of social well-being for those children who were implanted prior to 18 months and those using spoken language compared with those who were implanted after 18 months and used sign supported systems or signs only. However, due to the wide age range of 1-year to 18-years of age and the lack of any breakdown by age, it is not possible to determine if the results for older participants were similar to those of younger participants. Percy-Smith et al. (2008b) also compared the social well-being of 164 kindergarten and school-children with cochlear implants, this time based on parent questionnaires, with a larger cohort of hearing peers. They reported no difference between the two cohorts in overall self-esteem, number of friends, confidence, independence, social aspects, and happiness.

Although parent perceptions provide valuable information, observation studies and studies that directly ask children with cochlear implants about their experiences can provide more nuanced information. The observation studies reviewed for this chapter indicate that children with cochlear implants being observed in group situations or classroom discourse with hearing peers struggle in their attempts to become active participants (e.g., Boyd, Knutson, & Dahlstrom, 2000; Knutson, Boyd, Reid, Mayne, & Fetrow, 1997; Martin, Bat-Chava, Lalwani, & Waltzman, 2011; Preisler, Tvingstedt, & Ahlström, 2005). Generally, one-on-one interactions are less problematic than interactions involving more peers due to, for example, ambient noise and rapid dialogue.

In looking at the children themselves, a variety of studies demonstrate positive psychosocial adjustment via interview, questionnaire studies, or psychological measures. In a study of 37 children with cochlear implants who were spoken language users and in mainstream education, Schorr, Roth, and Fox (2009) used a self-report quality of life questionnaire and found that children reported significant improvement in their quality of life.

In the Nicholas and Geers (2003) study of 181 children with cochlear implants, the researchers noted that these children tended to appear competent and well-adjusted in the cognitive, physical, socioemotional, school performance, and communication domains based on self-reports. Interestingly, younger children and those using the most updated speech processors gave themselves higher ratings, therefore leading to the question of whether these ratings would be maintained in adolescence when there is greater awareness of difficulties in communicating, particularly in noisy group situations (e.g., Sheridan, 2008).

In an investigation of 150 children with cochlear implants divided into three groups aged 4–7, 8–11, and 12–16 who rated their physical, social, and emotional quality of life, the youngest group rated themselves higher than their parents did (Loy, Warner-Czyz, Roland, & Tobey, 2009). The middle group also rated themselves positively, but interestingly, in the group of children aged 12–16, their parents tended to view their children's school quality of life higher than the adolescents themselves did. This again suggests the possibility that the complex issues of adolescence might make adolescent perceptions of their quality of life less idealistic and reminds us that parents' perceptions of their children do not always match the children's perceptions of themselves. Otherwise, the results were similar to those of the younger groups and to nondeaf children, thus attesting to the resilience of these children.

A study of the psychosocial adjustment of 57 adolescents with and without cochlear implants suggested that despite some differences in background characteristics between the two groups, there were no differences between them on the psychosocial variables assessed in this study as indicated on measures of self-perception, satisfaction with life, and loneliness (Leigh, Maxwell-McCaw, Bat-Chava, & Christiansen, 2009). Considering that the adolescents without cochlear implants who participated in this study were primarily in schools for the deaf and preferred signed language whereas adolescents with cochlear implants were primarily spoken language users and in the mainstream, the study strongly supports the earlier mentioned studies affirming psychosocial health. For example, in terms of loneliness, the adolescents in this study were no lonelier than the hearing sample used for the loneliness measure. This result is also supported by Schorr (2006), who found that loneliness levels among her 37 children and youth with cochlear implants were similar to levels noted in hearing peers, even with variability factored in. These participants were spoken language users.

To conclude regarding psychosocial health, contrary to what some Deaf persons predicted, cochlear implants per se are not necessarily creating maladjusted individuals, although the possibility of frustrating communication situations does exist. Supportive environments and individual attributes, including resilience, are factors that need to be considered in ensuring positive psychosocial stability. But the fact that many of the participants with cochlear implants in the studies mentioned earlier rely on spoken language raises questions about how they label themselves in the Deaf-hearing identity domain.

STUDIES OF IDENTITY

The focus of the information presented by cochlear implant centers in their informed consent documents is primarily on medical, audiological, communication, and educational aspects (Berg, Ip, Hurst, & Herb, 2007). In this study, less than half of the 121 centers responding to a nationwide survey included information on Deaf culture and ASL. This strongly suggests an emphasis on developing hearing-acculturated identities. Whether this identity continues to be paramount depends on the individual attributes of the children themselves, the environment in which they are reared, and the quality of their social interactions with peers.

In terms of language choice, a number of studies indicate that parents tended to be practical regarding the necessity of using signed languages, particularly pre-implantation, and as needed postimplantation (Christiansen & Leigh, 2002/2005; Watson, Hardie, Archbold, & Wheeler, 2008; Zaidman-Zait, 2008). This would most certainly appear to set the stage for at least acceptance of bilingualism in cochlear implant users, thereby suggesting the possibility that children with cochlear implants should not be automatically inferred to function solely using a spoken language mode.

Wald and Knutsen's (2000) study of 45 deaf adolescents with and without cochlear implants not surprisingly found that hearing identity as measured by Glickman's (1996) Deaf Identity Development Scale was more frequently endorsed by adolescents with cochlear implants than those without implants, possibly in part because of improved socialization with hearing peers. Interestingly, both groups similarly endorsed marginal, immersion, and, most particularly, the bicultural category. This similarity reappears in the Most, Wiesel, and Blitzer (2007) study in which 115 deaf Israeli adolescents participated, with only 10 of these having cochlear implants. Specifically, the two groups did not significantly differ in terms of Deaf Identity Development Scale classifications. The authors consider the endorsement of a bicultural identity for these implanted adolescents as allowing for the potential to benefit from this technology without having to sacrifice the Deaf experience.

Also, in the U.S. preliminary questionnaire study of 57 deaf adolescents with and without cochlear implants mentioned earlier (Leigh et al., 2009), results from an acculturation-based measure, the Deaf Acculturation Scale (Maxwell-McCaw & Zea, 2011) indicated that most of the adolescents with cochlear implants were in mainstream settings and affirmed a hearing-oriented identity. Yet, the number of cochlear-implanted adolescents with bicultural identity results were similar to those in deaf settings, again affirming the salience of this identity for the cochlear implant group.

Most of the 14 adolescent and young adult cochlear implant users interviewed in the Christiansen and Leigh (2002/2005) study reported viewing themselves as deaf and having deaf friends while also desiring contact with both the Deaf community and hearing peers. In another interview study, this time with younger children, Preisler et al. (2005) noted that these children saw the implant as a natural part of their lives and used signed as well as spoken languages. This suggested to the authors that the children would be better off claiming bicultural identities. In a semistructured questionnaire interview study involving 29 British young adolescents aged 13 to 16 with cochlear implants who were in both mainstreamed and specialized educational settings, it was found that most participants were flexible in terms of communication mode (spoken and signed languages) and endorsed a deaf identity that was neither culturally Deaf nor strong hearing (Wheeler, Archbold, Gregory, & Skipp, 2007). There was no clear relationship between identity status and educational environment.

Finally, it has been noted that increasing numbers of deaf students with cochlear implants attend specialized college programs for deaf students (Brueggemann, 2008; Ladd, 2007). This adds credence to the value attributed to bicultural identities and the need to explore the Deaf part of oneself, particularly in relevance to entering environments with significant numbers of Deaf peers.

In sum, all of the data presented here suggest that it is time to end the "either-or" paradigm: either cochlear implantee or culturally Deaf (Hintermair & Albertini, 2005). Despite pockets of resistance as mentioned earlier in this chapter, it appears that the fusion approach has some credibility. This is affirmed by Lisa Herbert (2008), who writes, "I'm grateful for the opportunities my cochlear implant offers me and I see it as completely compatible with being a signing Deaf person" (p. 139). Additionally, hearing parents often view the potential of cochlear implantation as a means of creating possibilities and not necessarily precluding the option of entering the Deaf community (Berg, Herb, & Hurst, 2005; Christiansen & Leigh, 2002/2005). In contrast, they may see the refusal to implant their deaf child as limiting the opportunity to participate in the world of their hearing families.

Conclusion

The information in this chapter suggests that children and adolescents with cochlear implants generally demonstrate positive psychosocial adjustment, whether their affirmed identity is bicultural, culturally Deaf, or culturally hearing. Cochlear implantation is not necessarily creating children stuck between the deaf and hearing worlds; they can and do often have a clear identity and can shift between identity categorizations as the situation demands. This ability to shift appears to be conducive to psychosocial health. These findings have implications for professionals who work with cochlear-implanted children, specifically, professionals who are flexible, parent centered, and comfortable with D/deaf, auditorily deaf, or hard of hearing role models. It is noteworthy that the different identity possibilities for children with cochlear implants tend to be more appreciated by parents (Christiansen & Leigh, 2002/2005; Meadow-Orlans, Mertens, & Sass-Lehrer, 2003). This flexibility will also allow more positive self-images for these children themselves as they explore who they are in terms of identity. This has the potential to create better opportunities for parents to move from a dysfunctional child image to a more affirmative image of unique identity and positive self-esteem.

References

Abrams, J. (1998). *Judaism and disability.* Washington, DC: Gallaudet University Press.

Bahan, B. (2008). Upon the formation of a visual variety of the human race. In H. D. Bauman (Ed.), *Open your eyes: Deaf studies talking* (pp. 83–99). Minneapolis: University of Minnesota Press.

Bain, L., Scott, S., & Steinberg, A. (2004). Socialization experiences and coping strategies of adults raised using spoken language. *Journal of Deaf Studies and Deaf Education, 9,* 120–128.

Bat-Chava, Y. (2000). Diversity of deaf identities. *American Annals of the Deaf, 145,* 420–428.

Bat-Chava, Y., & Deignan, E. (2001). Peer relationships of children with cochlear implants. *Journal of Deaf Studies and Deaf Education, 6,* 186–199.

Bat-Chava, Y., Martin, D., & Kosciw, J. (2005). Longitudinal improvements in communication and socialization of deaf children with cochlear implants and hearing aids: Evidence from parental reports. *Journal of Child Psychology and Psychiatry, 46*(12), 1287–1296.

Bauman, H.-D. (2008). On the disconstruction of (sign) language in the Western tradition: A Deaf reading of Plato's *Cratylus.* In H.-D. Bauman (Ed.), *Open your eyes: Deaf Studies talking* (pp. 127–145). Minneapolis: University of Minnesota Press.

Berg, A., Herb, A., & Hurst, M. (2005). Cochlear implants in children: Ethics, informed consent, and parental decision-making. *The Journal of Clinical Ethics, 16*(3), 239–250.

Berg, A., Ip, S., Hurst, M., & Herb, A. (2007). Cochlear implants in young children: Informed consent as a process and current practices. *American Journal of Audiology, 16,* 13–28.

Blume, S. (1999). Histories of cochlear implantation. *Social Science and Medicine, 49*(9), 1257–1258.

Boyd, R., Knutson, J., & Dahlstrom, A. (2002). Social interaction of pediatric cochlear implant recipients with age-matched peers. *Annals of Otology, Rhinology & Laryngology, 109*(Suppl. 185), 105–109.

Branson, J., & Miller, D. (2002). *Damned for their difference: The cultural construction of deaf people as disabled.* Washington, DC: Gallaudet University Press.

Brueggemann, B. J. (2008). Think-between: A Deaf studies commonplace book. In H.-D. Bauman (Ed.), *Open your eyes: Deaf Studies talking* (pp. 177–188). Minneapolis: University of Minnesota Press.

Burch, S. (2002). *Signs of resistance: American Deaf cultural history, 1900 to 1942.* New York: New York University Press.

Cherney, J. L. (1999). Deaf culture and the cochlear implant debate: Cyborg politics and the identity of people with disabilities. *Argumentation and Advocacy, 36,* 22–34.

Chmiel, R., Sutton, L., & Jenkins, H. (2000). Quality of life in children with cochlear implants. *Annals of Otology, Rhinology & Laryngology. Supplement, 185*, 103–105.

Christiansen, J. B., & Leigh, I. W. (2002/2005). *Cochlear implants in children: Ethics and choices.* Washington, DC: Gallaudet University Press.

Cornell, S., & Lyness, K. (2004). Therapeutic implications for adolescent deaf identity and self-concept. *Journal of Feminist Family Therapy, 16*, 31–49.

Crouch, R. (1997). Letting the deaf be Deaf. *Hastings Center Report, 27*(4), 14–21.

Eriksson, P. (1993). *The history of Deaf people.* Örebro, Sweden: SIH Läromedel.

Glickman, N. (1996). The development of culturally Deaf identities. In N. Glickman & M. Harvey (Eds.), *Culturally affirmative psychotherapy with deaf persons* (pp. 115–153). Mahwah, NJ: Erlbaum.

Herbert, L. (2008). Deaf, signing and oral: My journey. In D. Napoli, I. W. Leigh, D. DeLuca, & K. Lindgren (Eds.), *Access: Multiple avenues for Deaf people* (pp. 122–139). Washington, DC: Gallaudet University Press.

Hintermair, M. (2008). Self-esteem and satisfaction with life of deaf and hard-of-hearing people: A resource-oriented approach to identity work. *Journal of Deaf Studies and Deaf Education, 13*(2), 278–300.

Hintermair, M., & Albertini, J. (2005). Ethics, deafness, and new medical technologies. *Journal of Deaf Studies and Deaf Education, 10*(2), 185–192.

House, W. F. (1995). *Cochlear implants: My perspective.* Retrieved July 3, 2009, from http://www.allhear.com/pdf/my_perspective.pdf

Jambor, E., & Elliott, M. (2005). Self-esteem and coping strategies among deaf students. *Journal of Deaf Studies and Deaf Education, 10*(1), 63–81.

Kegan, R. (1982). *The evolving self.* Cambridge, MA: Harvard University Press.

Kluwin, T., & Stewart, D. (2000). Cochlear implants for younger children: A preliminary description of the parental decision and outcomes. *American Annals of the Deaf, 145*(1), 26–32.

Kluwin, T., & Stinson, M. (1993). *Deaf students in local public high schools: Background, experiences, and outcomes.* Springfield, IL: Charles C Thomas.

Knutson, J., Boyd, R., Reid, J., Mayne, T., & Fetrow, R. (1997). Observational assessments of the interaction of implant recipients with family and peers: Preliminary findings. *Otolaryngology—Head and Neck Surgery, 117*(3), 196–207.

Ladd, P. (2007). Cochlear implantation, colonialism, and Deaf rights. In L. Komesaroff (Ed.), *Surgical consent: Bioethics and cochlear implantation* (pp. 1–29). Washington, DC: Gallaudet University Press.

Lane, H., Hoffmeister, R., & Bahan, B. (1996). *A journey into the Deaf-World.* San Diego, CA: DawnSignPress.

Leigh, I. W. (1999). Inclusive education and personal development. *Journal of Deaf Studies and Deaf Education, 4*, 236–245.

Leigh, I. W. (2002) *Cochlear implants and Deaf pride: Possible?* Presented at ASL/Deaf Culture Lecture Series Panel Discussion, University of Virginia, Charlottesville.

Leigh, I. W. (2009). *A lens on Deaf identities.* New York: Oxford University Press.

Leigh, I. W., Maxwell-McCaw, D., Bat-Chava, Y., & Christiansen, J. B. (2009). Correlates of psychosocial adjustment in deaf adolescents with and without cochlear implants: A preliminary investigation. *Journal of Deaf Studies and Deaf Education, 14*(2), 244–259.

Loy, E., Warner-Czyz, A., Roland, P., & Tobey, E. (2009). *Cochlear implants offer kids a gift beyond hearing.* Retrieved July 5, 2009, from http://www.utdallas.edu/news/2009/02/18-002.php

Martin, D., Bat-Chava, Y., Lalwani, A., & Waltzman, S. (2011). Peer relationships of deaf children with cochlear implants: Predictors of peer entry and peer interaction success. *Journal of Deaf Studies and Deaf Education, 16*(1), 108–120.

Maxwell-McCaw, D. (2001). Acculturation and psychological well-being in deaf and hard-of-hearing people (Doctoral dissertation, The George Washington University). *Dissertation Abstracts International, 61*(11-B), 6141.

Maxwell-McCaw, D., & Zea, M. C. (2011). The Deaf Acculturation Scale (DAS): Development and validation of a 58-item measure. *Journal of Deaf Studies and Deaf Education.* [Epub ahead of print]. doi: 10.1093/deafed/enq061.

Meadow-Orlans, K., Mertens, D., & Sass-Lehrer, M. (2003). *Parents and their deaf children: The early years.* Washington, DC: Gallaudet University Press.

Miles, M. (2000). Signing in the Seraglio: Mutes, dwarfs, and jesters at the Ottoman Court 1500–1700. *Disability and Society, 15*(1), 115–134.

Moores, D. F. (2001). *Educating the deaf: Psychology, principles, and practices* (5th ed.). Boston: Houghton Mifflin.

Most, T., Wiesel, A., & Blitzer, T. (2007). Identity and attitudes towards cochlear implant among deaf and hard of hearing adolescents. *Deafness and Education International, 9*(2), 68–82.

Mottez, B. (1993). The deaf-mute banquets and the birth of the Deaf movement. In J. Van Cleve (Ed.), *Deaf history unveiled* (pp. 27–39). Washington, DC: Gallaudet University Press.

Nicholas, J., & Geers, A. (2003). Personal, social, and family adjustment in school-aged children with a cochlear implant. *Ear & Hearing, 24,* 69S–80S.

Oliva, G. (2004). *Alone in the mainstream.* Washington, DC: Gallaudet University Press.

Padden, C., & Humphries, T. (1988). *Deaf in America: Voices from a culture.* Cambridge, MA: Harvard University Press.

Percy-Smith, L., Jensen, J., Cayé-Thomasen, P., Thomsen, J., Gudman, M., & Lopez, A. (2008a). Factors that affect the social well-being of children with cochlear implants. *Cochlear Implants International, 9*(4), 199–214.

Percy-Smith, L., Jensen, J., Cayé-Thomasen, P., Thomsen, J., Gudman, M., & Lopez, A. (2008b). Self-esteem and social well-being of children with cochlear implant compared to normal-hearing children. *International Journal of Pediatric Otorhinolaryngology, 72,* 1113–1120.

Percy-Smith, L., Jensen, J., Josvassen, J., Jonsson, M., Andersen, J., Samar, C., et al. (2006). *Ugeskr Laeger, 168*(33), 2659–2664.

Preisler, G., Tvingstedt, A., & Ahlström, M. (2005). Interviews with deaf children about their experiences using cochlear implants. *American Annals of the Deaf, 150*(3), 260–267.

Quartararo, A. (2008). *Deaf identity and social images in nineteenth-century France.* Washington, DC: Gallaudet University Press.

Rée, J. (1999). *I see a voice.* New York: Metropolitan Books.

Schindler, R. (1999). Personal reflections on cochlear implants. *Annals of Otology, Rhinology & Laryngology, 108*(Suppl. 177), 4–7.

Schorr, E. (2006). Early cochlear implant experience and emotional functioning during childhood: Loneliness in middle and late childhood. *The Volta Review, 106*(3), 365–379.

Schorr, E., Roth, F., & Fox, N. (2009). Quality of life for children with cochlear implants: Perceived benefits and problems and the perception of single words and emotional sounds. *Journal of Speech, Language, and Hearing Research, 52*(1), 141–152.

Sheridan, M. (2008). Deaf adolescents: Inner lives and lifeworld development. Washington, DC: Gallaudet University Press.

Tatum, B. (1997). *Why are all the Black kids sitting together in the cafeteria?* New York: Basic Books.

Tellings, A. (1996). Cochlear implants and deaf children. The debate in the United States. *Journal of the British Association of Teachers of the Deaf, 20*(1), 24–31.

Van Cleve, J., & Crouch, B. (1989). *A place of their own: Creating the Deaf community in America.* Washington, DC: Gallaudet University Press.

Wald, R., & Knutsen, J. (2000). Deaf cultural identity of adolescents with and without cochlear implants. *Annals of Otology, Rhinology & Laryngology. Supplement, 185*, 87–89.

Watson, L., Hardie, T., Archbold, S., & Wheeler, A. (2008). Parents' views on changing communication after cochlear implantation. *Journal of Deaf Studies and Deaf Education, 13*(1), 104–116.

Wheeler, A., Archbold, S., Gregory, S., & Skipp, A. (2007). Cochlear implants: The young people's perspective. *Journal of Deaf Studies and Deaf Education, 12*(3), 303–316.

Woll, B., & Ladd, P. (2003). Deaf communities. In M. Marschark & P. E. Spencer (Eds.), *Oxford handbook of deaf studies, language, and education* (pp. 151–163). New York: Oxford.

Zaidman-Zait, A. (2008). Everyday problems and stress faced by parents of children with cochlear implants. *Rehabilitation Psychology, 53*(2), 139–152.

PART II

Language and Auditory Processing

7

BIMODAL PROCESSING OF LANGUAGE FOR COCHLEAR IMPLANT USERS

Donna A. Morere

It is not uncommon for implant teams or therapists to request that families of individuals receiving cochlear implants (CIs) cease or limit use of visual modes of communication following implantation (Moores, 2009). However, research with hearing participants indicates that speech is perceived through a combination of vision and audition (Bernstein, Auer, Wagner, & Ponton, 2008; Möttönen, Schürmann, & Sams, 2004). Information from speechreading speeds up the processing of the speech signal (Van Wassenhove, Grant, & Poeppel, 2005). Further, the auditory signal is supported by visual input (especially when the auditory signal is unclear) and processed in the auditory area of the brain (Calvert & Campbell, 2003). These findings indicate that both auditory and visual processing are important for language reception regardless of hearing status. They further suggest that the use of prior skills in visual communication, if properly applied, could enhance both the development of auditory linguistic skills in recent implant recipients and the optimal use of implants by skilled users. This chapter will review the literature on the cognitive processing of bimodal linguistic input and its relation to implant use.

Speechreading and Bimodal Speech Processing in the Hearing Listener

Research into the reception of spoken language has historically focused on auditory speech reception. However, it has been known for more than half a century that visual information can increase the listener's ability to understand speech, particularly in noisy situations (Sumby & Pollack, 1954). Over the past several decades, it has become clear that, rather than a unimodal auditory process, speech perception is multimodal. Even hearing listeners naturally integrate the available visual information with the auditory signal, although the mechanism of this integration continues to be debated (Bernstein & Benoît, 1996; Rosenblum, 2008; Woodhouse, Hickson, & Dodd, 2009). Although the information available through the auditory signal is less ambiguous, speech can be understood with varying accuracy based solely on the more limited visual information (Bernstein, 2006). Speechreading is commonly thought to depend on the information available on the lips (lipreading); however, Bernstein cited research indicating that visual cues to speech can additionally be observed on the cheeks, jaw, and other areas of the lower face. Furthermore, she noted that among deaf and hearing speechreaders, the best quartile among the hearing participants are significantly outperformed by the best quartile of the deaf speechreaders. This suggests that reliance on visual reception of speech has resulted in enhanced visual phonetic processing in successful deaf speechreaders. Even so, speechreading also appears to be a natural skill for hearing people (Paulesu et al., 2003).

The capacity to understand speech through vision varies depending on the type of speech stimulus involved. Some phonemes are harder to speechread than others due to the greater ambiguity of the signal. Speechreading research using hearing individuals has indicated that consonants in isolation are difficult to discriminate due to lack of specificity of the visual signal (Lidestam & Beskow, 2006). However, it was found that the accuracy of identification improved for words and sentences and that the provision of cues related to the topic of the stimulus further improved accuracy. Additionally, in comparing speechreading accuracy for stimuli produced by a human speaker with that from a computer-generated speechreadable avatar, they found that although accuracy of consonant identification did not differ significantly between the two, the human speaker produced better results for both sentence and word identification. This is consistent with the contention that information from multiple aspects of the face, rather than simply the mouth, provides important clues to visible speech. This has implications for the complexity of avatars needed to produce adequately readable speech.

Early research in speechreading expanded during the 1970s, with numerous studies investigating the bimodal visual-auditory perception of speech. Adults (Binnie, Montgomery, & Jackson, 1974) and adolescents (Dodd, 1977) with normal hearing were able to use speechreading to support consonant identification in the bimodal stimulus presentation, with increasing visual contribution to the discrimination as the signal to noise ratio (SNR) declined (i.e., as noise levels increased). One of the most innovative and widely cited studies was that of McGurk and MacDonald (1976). They generated visual-auditory mismatches, with hearing participants presented with the video of a speaker saying /ga/ dubbed over with the auditory stimulus of /ba/. This was perceived by most participants as /da/. The perceptual fusion does not occur for all visual-auditory pairings. For example, the authors found that the audio /ga/ dubbed on the video /ba/ was perceived as a sequence of the two consonants in the stimuli followed by the vowel rather than a fused consonant-vowel (CV) pair. The integration of the visual and auditory information to produce a fused, third perceived phoneme has been labeled the "McGurk effect." When users of cued speech[1] were presented with speechreading stimuli paired with congruent and incongruent cued speech manual cues, a similar phonological fusion effect within the visual system resulted (Alegria & Lechat, 2005).

The audiovisual fusion demonstrated in the McGurk effect provided clear evidence of visual-auditory integration and was found to occur even when the visual and auditory stimuli were produced by speakers of different genders (Green, Kuhl, Meltzoff, & Stevens, 1991). Although this effect occurs across languages, the degree of impact of visual information has been found to differ among languages, such as French (Werker, Frost, & McGurk, 1992) and Japanese (Sekiyama & Burnham, 2008). Werker and colleagues found that linguistic experience affected the ability to identify both auditory and visual phonemes in nonnative languages. Sekiyama and Burnham found that visual impact was greater for English than Japanese, and this difference appeared to emerge between 6 and 8 years of age. Jerger, Damian, Spence, Tye-Murray, and Abdi (2009) note that, based on the literature investigating the McGurk effect in infants, "the evidence as a whole continues to suggest that visual speech may play an important role in learning the phonological structure of spoken language" (p. 41). Consistent with previous studies, Jerger and colleagues found that whereas older and younger children were influenced by the visual component of audiovisual speech, those in the 5- to 9-year-old age range showed a diminished impact of visual speech. They suggested that this change may relate to "the proposal that phonological representational knowledge reorganizes during the kindergarten–early elementary school years" (p. 54).

Sommers, Spehar, and Tye-Murray's (2005) investigation of audiovisual integration across different SNRs supported a combination of unimodal processing and integration of the bimodal (audiovisual) sensory information working together to produce the final speech perception. Indeed, experience in speechreading a specific person improves the ability to understand the audio-only speech of the same speaker in a noisy environment (Rosenblum, Miller, & Sanchez, 2007). This suggests that visual practice in receiving a specific person's speech can produce cross-modal enhancement of auditory reception of that person's speech in the noise similar to the unimodal enhancement seen with experience listening to the speaker. This suggests that some type of interactive/integrative process involving the auditory and visual signals occurs during the early stages of processing.

1. Cued speech is a phonemically based system of handshapes and placements that clarifies the ambiguous information available through speechreading, allowing the "listener" to determine which member of each set of visually similar phonemes is being spoken.

Brain Imaging and Electrophysiological Studies With Hearing Participants

Speechreading and Speech Perception

Kislyuk, Möttönen, and Sams (2008) combined the McGurk effect with electroencephalogram measurement of responses in the auditory cortex to the introduction of a deviant stimulus in a sequence of repetitive speech stimuli (e.g., /ba/ inserted into a string of /va/), resulting in a change in the electroencephalogram response in the auditory cortex labeled "mismatch negativity" (MMN). The participants demonstrated typical MMN to the auditory stimuli, but when the deviant auditory stimulus (which would typically produce the MMN) was dubbed over a visual speech stimulus that continued to reflect the repetitive stimulus, the MMN was absent. In essence, the stimulus was perceived as the fused audiovisual stimulus rather than the actual auditory stimulus within the auditory cortex, and the participants "heard" the audiovisual phoneme rather than the actual auditory stimulus. Electrophysiological data from children as young as 5 months old have demonstrated this audiovisual fusion (the McGurk effect), whereas audiovisual combinations not perceived as fused phonemes by adults were perceived as discordant even by infants (Kushnerenko, Teinonen, Volein, & Csibra, 2008). It appears that audiovisual integration develops in infancy, with similar constraints to those seen in adults.

This differential response to sets of visual and auditory stimulus combinations, with some being perceived as fused, whereas others are not, suggests that some type of analysis of the match between the two occurs during processing. Bernstein, Lu, and Jiang (2008) imaged the brains of participants during responses to a set of stimuli with varying degrees of match between the two modalities. They found that when the two were highly matched, the response was consistent with an auditory response. With a moderate mismatch, a high level of fusion (McGurk effect) responses occurred. However, with a high degree of mismatch between the visual and auditory stimuli, the responses varied, with most responses favoring the auditory stimulus, whereas others were fused, visual, or reflected sequential reporting of the auditory and visual consonants. The imaging data indicated that the overall level of activity increased with increasing incongruity between the audio and visual portions of the stimuli. Additionally, the left supramarginal gyrus, which has been implicated in auditory processes such as phonological memory, detection of phonological change, and learning nonnative phonemes, was differentially active across the degrees of mismatch. This was hypothesized to reflect supramarginal gyrus involvement in the detection of multisensory incongruity, and the comparison of the data perceived with the "stored knowledge of the normal relationships between auditory and visual patterns" (Bernstein et al., 2008, p. 179). This process could allow the determination of the most likely candidate for the discordant perceptual information.

Consistent with previous research, Van Wassenhove et al. (2005) found that bimodal presentation of speech information improves accuracy over either unimodal (auditory or visual) stimulus presentation. They investigated the timing of neural activation using surface (scalp) electrodes. They found that the auditory cortex responded more quickly and more accurately in the audiovisual condition than in the auditory-only condition, with the degree of the facilitation varying based on the accuracy with which the individual phonemes were speechread in the visual-only condition. Thus, in the bimodal condition the visual contribution appeared to "speed up" the auditory response, with greater facilitation for the more visually unambiguous phonemes. The authors note that the visual aspects of speech precede the auditory signal in natural speech and suggest that the visual information may predict the most likely set of potential phonemes, allowing the auditory system to respond with increasing speed due to a reduced range of potential responses. That is, if closed lips as in /b/ are seen, the auditory system can focus on comparing the incoming signal to consonants such as /b/, /p/, and /m/, which have that configuration, and not waste resources on those such as /k/, /h/, and /g/, which have an open-mouthed configuration.

Presurgery evaluations of epilepsy patients using implanted electrodes have allowed precise recordings of electrophysiological responses to speech stimuli through analysis of event-related potentials in the auditory and visual cortex. Auditory speech stimuli produced initial activation in the primary auditory cortex followed by activation of secondary auditory and linguistic areas. Although there was more interpatient variability in the responses, visual speech stimuli produced initial activation of the area involved in the processing of visual motion, immediately followed by activation in the secondary auditory cortex (Besle et al., 2008). Consistent with Van Wassenhove et al. (2005), audiovisual stimuli appeared to produce a decrease in the auditory response followed by a suppression of the visual response and had characteristics similar to the response to the auditory-only stimulus. Although the primary auditory cortex was not activated by the unimodal visual stimulus in most patients, they were only asked to look at the faces, not speechread. Thus, these data do not conflict with the imaging studies that have demonstrated speechreading activation in the primary auditory cortex. However, they do offer some insights into the timing and characteristics of bimodal speech perception.

Neuroimaging techniques allow observation of the functioning of the brain during various activities, including speech perception. Functional magnetic resonance imaging (fMRI) analysis of activation during speechreading indicated that speechreading in the absence of accompanying auditory stimuli can produce activation of the auditory cortex in hearing individuals (Hall, Fussell, & Summerfield, 2005). Furthermore, although not all participants had enhanced activation of the left auditory cortex during speechreading, there was a positive correlation between speechreading skill and the level of auditory cortex activation for the group who did. That is, even in hearing individuals, the better speechreaders have greater auditory cortex involvement in processing speechreading.

Calvert and Campbell (2003) found that both dynamic speech images such as videos of speech without sound and still images of speech (to a lesser degree) activate brain regions associated with speech processing. Their analysis of fMRI data on hearing participants indicated that the presentation of sequences of still photographs of speech (e.g., a lower face producing /v/ followed by one during /oo/) resulted in activation of areas associated with biological movement, whereas a letter stimulus superimposed on the lips of a neutral face did not. However, although both the static and dynamic visual speech stimuli activated visual brain regions, including those for biological movement, the degree of activation varied and dynamic speech also activated the auditory cortex, whereas the static stimuli produced greater activation of motor areas. These data suggest that although the dynamic visual speech stimuli directly accessed the auditory cortex for the phonemic analysis, the identification of the static phonemes may be through an alternative circuit that analyzes the stimulus and then internally models the movements involved in its reproduction.

This distinction in the neurological processing of still and dynamic speech is consistent with the observations of patients with cortical visual disturbances. Campbell, Zihl, Massaro, Munhall, and Cohen (1997) found that a patient who was unable to process visual movement was still able to identify phonemes from static speech stimuli but was able to perform only minimal dynamic speechreading and did not demonstrate audiovisual fusion. In contrast, Campbell (1992) studied a patient with visual agnosia who was unable to perceive static faces but was nevertheless able to speechread dynamic speech and demonstrate audiovisual fusion.

Möttönen et al. (2004), using magnetoencephalography, found that the audiovisual integration processing of dynamic speech resulted in activation in the auditory cortex prior to activation of the multisensory regions involved in biological motion analysis. This supports the direct processing of audiovisual integration within the auditory cortex. In contrast, during a task involving simply viewing facial stimuli involving production of CV syllables without attempted speechreading by hearing participants, areas involved in speech production were activated (Fridriksson et al., 2009). However, Skipper, van Wassenhove, Nusbaum, and Small (2007) reported activation of speech production areas during McGurk illusions as well as during congruent audiovisual tasks. They suggest that the visual input in the bimodal stimulus is used in analysis through the speech production system to determine which of a subset of possible phonemes is being heard. Thus, there appears to be support for both a direct auditory analysis and a "top-down" speech production analysis of audiovisual speech stimuli.

Sekiyama, Kannoc, Miura, and Sugita (2003) investigated bimodal processing of speech using both fMRI and positron emission tomography during a McGurk audiovisual fusion task at various SNRs using native speakers of Japanese, whose weaker McGurk effects allowed the investigation of the relative degree of fusion across listening conditions. Fusion was greater in the noisier conditions, and the percentage of responses based on the auditory component of the stimulus increased as the SNR increased. That is, visual input had a greater influence as the auditory input became more difficult to hear. Similarly, bilateral responses were seen in auditory regions for the auditory-only condition and responses in brain regions associated with visual motion processing for the visual condition, whereas the areas of activation shifted for bimodal stimuli depending on the SNR, with more auditory area activation in the high SNR (clear speech) conditions and a shift to more posterior (visual) areas as the noise levels increased relative to the speech. The focus of activation during the audiovisual task appeared to be in the areas receiving multisensory input, which are involved in the analysis of biological motion. Sekiyama et al. noted that the greater activation in this area during the audiovisual task was confined to the left hemisphere, suggesting that "the cross-modal binding occurred as a linguistic event" (p. 285). Interestingly, speech production areas were activated across conditions (auditory, visual, and bimodal), suggesting that the top-down analysis of speech input involving the speech production mechanism may run parallel to the sensory analysis regardless of the modality of the input. The authors also noted that the variability in the literature, particularly as it relates to the inconsistent finding of primary auditory cortex activation for bimodal conditions, could be related to methodological differences; however, activation of the areas involved in the processing of biological motion has been generally found for bimodal listening tasks.

Not only is there fMRI evidence of activation of cortical areas associated with audition during speechreading in hearing individuals but also activation of areas associated with visual word form processing has been noted during a task involving auditory attention to phonological rather than melodic aspects of complex auditory stimuli (Yoncheva, Zevin, Maurer, & McCandliss, 2010). This further supports the proposal that the visual and auditory processing of speech information is an interactive, rather than parallel, process.

Gesture

Although the primary focus of research into the bimodal processing of speech has focused on speechreading, the facial features associated with speech provide only a portion of the visual information available to the listener during normal interaction. Straube, Green, Weis, Chatterjee, and Kircher (2009) found differential fMRI activation for gestures related to the speech and unrelated gestures. This supports semantic integration of related gestures and speech in hearing listeners. Furthermore, the participants' later recognition of the sentences was most accurate for the sentences presented with related meaningful gestures, suggesting that the bimodal content was integrated and that it supported later memory performance for the sentences.

Willems, Ozyurek, and Hagoort (2007) also found semantic integration of gestures and speech. They studied the processing of speech with concurrent iconic gestures (e.g., fingers walking to represent "walking across"). In a design similar to those using the McGurk effect, the participants were presented with speech-gesture pairs that represented either a semantic match or a mismatch. Furthermore, in one condition the mismatched gesture better fit the context of the sentence (speech mismatch), in another condition the spoken component best fit the sentence (gesture mismatch), and in a third mismatch condition (double mismatch), neither the word nor the gesture fit readily into the sentence. Overlapping activation of the left inferior frontal cortex for both speech and gestures was found, which "is consistent with a theory of language comprehension in which the left inferior frontal cortex serves as the general (i.e., not domain-specific) unification site for language comprehension" (p. 2329). The semantic intent of the gesture and speech would be integrated to arrive at meaning in this area, which produced greater activation when the sentences contained words that were semantically ambiguous, suggesting the involvement of analysis of the stimuli for semantic associations to most accurately integrate the information. The authors noted, "Our results also show overlap with sign language comprehension with regard to the involvement of left inferior frontal and temporal cortices" (p. 2329). This has potential implications for simultaneous use of speech and signs. If nonlinguistic gestures are integrated with speech at the semantic level, one would expect at least that level of interaction from concurrently presented signs and speech, particularly if signs and linguistically relevant gestures share some areas of processing.

Kelly, Kravitz, and Hopkins (2004) used a similar match–mismatch between speech and gesture but added a complementary gesture condition. In their study an actor gestured to one of two items while the voice-over presented a word. In the match condition, a gesture corresponded to the specific word used, supporting the exact information provided by the speech. In the complementary condition, the gesture reflected another characteristic of the same item to which the spoken word referred, elaborating on the speech-based information. In the mismatch condition, the speech referred to a characteristic of one item, whereas the gesture indicated a characteristic of the other item, offering information conflicting with the speech. These authors again found that accompanying gestures affect the processing of speech reflected in event-related potentials, with the influence appearing in the early stages of the auditory linguistic processing. Consistent with Willems et al. (2007), there was a difference between the impact of matching and conflicting gestures. However, there was also a difference in the electrophysiological impact of matching and complementary gestures. This suggests that even when the referent of the gesture is consistent between the speech and the gesture, the specific content of the gesture is also analyzed and combined with the speech-based information to arrive at meaning.

Although the complementary gestures were distinguished from the matching early in processing, eventually the complementary information was processed as more consistent with the matching gesture and the mismatch condition was seen as discrepant. This suggests that in later processing, the related information was seen as having some degree of semantic consistency with the speech. Thus, this study supports the presence of the integrated processing of speech and gesture that begins early with the relationship to specific information. Gestural information then continues to be analyzed for relevant content during semantic analysis in the pursuit of meaning. Kelly and colleagues concluded, "Language naturally occurs in a rich communicative and audiovisual context. The results from the present study demonstrate that one aspect of this context—hand gesture—significantly impacts the comprehension of accompanying speech at multiple stages of language comprehension" (2004, p. 259). They saw this as a reflection of how the brain processes language in "natural discourse." Considering the very basic, simple nature of the stimuli in this study (single word/gesture combinations), this has significant implications for the complex integration of "meaningful gesture" and speech reflected in the simultaneous production of speech and signs.

Gesture can even affect language reception when it does not carry information about the content but merely reflects the speech prosody of the speaker. When listeners were able to see associated beat gestures, nonsense hand movements, or still bodies, the activation of the auditory cortex was increased compared with an auditory-only condition solely for the beat gesture condition, suggesting that visual information related to beat supports auditory speech reception (Hubbard, Wilson, Callan, & Dapretto, 2009).

Summary

Overall, the research on bimodal processing of speech supports the contention that, when available, both visual and auditory (and likely also somatosensory) information is used to process incoming linguistic stimuli. Although the exact nature of this process remains unclear, it appears to occur automatically, with the decision about what has been "heard" based on an integration of the available information. The degree of impact of the various sensory modalities appears to depend on the relative clarity of each modality, with increasing influence as the relative clarity of one type of input exceeds that of the other(s). Although there remains some uncertainty as to whether visual linguistic input is normally processed in the primary auditory cortex during either unimodal or bimodal visual reception, secondary areas associated with audition do appear to be involved in the processing of visual speech. Also implicated in the processing of visual speech is the multisensory area involved in the analysis of biological motion, which has been implicated in the processing of social interactions and social cognition. Dysfunction in this area has been related to autism spectrum disorders, in which social cognition is deficient (Zilbovicius et al., 2006).

Thus, visual support of receptive language processing appears to provide vital additional cues to the intent, as well as the words, of the speaker.

In addition to the direct impact of visual information from speechreading on the processing of the auditory speech stimulus, some authors have found support for the use of visual speech information through an alternative route that involves cognitive modeling of the speech production process (Calvert & Campbell, 2003). Furthermore, the studies reviewed in the preceding section found that even manual gestures related to the speech can affect the processing of auditory linguistic information at both the early stages of auditory analysis and later semantic analysis, affecting both comprehension and retention of the spoken material.

Brain Imaging and Electrophysiological Studies with Deaf or Hard of Hearing Participants

Speechreading and Speech Perception

Lee, Truy, Mamou, Sappey-Marinier, and Giraud (2007) used fMRI data to investigate the neural circuits involved in speechreading in adults with normal hearing and nonsigning adults who became profoundly deaf after developing language. Consistent with previous research (Auer & Bernstein, 2007; Bernstein, Auer, & Tucker, 2001), the deaf participants were the more accurate speechreaders; however, speechreading skill did not increase with longer duration of deafness. Consistent with outcomes for hearing speechreaders (Hall et al., 2005), the speechreading tasks produced increased activation in the deaf participants relative to controls in areas associated with audition, and the level of activation correlated positively with speechreading skill. The data support greater processing of speechreading within the auditory cortex for individuals who became deaf prior to language development, and the degree of auditory cortex involvement appears to relate to speechreading fluency.

The above results were consistent with those of Capek et al. (2008), who compared fMRI data during speechreading from congenitally deaf native signers and hearing nonsigners. They also found significant overlaps in activation, particularly in areas involved in the analysis of biological motion and primary and secondary auditory processing. Again the degree of activation varied depending on both hearing status and speechreading skill, with higher levels of activation in some areas associated with both increased speechreading skill and decreased residual hearing. The authors related their results to those of Bergeson, Pisoni, and Davis (2005), who found that children with more developed preimplantation speechreading skills develop better auditory speech reception after receiving

CIs. They then suggested that the brain areas activated during speechreading in this study, which are typically associated with processing auditory speech, "once tuned to visible speech, may then more readily adapt to perceiving speech multimodally" and added that this "should be seriously considered when recommendations concerning pediatric cochlear implantation procedures are being developed" (p. 2139).

Spatial Localization

Investigation of audiovisual integration has not been limited to speech perception. In his review of the data on visual influences on auditory spatial learning, King (2009) noted that visual localization (e.g., where the dog you see is located) is more precise than that based on auditory information (e.g., where the dog you hear barking is located) and can provide calibration for the auditory localization system even at subcortical levels. He concluded that bilateral CI users should receive training in auditory localization, and for those who are able to integrate multisensory inputs, "training with congruent auditory and visual stimuli should be particularly useful for promoting adaptive plasticity in the auditory system of these individuals" (p. 337).

Sign Language and Speech

Although many deaf individuals use a combination of signs and speech, this has not been an area of interest in research. Rather, the research into the neurological correlates of signing has focused on the relationship of signed languages to the brain. This is not the focus of the current chapter; however, Campbell, MacSweeney, and Waters (2008) provide a current review of the research related to that topic. Although there is little, if any, research on the neurological processing of simultaneous communication (SimCom—speech while simultaneously producing a compatible sign, typically in the syntactic order of the spoken language), the above discussed studies on the neural integration of speech and gesture in hearing individuals (Willems et al., 2007; Straube et al., 2009) suggest that even if the signs were processed as iconic gestures, they would be incorporated into the understanding of the linguistic message at the level of semantic processing. However, based on the research into the neural processing of signed *languages,* it appears likely that signs produced during SimCom would be processed linguistically at some level and integrated with the auditory speech at the semantic level. Since almost half of the deaf children in the United States, including those with CIs, are educated with some form of SimCom (typically labeled "total communication" [TC]; Karchmer & Mitchell, 2003), this is an important area of research that has yet to be tapped.

Speechreading and Bimodal Language Processing in the Deaf or Hard of Hearing Listener

Unisensory Auditory Processing in the Deaf or Hard of Hearing Individual

How do the brains of individuals with acquired deafness process language through hearing? Despite comparable performance on speech reception tasks, differences in cerebral activation were observed during auditory speech reception of adult CI users with an average of 2 years of deafness prior to implantation compared with hearing controls (Giraud et al., 2000). Based on positron emission tomography data, the CI users appeared to consume more neuronal resources in the early stages of analysis (acoustic and early phonemic) compared with the controls. This could represent either the use of adaptive strategies comparable to those of hearing individuals listening to degraded auditory input or neural reorganization due to the hearing loss and subsequent restoration of access to sound. The authors noted that although the CI users do receive an auditory stimulus, the speech signal produced by the CI is limited compared with "normal" hearing and the differences observed may represent long-term adaptations due to an ongoing need for increased analysis of the incoming speech signal.

This contention was supported by the results of Giraud, Price, Graham, and Frackowiak (2001), who also studied differential activation of implantees deafened after the development of language compared with controls. They found decreased differentiation in the processing of speech and nonspeech sounds in the CI users compared with the controls. The CI users seemed to actively analyze all incoming auditory stimuli to see if they represented speech input requiring further analysis. Areas involved in memory were also recruited more in the CI users. Furthermore, the authors also noted that despite the auditory nature of the stimuli, the CI users consistently responded with increased activation in the visual areas, which they suggested "might reflect learned expectancy (e.g., from lipreading experience) to process auditory and visual stimuli simultaneously" (p. 1313). Such an expectation makes sense when one considers that when using open set measures, even after 2 years of use, CI users who became deaf after spoken language development are still able to recognize consonants with about 71% accuracy (Valimaa, Maatta, Lopponen, & Sorri, 2002b) and vowels with 68% accuracy (Valimaa, Maatta, Lopponen, & Sorri, 2002a). Giraud and colleagues (2001) concluded that the CI recipients use alternate resources, including memory, visual attention, and available visual input to clarify the less clear auditory signal. They proposed that, rather than the typical sequence of first analyzing the phonological properties of the stimuli and then performing semantic analysis, the CI users "probably go through a series of concurrent and interactive steps before reaching stable sound recognition" (p. 1315) and that these steps include a number of areas outside the standard language system.

Taken together, these studies suggest that, in contrast to the typical hearing person, multichannel CI users who become deaf after developing spoken language may need to actively investigate whether each sound heard is a speech sound or not. If they determine it to be a speech sound, they must then analyze it at the phonemic level, after which they can determine if it is a word or not, and so forth. This may consume cognitive resources that the control participants in the latter study used for semantic analysis and other processing not required for the research tasks, which involved the simple naming of environmental sounds and the repetition of speech stimuli. However, this does raise the question of whether increased consumption of resources for lower level analysis might affect performance of higher level language tasks. If this is the case, it is possible that if the CI user could support auditory reception with the visual analysis apparently anticipated by the participants in the latter study, cognitive resources might be released for further, higher level linguistic analysis.

The above studies presented the stimuli without background noise. Considering the difficulty discriminating between speech and nonspeech sounds apparent in this study, it is not surprising that even highly successful adult CI users, who are able to achieve a median 92.5% correct keywords in sentences presented in quiet, had difficulty with the same task presented with background noise (Donaldson et al., 2009). They required an SNR of 11.9 dB to achieve 50% correct responses in noise, compared with a SNR of –1.6 dB for the hearing controls. This would make communication through audition alone difficult in many environments, even for highly effective CI users.

Bimodal Speech Reception and Deaf and Hard of Hearing Adults

Although it has been generally accepted that speechreading is an unclear art, with more advanced deaf speechreaders achieving only about 48% to 85% accuracy of identifying words in sentences (Bernstein, 2006), the fact that even hearing listeners use visual input to support their auditory reception of language, particularly as the auditory signal becomes less clear, suggests that audiovisual integration may provide a significant contribution even to individuals with relatively minor hearing loss. This is supported by the work of Grant and Seitz (1998), who found that adults with sloping mild to severe (pure tone average 39 dB) acquired hearing loss benefited significantly from visual speech information during low context sentence (meaning could not be derived from isolated words) and consonant identification tasks presented in noise. However, they noted that the amount of benefit varied. Audiovisual benefit (increased audiovisual accuracy relative to audio-only accuracy) for both sentence and consonant identification was correlated with susceptibility to the McGurk effect, reflecting the degree of audiovisual integration. This was interpreted as indicating that individuals who performed audiovisual integration automatically were more able to take advantage of the bimodal information to enhance receptive language processing. The authors suggested that "some form of integration training would be beneficial" for those with weaker integration skills (p. 2444). Surprisingly, enhanced consonant identification had little relation to the audiovisual benefit for the sentence identification task in this study.

Individuals in a similar study who had adult onset, primarily noise-related, sloping mild to moderate (pure tone average 33 dB) acquired hearing loss also benefited significantly from audiovisual (vs. unimodal auditory) stimuli despite minimal accuracy in the unimodal visual (speechreading) condition for both consonant and sentence recognition tasks (Grant, Walden, & Seitz, 1998). It was noted that for sentence recognition, "Every subject's AV [audiovisual] score was better than his/her A [auditory-only] score, even when the V [visual-only] score was 0% correct" and "The average relative benefit was 44% (s.d. = 17.8%) with a maximum of 83% and a minimum of 8.5%" (p. 2686). Thus, even individuals with late-onset hearing loss who are minimally skilled at speechreading are able to make significant use of speechreading information to support their language reception. In contrast to the above study, approximately half of the variance in the sentence recognition was accounted for by the consonant recognition performance. Variability in sentence recognition may be affected by a range of factors, such as top-down processes, including lexical, grammatical, and contextual analysis, and memory processes. Regardless of the relationship between benefit at the phonemic and sentence level, it is clear that even very weak speechreaders with hearing loss can benefit significantly from bimodal, audiovisual analysis of receptive language.

Although the above studies investigated the audiovisual benefit for hard of hearing individuals whose hearing loss occurred after spoken language development, Rouger and colleagues (2007) studied audiovisual benefits in French-speaking CI users who became deaf after spoken language development. Prior to implantation, the participants used their minimal auditory capacity (10.0% accuracy on open set speech recognition) to support the information received through speechreading (30.1%), resulting in a significantly enhanced audiovisual performance (55.8%). Although the speechreading skills remained relatively stable over the 8 years of data, as the auditory performance improved, the audiovisual scores increased, presumably due to the increased auditory input. The CI users demonstrated significantly better speechreading and audiovisual integration than hearing individuals tested with degraded auditory components of the signal. The authors concluded that the CI users were better multisensory integrators than the hearing controls.

Desai, Stickney, and Zeng (2008) compared the auditory, visual, and audiovisual performances of English-speaking CI users who became deaf after developing spoken language and hearing controls. They also included trials of the control participants during which the auditory component of the stimuli was processed to simulate the input received through four- and eight-channel (representing the number of electrodes used to stimulate the auditory nerve) CIs.

The stimuli were CV pairs presented via a computer-generated speechreadable avatar. The pairs were presented with the consonant stimuli manipulated to produce multiple slightly different CV pairs with formant frequencies transitioning stepwise across the ranges from those representing the model for /ba/ through /da/ to the model for /ga/ to investigate the relative ability to categorize more ambiguous stimuli; that is, to determine the "cutoff" between /ba/ and /da/.

Using a forced-choice response format, the hearing participants listening to unprocessed auditory-only stimuli responded with fairly pronounced and consistent boundaries between the consonants, with some ambiguity during the transitional stimuli. In contrast, both the CI users and the hearing "simulated CI users" had difficulty on this task. They were only moderately accurate even with the reference stimuli (precise formant frequency representation of the phonemes). Indeed, despite the availability of only three response choices, the best response accuracy for the CI users was only 50% for the CV pair /ba/. Both the CI users and simulated users did categorize the stimuli. With the exception of the four-channel simulation, during which both typical /da/ and /ga/ stimuli produced a greater percentage of /da/ responses, the actual and simulated CI users produced a relatively greater proportion of the responses generally consistent with the pattern of the controls. However, all three groups also responded with a high percentage of errors across the auditory stimuli, and the boundaries of the phonemes differed from those of the controls. Thus, degraded auditory signals, be they through a CI or simulation thereof, make accurate consonant identification difficult.

All three of these groups appeared to depend heavily on the visual stimulus component during the bimodal tasks, whereas the controls depended more heavily on the auditory component. However, given congruent audiovisual information, the actual CI users demonstrated a significant audiovisual benefit. In contrast, the simulated CI users appeared to achieve little benefit from the audiovisual presentation and performed best in the visual-only condition, suggesting that they were focusing on the visual aspects of the stimuli in the audiovisual task. On a side note, despite the advanced technology (most having 22- or 24-channel devices) of the CI participants, the hearing listeners in the 8-channel simulation (63% correct identifications) outperformed the CI users (51%) in the auditory condition, whereas results for the 4-channel simulation (48%) were only slightly below those of the CI users.

Among the CI users in the study by Desai et al. (2008), duration of experience with the CI, rather than duration of deafness prior to implantation with the CI, correlated with the ability to integrate audiovisual information. This may be why the hearing participants in the simulated CI conditions did not produce audiovisual integration, as this represented a novel situation for them. Indeed, these results may more closely reflect the experiences of newly implanted individuals who became deaf after developing spoken language rather than the experienced users in the study. This study indicates that even experienced CI users who became deaf after developing spoken language have difficulty with speech perception through audition alone even in the absence of noise and with a very limited response set. Although they do benefit significantly from audiovisual integration, this appears to represent a skill that must be developed over time.

Individuals who became deaf after developing spoken language are typically considered good candidates for CIs, whereas implantation of congenitally deaf adults has been more controversial due to a lack of "auditory memory" to which the new speech sounds can be related. However, Moody-Antonio and colleagues (2005) found that even congenitally deaf adults who, at least 1 year postimplantation, had fairly poor speech perception scores with either the auditory (median score 5.2%) or visual (25.9%) unisensory presentation were able to benefit significantly from the bimodal presentation (50.7%). Thus, despite a lack of "auditory memory" from preimplantation hearing, these individuals were able to support their speechreading with the newly acquired auditory signal, and at least some of the participants were able to integrate the audiovisual signal to produce greater benefit than simple additive effects of the auditory and visual input combined. Considering the results of Desai et al. (2008), the relatively short duration of implant use for some of the implantees may have accounted for some of the variability in the bimodal integration seen in this study.

The use of minimal auditory speech identification skills to support speechreading by the participants in the Moody-Antonio et al. (2005) study mirrors the use of minimal speechreading skills to support the diminished auditory capacity of individuals with mild to moderate late-onset hearing loss in the previously discussed study by Grant et al. (1998). Thus, although the audiovisual benefit in hearing individuals and those with less severe hearing loss (and perhaps some CI users who became deaf after developing spoken language) may be thought of as using the visual information to support a degraded auditory signal, it also appears that for deaf individuals even a very limited auditory signal may be used to support the ambiguous visual speech signal. This may be especially true for those with recently activated CIs, as suggested by the above study. The ability to integrate audiovisual speech information automatically appears to produce the best receptive outcomes. For those who are learning to process the combined auditory and visual signal, training to integrate the two may provide the best outcome (Grant & Seitz, 1998).

Bimodal Speech Reception and the Child Who Is Deaf or Hard of Hearing

The above studies addressed unisensory and audiovisual integration of incoming spoken language in adults with previously developed language. This is not the case with the child with early-onset hearing loss who must learn language through whatever signals are available, even if they are ambiguous or degraded. This chapter will not address the controversy over the appropriateness of spoken language for deaf children. Lynas (2005) provides a review of the oral, bilingual, and TC debate. This chapter will simply focus on the impacts of unimodal and bimodal access on spoken language development of children using some form of access to sound.

Profoundly deaf hearing aid users ages 8 to 18 have been shown to benefit from audiovisual speech presentation compared with both audio-only and visual-only presentation (Lamoré, Huiskamp, van Son, Bosman, & Smoorenburg, 1998). The authors analyzed the phonemic feature information available through audition and vision for each of the phonemes presented and found that the increased accuracy of the children under the audiovisual presentation was significantly greater than the simple additive properties of the visual and auditory information. They termed this the "synergistic effect AV-enhancement (ENH_{AV})." Thus, although the children's overall average scores improved from 53.7 (audio only) and 52.7 (video only) to 81.7 (audiovisual), resulting in an improvement from the unimodal to bimodal condition of more than 50% for either comparison, the ENH_{AV} (added accuracy not explained by the combined information provided) was 3.7%. This enhancement was greatest for final consonants (ENH_{AV} 7.1), followed by initial consonants (ENH_{AV} 5.5) and had the least impact on vowels (ENH_{AV} 1.6). The degree of enhancement appeared to be related to the accuracy in the auditory-only condition. This study is important, as it demonstrates that the audiovisual interaction, even in children with early-onset profound hearing loss, represents more than simply the additive effects of the perceptible visual and auditory speech features and is indicative of integration of this information to form a more accurate audiovisual gestalt. This is consistent with the proposed interactive model in which unimodal processing is combined with integrative bimodal processing to produce the final speech perception (Sommers et al., 2005).

Schorr, Fox, van Wassenhove, and Knudsen (2005) studied 5- to 14-year-old hearing children and congenitally deaf CI users who were able to perceive speech through the implant alone. They were presented with CV pairs through audition, vision, and audiovisual sets that were congruent or incongruent. McGurk effects were observed in both the hearing children and the CI users, but there were inconsistencies in both groups. Whereas some children in each group demonstrated consistent audiovisual integration, others (more frequently hearing children) tended to use the auditory information more, and a third group (more often the CI users) focused more on the visual aspects of the stimuli. Bearing in mind the results of Jerger et al. (2009) and the age range of the participants, the variability within the hearing group and the tendency to focus on the auditory signal when fusion did not occur is not surprising. For the CI users who produced consistent responses to the auditory-only stimuli, 20% (compared with 57% of the hearing participants) demonstrated consistent audiovisual integration (fusion).

Although only a minority of the CI users demonstrated consistent bimodal integration of the stimuli, within that subgroup, the performances were indistinguishable from those of the hearing bimodal processers. All of the CI users who demonstrated consistent bimodal fusion received their implants prior to 30 months of age; however, duration of CI use and age at the time of testing were not significant predictors of fusion. Thus, early bimodal language experience—and therefore early implantation—appears to be the primary force affecting automatic bimodal processing of speech stimuli in congenitally deaf pediatric CI users. Although most CI users did benefit significantly from bimodal presentation of the stimulus compared with either unimodal condition (i.e., their accuracy was greater in the audiovisual condition), for automatic bimodal processing of speech information, early bimodal language exposure appears to be critical. Whereas for the hearing aid users in the study by Lamoré and colleagues (1998) this was apparently possible through residual hearing, for profoundly deaf children this would appear to support early implantation if the goal is the development of auditory-oral language.

Deaf Children, CIs, and the Bimodal Reception of Language

Language Development and the Pediatric CI User

Recent research has demonstrated that children with early-onset profound deafness are able to develop language through audition using CIs (Geers, Nicholas, & Sedey, 2003; Geers, Tobey, Moog, & Brenner, 2008; Svirsky, Robbins, Kirk, Pisoni, & Miyamoto, 2000). Svirsky and colleagues demonstrated that with adequate intervention not only did the language development of the CI users exceed expectations for similar deaf children using hearing aids, but also, over the first 2 and a half years following implantation, they were comparable to the gains expected in hearing children. Thus, although on average the children did not "catch up," they did not demonstrate the increasing spoken language delays typically observed with deaf children. However, their outcomes varied, and some children appeared to have an increased learning trajectory whereas others did not demonstrate significant language growth. Within the group, a significant correlation between auditory word recognition and language quotient was seen for those who were primarily oral but not for those who used TC despite comparable language development for the two subgroups. This suggests that the children using TC may be learning language through either a visual or an audiovisual process, whereas the oral children are doing so primarily through audition or a more "auditorily oriented" audiovisual process.

Investigation of language development in early implanted children with hearing loss prior to language development suggests that both children who are primarily oral and those who use TC can develop language and perform on measures of language development within expectations. However, whereas some suggest that the oral children performed better on some of the expressive language measures even for the TC administration (Geers et al., 2003), others suggest that use of TC may support greater language development in children implanted early (Connor, Hieber, Arts, & Zwolan, 2000). Thus, the data are not consistent, and further study is needed to determine if there are advantages or disadvantages to either approach. This type of research is important, as there may be subgroups of children who have better outcomes using different approaches. If this is the case, early identification of such subgroups may decrease the frequency of severe language delays too often seen in deaf children.

Eighty-five children from the study by Geers et al. (2003) were followed and reevaluated at ages 15 to 18 to investigate long-term CI outcomes (Geers et al., 2008). Although most of the children reported using speech for communication in their school setting, 38% continued to report using a combination of speech and signs. In general, the children appeared to continue on the trajectory observed in the earlier study. That is, the children who performed better on measures of language and reading in elementary school continued to perform well at the high school assessment. Overall, speech perception through the CI improved with the increased duration of CI use. Average language scores of the participants increased at a faster rate than those of their hearing peers, reflecting some degree of "catching up" that was not seen in the short-term follow-up reported by Svirsky et al. (2000). However, despite adequate development, reading skills did not generally reflect such "catching up." As seen in other studies, these skills varied widely, with some children excelling whereas others made little progress over the years. The best predictors of reading and language performance at the older ages were skill levels on the measures when tested during elementary school and scores on nonverbal intelligence measures. Age at implantation was also a significant, but weak, predictor of reading outcomes.

Most of the students were fully mainstreamed (77%) and in age appropriate grades (Geers et al., 2008). One disadvantage of mainstreaming is the noisy acoustic environment in most schools, which affects academic achievement and social development as well as speech perception (ASHA Working Group on Classroom Acoustics, 2005; Crandell & Smaldino, 2000; Nelson & Soli, 2000). Since the majority of these students reported using oral communication, enhancing their ability to do so through optimizing both visual supports and acoustic environments should be a priority. Speech perception outcomes in this study were again best predicted by the scores from the assessment during the primary school years, but pure tone average with the CI was also a significant, if weak, predictor. This suggests that early language skills contribute more to the child's ability to accurately perceive speech than the degree of "hearing" available. For these students, it appears that audiovisual integration would provide important support for their daily communication.

Bimodal Speech Reception and the Pediatric CI User

Electrophysiological investigation of auditory perception has suggested that early implantation (before age 3.5) may be required for appropriate development of the central auditory pathway in congenitally deaf children who did not receive significant benefit from amplification (Sharma, Dorman, & Spahr, 2002). These data are consistent with the relative lack of audiovisual fusion in children implanted after 30 months of age, which suggests that an even earlier age may be required for optimal outcomes (Schorr et al., 2005). However, nonverbal intelligence also correlates with speech perception in early implanted children with at least 4 years of CI use (Geers, Brenner, & Davidson, 2003). Despite extended CI use, the average accuracy in open set speech recognition was only 50% for unimodal auditory reception and 40% for unimodal visual (speechreading) reception. Bimodal (audiovisual) reception improved accuracy to 80%. It was noted that the auditory perception of vowels and consonants was "roughly equivalent to that of a severely hearing-impaired child using hearing aids" (p. 33S). Use of the most up-to-date speech external equipment and processing strategy appeared to have a significant impact on performance, and the authors noted that these results emphasize the importance of ensuring that children have the most current technology to optimize their auditory-oral functioning. Oral education appeared to best support development of auditory speech perception.

Lachs, Pisoni, and Kirk (2001) studied children ages 4 to 8 who had had their CIs for at least 2 years. Most were congenitally deaf and the average age at implantation was 4.5. They were tested using the Common Phrases Test, which presents well-known phrases such as "It is cold outside." The child then repeats what was heard and the score is the number of correct repetitions. The children were tested in audio-only, video-only, and audiovisual conditions. The authors measured audiovisual gain (improvement over the unimodal conditions) and found that greater audiovisual gain was correlated with better speech intelligibility, suggesting a relationship between speech reception and production. They also compared children in primarily oral and TC educational settings and found that the oral children demonstrated greater speech intelligibility, audiovisual gain, and spoken word recognition.

Although, most children in both settings showed audiovisual gain over either unimodal condition, a few appeared to experience audiovisual interference compared with their best unimodal score. However, even when those children were included in the calculation, the average positive difference from the better unimodal to the bimodal condition comparison was a gain of 7.50%. Unimodal scores ranged from 0.00% to 90.00% for audio alone (mean 27.78%) and 0.00% to 80.00% for visual alone (mean 32.50%). Surprisingly, even 1 of the 2 children who received scores of 0.00% for both unimodal conditions was able to demonstrate an audiovisual benefit, achieving 20.00% in the bimodal condition. This suggests that the combined information provides an enhanced receptive experience even for the weakest speechreaders/listeners. Three children, who were among the high scorers on the unimodal conditions, achieved 100.00% in the bimodal condition, suggesting a possible ceiling effect for the task. The authors note that children with CIs are often tested using audition alone and promote the idea of audiovisual testing to obtain more accurate information about actual development of spoken language skills. They also pointed out the significant individual differences observed and advocated investigation of these differences in outcomes.

Eight- to 10-year-old children with congenital or early-onset hearing loss who were experienced CI users (minimum 3.8 years, mean 5.4 years) were able to repeat only 5% of the "words" accurately when presented with audiotapes of nonwords to avoid access to speechreading and known vocabulary to support perception (Carter, Dillon, & Pisoni, 2002). Although some of the errors may have reflected limitations in articulation, this would not account for the fact that less than two thirds (64%) of the responses had the correct number of syllables and only 61% of the responses had the correct placement of stress. Furthermore, only half of the responses contained both the correct number of syllables and the correct stress. The study included both children who use TC and oral children, and language scores based on TC administration correlated significantly with both syllable and stress accuracy. These data suggest that even children with relatively early implantation and significant experience with their CIs depend on their knowledge of the language and visual supports to clarify ambiguous auditory signals.

Bergeson, Pisoni, and Davis (2003) investigated audiovisual speech perception in prelingually deaf children implanted either before 53 months of age (early implanted) or between 54 and 108 months (late implanted) over a 3-year period. Comparisons between children using primarily oral communication and TC were also made. The oral children performed consistently better in the auditory-only conditions on both word and sentence tasks over the 3 years of study despite comparable hearing histories. Although they also initially surpassed the TC group on the visual-only task, by the second year postimplant, the TC group was somewhat better in this condition and their relative skill improved further by year 3. Similarly, through the first year postimplantation, the oral group performed better on the audiovisual task, but by year 2 postimplant the performances were comparable, and both groups continued to improve to a near perfect performance by year 3. On the sentence task, despite dramatic improvement between the first and second years postimplantation by the TC group for both the visual-only and audiovisual tasks, the oral group continued to outperform the TC group through year 3, although on the bimodal task both performed quite well by the final evaluation. When the early implanted children were compared with the later implantees on both sentence and word recognition, the later implanted children initially performed better on the auditory tasks but were surpassed by the early implanted children by year 2.

Although both groups made significant gains over the years on the visual-only task, the late implanted children continued to perform better during the postimplant period. Despite initial relative limitations, the early implanted children made steady gains on the audiovisual task, and by year 2 the groups performed comparably. However, although the late implanted children appeared to depend more on their visual receptive skills, the early implantees appeared to use the auditory information more effectively. Regardless of how the participants were grouped, all groups performed best in the audiovisual condition. These data suggest that for development of spoken language reception, oral immersion produces better outcomes; however, overall language skills can be achieved using either approach. Although the children in the TC group developed their auditory-receptive language skills more slowly than those in the oral group, over time they were able to achieve results comparable to their orally trained peers.

A later study by this group (Bergeson et al., 2005) investigated 80 children deaf before 36 months and implanted before age 9. They again found that these deaf children using CIs performed better in the bimodal (audiovisual condition) than in either of the unimodal (auditory-only or visual-only) conditions. In this study, the bimodal sentence comprehension skills were highly correlated with a number of factors associated with speech perception, speech intelligibility, and language, and the best speechreaders prior to implantation had the best postimplantation outcomes on these skills. Thus, children with stronger speechreading skills before implantation were better able to access speech and language through their CIs 3 years after implantation.

Taken as a whole, although the data appear to support a more oral orientation if the desired outcome is primarily oral functioning, spoken *language* development for early-onset deaf children with CIs appears to be accessible through both oral and TC approaches. Furthermore, although the manner in which they use the audiovisual signal varies, children using both approaches appear to benefit significantly from audiovisual integration of the speech signal and would likely require such integration for functioning in daily life.

Applications of Bimodal Processing to CI Recipients

Based on the studies reviewed above, a few things are clear. First is the fact that although many CI users are able to perceive speech relatively well with their CIs regardless of the quality of the input from the device, the signal received from the implant is still a degraded stimulus compared with "normal" hearing. Furthermore, noise is extremely difficult to filter out, especially speech-based noise, and CI users appear to require additional initial processing of nonspeech signals compared with hearing listeners to determine that the stimuli do not represent speech. The impact of extraneous noise (both speech and nonspeech) is particularly relevant for children using CIs, as they appear to be educated primarily in the mainstream, and classrooms have notoriously bad acoustics. In their review of the literature, Crandell and Smaldino (2000) noted that for children with only mild to moderate hearing loss, even in classrooms with optimal acoustics, "children with hearing impairment obtained perception scores of only 60% as compared to 83% for the normal hearers" and in more typical classroom environments, "children with SNHL [sensorineural hearing loss] obtained perception scores of just 11% as compared to 21% for children with normal hearing" (p. 366). They cited studies indicating that even mild or unilateral hearing loss can be exacerbated significantly by classroom acoustics and that the differential impacts on children with normal hearing compared with those with hearing loss increase as the acoustic environment deteriorates. Anyone who has ever been in a school cafeteria (or a fast food restaurant) can understand that a child listening through a CI, even one with exceptional speech perception, will have to use visual support for communication to function adequately.

These outcomes indicate the need for visual supports for communication. The data from the studies of both hearing and deaf or hard of hearing listeners indicate that the auditory and visual signals can (and some say *must*) be used in an integrative fashion to clarify the perception of spoken language. This appears to occur through a combination of the additive effects of the information provided by the two unimodal signals and an integrative process that provides enhancement of the perception above that of the simple additive effects. The data indicate that even minimal ability to use either signal can provide significant enhancement of the bimodal perception of speech. In their review of visual speech perception in both hearing and deaf or hard of hearing individuals, Woodhouse et al. (2009) noted that due to the multimodal nature of speech perception, speech and language therapists need to include speechreading "as an integral part of intervention for speech and language disorders" (p. 266) and suggest that the view of speech assessment and intervention as an exclusively auditory process is outdated. They concluded that "given the mandatory aspect of bimodal speech processing, an obvious avenue for intervention should be an awareness of speech-reading skills" (p. 266).

Although there are clear data supporting enhanced speech perception through bimodal access to the speech signal itself (via hearing and speechreading), there is less information concerning the bimodal enhancement of speech perception—and language comprehension—through a combination of speech and signs (e.g., SimCom or TC). However, available data from the research on gestures and the clarification of language reception suggest that this is a viable option. Furthermore, although the research on children with early-onset deafness using CIs suggests that *oral* language skills may be optimized by an oral educational approach, language as a whole appears to be comparably accessible through either approach. Although proponents of oral education for pediatric CI users press for limitation or elimination of signing, the reality is that not all children are able to learn language through their CIs or even CI plus speechreading alone.

Some in the field have suggested that language and speech perception can be developed through enhanced visual access to spoken language through cued speech (Leybaert & Alegria, 2003). Research in France suggests that this may be the case (Cochard et al., 2003; Vieu et al., 1998). Vieu and colleagues found that of pediatric CI users with early-onset deafness using oral, TC, or cued speech approaches, those using cued speech outperformed the other two groups on both speech intelligibility and syntactic accuracy, and the language level of the output was comparable to that of the oral children postimplant despite weaker speech skills of the cuers prior to implantation. Cochard and colleagues found that children using cued French, who had comparable speech to the children using oral or signed French prior to implantation, far outdistanced their oral and signing peers by 3 years postimplantation. They also outperformed the other groups on both closed and open set speech perception by the third year of implant use, with the greatest impact on open set perception. Currently, this method is used in Spain as a support for CI rehabilitation as well as for language development in deaf children, and one case study reflecting its use for language development in a child with a CI has supported its use (Moreno-Torres & Torres, 2008).

These data suggest that cued speech may be another visual option for those for whom the CI combined with speechreading alone does not provide adequate oral language access. Regardless of the approach used, bimodal processing of language appears to be not only possible but also critical for the successful use of the CI.

REFERENCES

Alegria, J., & Lechat, J. (2005). Phonological processing in deaf children: When lipreading and cues are incongruent. *Journal of Deaf Studies and Deaf Education, 10*(2), 122–133.

ASHA Working Group on Classroom Acoustics. (2005). Acoustics in educational settings: Technical report. *American Speech-Language-Hearing Association.* Retrieved August, 18, 2009, from http://www.asha.org/docs/pdf/TR2005-00042.pdf

Auer, E. T., & Bernstein, L. E. (2007). Enhanced visual speech perception in individuals with early-onset hearing impairment. *Journal of Speech, Language, and Hearing Research, 50*(5), 1157–1165.

Bergeson, T. R., Pisoni, D. B., & Davis, R. A. O. (2003). A longitudinal study of audiovisual speech perception by children with hearing loss who have cochlear implants. *The Volta Review, 103*(4), 347–370.

Bergeson, T. R., Pisoni, D. B., & Davis, R. A. O. (2005). Development of audiovisual comprehension skills in prelingually deaf children with cochlear implants. *Ear and Hearing, 26*(2), 149–164.

Bernstein, L. E. (2006). Visual speech perception. In E. Vatikiotis-Bateson, G. Bailly, & P. Perrier (Eds.), *Audio-visual speech processing* (pp. 20–40). Cambridge: Massachusetts Institute of Technology Press.

Bernstein, L. E., Auer, E. T., Jr., Tucker, P. E. (2001). Enhanced speechreading in deaf adults: Can short-term training/practice close the gap for hearing adults? *Journal of Speech, Language, and Hearing Research, 44*, 5–18.

Bernstein, L. E., Auer, E. T., Jr., Wagner, M., & Ponton, C. W. (2008). Spatiotemporal dynamics of audiovisual speech processing. *Neuroimage, 39*(1), 423–435.

Bernstein, L. E., & Benoît, C. (1996). For speech perception by humans or machines, three senses are better than one. In University of Delaware, Alfred I. DuPont Institute, & Acoustical Society of America (Eds.), *Proceedings of the Fourth International Conference on Spoken Language Processing* (pp. 1477–1480). New York: Institute of Electrical and Electronics Engineers.

Bernstein, L. E., Lu, Z. L., & Jiang, J. (2008). Quantified acoustic-optical speech signal incongruity identifies cortical sites of audiovisual speech processing. *Brain Research, 1242*, 172–189.

Besle, J., Fischer, C., Bidet-Caulet, A., Lecaignard, F., Bertrand, O., & Giard, M. (2008). Visual activation and audiovisual interactions in the auditory cortex during speech perception: Intracranial recordings in humans. *The Journal of Neuroscience, 28*(52), 14301–14310.

Binnie, C. A., Montgomery, A. A., & Jackson, P. L. (1974). Auditory and visual contributions to the perception of consonants. *Journal of Speech and Hearing Research, 1*(17), 619–630.

Calvert, G. A., & Campbell, R. (2003). Reading speech from still and moving faces: The neural substrates of visible speech. *Journal of Cognitive Neuroscience, 15*(1), 57–70.

Campbell, R. (1992). The neuropsychology of lipreading. *Philosophical Transactions of the Royal Society of London, Series B: Biological Sciences, 335*, 39–45.

Campbell, R., MacSweeney, M., & Waters, D. (2008). Sign language and the brain: A review. *Journal of Deaf Studies and Deaf Education, 13*(1), 3–20.

Campbell, R., Zihl, J., Massaro, D. W., Munhall, K., & Cohen, M. M. (1997). Speechreading in the akinetopsic patient, L.M. *Brain, 120*(10), 1793–1803.

Capek, C. M., MacSweeney, M., Woll, B., Waters, D., McGuire, P. K., David, A. S., et al. (2008). Cortical circuits for silent speechreading in deaf and hearing people. *Neuropsychologia, 46*(5), 1233–1241.

Carter, A., Dillon, C., & Pisoni, D. (2002). Imitation of nonwords by hearing impaired children with cochlear implants: Suprasegmental analyses. *Clinical Linguistics and Phonetics, 16*, 619–638.

Cochard, N., Calmels, M., Pavia, G., Landron, C., Husson, H., Honegger, A., et al. (2003). *L'impact du LPC sur l'évolution des enfants implantés. Unité édiatrique d'implantation cochléaire.* Retrieved August, 20, 2009, from http://www.alpc.asso.fr/rech01-a.htm

Connor, C., Hieber, S., Arts, H., & Zwolan, T. (2000). Speech, vocabulary, and the education of children using cochlear implants: Oral or total communication? *Journal of Speech, Language, and Hearing Research, 43*, 1185–1204.

Crandell, C. C., & Smaldino, J. J. (2000). Classroom acoustics for children with normal hearing and with hearing impairment. *Language, Speech, and Hearing Services in Schools, 31*, 362–370.

Desai, S., Stickney, G., & Zeng, F. (2008). Auditory-visual speech perception in normal-hearing and cochlear-implant listeners. *Journal of the Acoustical Society of America, 123*(1), 428–440.

Dodd, B. (1977). The role of vision in the perception of speech. *Perception, 6*(1), 31–40.

Donaldson, G. S., Chisolm, T. H., Blasco, G. P., Shinnick, L. J., Ketter, K. J., & Krause, J. C. (2009). BKB-SIN and ANL predict perceived communication ability in cochlear implant users. *Ear and Hearing, 30*(4), 401–410.

Fridriksson, J., Moser, D., Ryalls, J., Bonilha, L., Rorden, C., & Baylis, G. (2009). Modulation of frontal lobe speech areas associated with the production and perception of speech movements. *Journal of Speech, Language, and Hearing Research, 52*(3), 812–819.

Geers, A. E., Brenner, C., & Davidson, L. (2003). Factors associated with development of speech perception skills in children implanted by age five. *Ear and Hearing, 24*(Suppl. 1), 24S–53S.

Geers, A. E., Nicholas, J. G., & Sedey, A. L. (2003). Language skills of children with early cochlear implantation. *Ear and Hearing, 24*(Suppl. 1), 46S–58S.

Geers, A., Tobey, E., Moog, J., & Brenner, C. (2008). Long-term outcomes of cochlear implantation in the preschool years: From elementary grades to high school. *International Journal of Audiology, 47*(Suppl. 2), S21–S30.

Giraud, A., Price, C. J., Graham, J. M., & Frackowiak, R. S. J. (2001). Functional plasticity of language-related areas after cochlear implantation. *Brain, 124*, 1307–1316.

Giraud, A., Truy, E., Frackowiak, R. S. J., Gregoire, M., Pujol, J., & Collet, L. (2000). Differential recruitment of the speech processing mechanism in healthy subjects and rehabilitated cochlear implant patients. *Brain, 123*, 1391–1402.

Grant, K. W., & Seitz, P. F. (1998). Measures of auditory-visual integration in nonsense syllables and sentences. *Journal of the Acoustical Society of America, 104*(4), 2438–2450.

Grant, K. W., Walden, B. E., & Seitz, P. F. (1998). Auditory-visual speech recognition by hearing-impaired subjects: Consonant recognition, sentence recognition, and auditory-visual integration. *Journal of the Acoustical Society of America, 103*(5, Pt. 1), 2677–2690.

Green, K., Kuhl, P., Meltzoff, A., & Stevens, E. (1991). Integrating speech information across talkers, gender, and sensory modalities: Female voices and male voices in the McGurk effect. *Perception and Psychophysics, 50*, 524.

Hall, D. A., Fussell, C., & Summerfield, A. Q. (2005). Reading fluent speech from talking faces: Typical brain networks and individual differences. *Journal of Cognitive Neuroscience, 17*, 939–953.

Hubbard, A. L., Wilson, S. M., Callan, D. E., Dapretto, M. (2009). Giving speech a hand: Gesture modulates activity in auditory cortex during speech perception. *Human Brain Mapping, 30*(3), 1028–1037.

Jerger, S., Damian, M. F., Spence, M. J., Tye-Murray, N., & Abdi, H. (2009). Developmental shifts in children's sensitivity to visual speech: A new multimodal picture-word task. *Journal of Experimental Child Psychology, 102*, 40–59.

Karchmer, M. A., & Mitchell, R. E. (2003). Demographic and achievement characteristics of deaf and hard-of-hearing students. In M. Marschark & P. E. Spencer (Eds.), *Deaf studies, language, and education* (pp. 21–37). New York: Oxford University Press.

Kelly, S. D., Kravitz, C., & Hopkins, M. (2004). Neural correlates of bimodal speech and gesture comprehension. *Brain and Language, 89*(1), 253–260.

King, A. J. (2009). Auditory spatial learning. *Philosophical Transactions of the Royal Society of London, Series B: Biological Sciences, 364*, 331–339.

Kislyuk, D. S., Möttönen, R., & Sams, M. (2008). Visual processing affects the neural basis of auditory discrimination. *Journal of Cognitive Neuroscience, 20*(12), 2175–2184.

Kushnerenko, E., Teinonen, T., Volein, A., & Csibra, G. (2008). Electrophysiological evidence of illusory audiovisual speech percept in human infants. *Proceedings of the National Academy of Sciences, 105*(32), 11442–11445.

Lachs, L., Pisoni, D. B., & Kirk, K. I. (2001). Use of audiovisual information in speech perception by prelingually deaf children with cochlear implants: A first report. *Ear and Hearing, 22*(3), 236–251.

Lamoré, P. J., Huiskamp, T. M., van Son, N. J., Bosman, A. J., & Smoorenburg, G. F. (1998). Auditory, visual and audiovisual perception of segmental speech features by severely hearing-impaired children. *International Journal of Audiology, 37*, 396–419.

Lee, H., Truy, E., Mamou, G., Sappey-Marinier, D., & Giraud, A. (2007). Visual speech circuits in profound acquired deafness: A possible role for latent multimodal connectivity. *Brain, 130*, 2929–2941.

Leybaert, J., & Alegria, J. (2003). The role of cued speech in language development of deaf children. In M. Marschark & P. E. Spencer (Eds.), *Deaf studies, language, and education* (pp. 261–274). New York: Oxford University Press.

Lidestam, B., & Beskow, J. (2006). Visual phonemic ambiguity and speechreading. *Journal of Speech, Language, and Hearing Research, 49*(4), 835–847.

Lynas, W. (2005). Controversies in the education of deaf children. *Current Paediatrics, 15*, 200–206.

McGurk, H., & MacDonald, J. (1976). Hearing lips and seeing voices. *Nature, 264*, 746–748.

Moody-Antonio, S., Takayanagi, S., Masuda, A., Auer, E. T., Jr., Fisher, L., & Bernstein, L. E. (2005). Improved speech perception in adult congenitally deafened cochlear implant recipients. *Otology & Neurotology, 26*(4), 649–654.

Moores, D. F. (2009). Cochlear failures. *American Annals of the Deaf, 53*(5), 423–424.

Moreno-Torres, I., & Torres, S. (2008). From 1-word to 2-words with cochlear implant and cued speech: A case study. *Clinical Linguistics & Phonetics, 22*(7), 491–508.

Möttönen, R., Schürmann, M., & Sams, M. (2004). Time course of multisensory interactions during audiovisual speech perception in humans: A magnetoencephalographic study. *Neuroscience Letters, 363*, 112–115.

Nelson, P. B., & Soli, S. (2000). Acoustical barriers to learning: Children at risk in every classroom. *Language, Speech, and Hearing Services in Schools, 31*, 356–361.

Paulesu, E., Perani, D., Blasi, V., Silani, G., Borghese, N. A., De Giovanni, U., et al. (2003). A functional-anatomical model for lipreading. *Journal of Neurophysiology, 90*, 2005–2013.

Rosenblum, L. D. (2008). Speech perception as a multimodal phenomenon. *Current Directions in Psychological Science, 17*(6), 405–409.

Rosenblum, L. D., Miller, R. M., & Sanchez, K. (2007). Lip-read me now, hear me better later: Cross-modal transfer of talker-familiarity effects. *Psychological Science, 18*(5), 392–396.

Rouger, J., Lagleyre, S., Fraysse, B., Deneve, S., Deguine, O., Barone, P. (2007). Evidence that cochlear-implanted deaf patients are better multisensory integrators. *Proceedings of the National Academy of Sciences, 104*, 7295–7300.

Schorr, E. A., Fox, N. A., van Wassenhove, V., & Knudsen, E. I. (2005). Auditory-visual fusion in speech perception in children with cochlear implants. *Proceedings of the National Academy of Sciences, 102*(51), 18748–18750.

Sekiyama, K., & Burnham, D. (2008). Impact of language on development of auditory-visual speech perception. *Developmental Science, 11*(2), 306–320.

Sekiyama, K., Kannoc, I., Miura, S., & Sugita, Y. (2003). Auditory-visual speech perception examined by fMRI and positron emission tomography. *Neuroscience Research, 47*, 277–287.

Sharma, A., Dorman, M. F., & Spahr, A. J. (2002). A sensitive period for the development of the central auditory system in children with cochlear implants: Implications for age of implantation. *Ear and Hearing, 23*(6), 532–539.

Skipper, J. I., van Wassenhove, J., Nusbaum, H. C., & Small, S. L. (2007). Hearing lips and seeing voices: How cortical areas supporting speech production mediate audiovisual speech perception. *Cerebral Cortex, 17*, 2387–2399.

Sommers, M. S., Spehar, B., & Tye-Murray, N. (2005). The effects of signal-to-noise ratio on auditory-visual integration: Integration and encoding are not independent. *The Journal of the Acoustical Society of America, 117*(4, Pt. 2), 2574.

Straube, B., Green, A., Weis, S., Chatterjee, A., & Kircher, T. (2009). Memory effects of speech and gesture binding: Cortical and hippocampal activation in relation to subsequent memory performance. *Journal of Cognitive Neuroscience, 21*(4), 821–836.

Sumby, H. W., & Pollack, I. (1954). Visual contribution to speech intelligibility in noise. *Journal of the Acoustical Society of America, 26*(2), 212–215.

Svirsky, M. A., Robbins, A. M., Kirk, K. I., Pisoni, D. B., & Miyamoto, R. T. (2000). Language development in profoundly deaf children with cochlear implants. *Psychological Science, 11*(2), 153–158.

Valimaa, T. T., Maatta, T. K., Lopponen, H. J., & Sorri, M. J. (2002a). Phoneme recognition and confusions with multichannel cochlear implants: Vowels. *Journal of Speech, Language, and Hearing Research, 45*(5), 1039–1054.

Valimaa, T. T., Maatta, T. K., Lopponen, H. J., & Sorri, M. J. (2002b). Phoneme recognition and confusions with multichannel cochlear implants: Consonants. *Journal of Speech, Language, and Hearing Research, 45*(5), 1055–1069.

van Wassenhove, V., Grant, K. W., & Poeppel, D. (2005). Visual speech speeds up the neural processing of auditory speech. *Proceedings of the National Academy of Sciences, 102*(4), 1181–1186.

Vieu, A., Mondain, M., Blanchard, K., Sillon, M., Reuillard-Artieres, F., Tobey, E., et al. (1998). Influence of communication mode on speech intelligibility and syntactic structure of sentences in profoundly hearing impaired French children implanted between 5 and 9 years of age. *International Journal of Pediatric Otorhinolaryngology, 44*(1), 15–22.

Werker, J. F., Frost, P., & McGurk, H. (1992). La langue et les lèvres: Cross-language influences on bimodal speech perception. *Canadian Journal of Psychology, 46*, 551–568.

Willems, R. M., Ozyurek, A., & Hagoort, P. (2007). When language meets action: The neural integration of gesture and speech. *Cerebral Cortex, 17*(10), 2322–2333.

Woodhouse, L., Hickson, L., & Dodd, B. (2009). Review of visual speech perception by hearing and hearing-impaired people: Clinical implications. *International Journal of Language & Communication Disorders, 44*(3), 253–270.

Yoncheva, Y. N., Zevin, J. D., Maurer, U., & McCandliss, B. D. (2010). Auditory selective attention to speech modulates activity in the visual word form area. *Cerebral Cortex, 20*(3), 622–632.

Zilbovicius, M., Meresse, I., Chabane, N., Brunelle, F., Samson, Y., & Boddaert, N. (2006). Autism, the superior temporal sulcus and social perception. *Trends in Neurosciences, 29*(7), 359–366.

8

LISTENING STRATEGIES TO FACILITATE SPOKEN LANGUAGE LEARNING AMONG SIGNING CHILDREN WITH COCHLEAR IMPLANTS

Ellen A. Rhoades

Deafness typically places children in the minority of communities. Less than 5% of children who are deaf have at least one parent who is deaf (Mitchell & Karchmer, 2004), and many parents with typical hearing do not communicate either effectively or typically with their children in signed language (Marschark, 2001; Mitchell & Karchmer, 2005; Surian, 2010). Some children with severe-profound deafness have poor language skills that are associated with poor executive capacities, low academic achievement, or problematic interpersonal behaviors (Barker et al., 2009; Bat-Chava, Martin, & Kosciw, 2005; Stevenson, McCann, Watkin, Worsfold, & Kennedy, 2010). Insufficient knowledge of language may hinder the literacy development of children (Archbold et al., 2008; Mayer, 2009; Wauters, Tellings, van Bon, & Mak, 2007).

Hearing and speaking the majority language has considerable advantages. Hearing can afford a sense of security in that listening children have access to warning signals and environmental conditions. Spoken language may enable children with severe-profound deafness to become part of the larger community of typically hearing peers, thus decreasing mainstreamed children's risk for social isolation and interference with the learning process (Eriks-Brophy et al., 2006). Hearing and understanding the prevailing spoken language can provide a sense of social connection with the larger community of typically hearing peers. Hearing the spoken language enables "overhearing" or eavesdropping as well as access to those acoustic cues that readily facilitate learning the pragmatic and linguistic units of the majority communication system (Fisher & Tokura, 1996; Floor & Akhtar, 2006; Mastropavlou, 2010). Furthermore, reading and writing are predicated on voice-based languages. Hearing the spoken language facilitates phonological awareness, a significant skill that, in turn, facilitates the reading process (Ormel et al., 2010; Shaywitz, Morris, & Shaywitz, 2008). Finally, in the case of typically hearing parents, learning the spoken language increases most children's accessibility to their family's cultural heritage.

Notwithstanding these advantages of hearing the spoken language, it should not be misconstrued that signed languages are rejected or devalued. As the International Congress on Education of the Deaf proclaimed, 21st-century interventions should reflect international collaboration to best meet the multilingual and multicultural educational needs of children with hearing loss (International Congress on Education of the Deaf, 2010). Signed language reflects such diversity in that it has its own grammar and a different word order from English (Woolfe, Herman, Roy, & Woll, 2010). Signed languages are legitimate language systems quite distinct from English and other spoken languages in several domains (Emmorey, 2002). Signed languages are considered part of the cultural heritage, not just of Deaf parents but also of some typically hearing parents whose families of origin included Deaf members using a signed language.

Multiculturalism is the recognition and celebration of cultural differences, including signed and spoken languages. *All* languages and cultures should be valued. Auditory-based practitioners have been charged with supporting each family's culture (Rhoades, Price, & Perigoe, 2004).

AUDITORY-VERBAL PRACTICE

Auditory-verbal (AV) practice is an evidence-informed intervention approach for children with severe-profound deafness. Its overriding goal is to enable each child to communicate in the prevailing spoken language(s) of home and school. This entails the facilitation of effective listening skills with optimal use of appropriate and consistently worn hearing devices. Restated, AV practice involves primacy of audition through the active facilitation of listening skills. Additionally, this practice involves active participation of each child's family members, usually at least one of the primary caregivers. Such partnerships between AV practitioners and parents mandate frequent and open communication, so that parents or other caregivers can become their children's best advocates and primary facilitators of spoken language. In this way, spoken language can become the natural or anchor language of children with severe-profound deafness. Mainstreaming young children with typically hearing peers beginning at the preschool level is also considered integral to the AV intervention model. Minimal support for children with severe-profound deafness in inclusive settings typically includes the use of assisted listening systems in regular classroom settings (Flexer, 1999). Additional support typically involves regular communication and consistently positive collaboration between parent, AV practitioner, and classroom teacher as well as administrators, peers, and all support personnel, such as itinerant/resource teacher or speech-language pathologist (Eriks-Brophy et al., 2006).

The strategy of sometimes focusing on auditory information while avoiding visual stimuli can serve as a gating mechanism; that is, filtering out nonauditory information can permit the listening brain to more strongly process auditory stimuli (Ciaramitaro, Buracas, & Boynton, 2007). Focusing on auditory input to the exclusion of visual input does not, however, imply that visual input is devalued. On the contrary, it is widely recognized that visual input complements auditory input (Bahrick, Lickliter, Castellanos, & Vaillant-Molina, 2010; Dick, Solodkin, & Small, 2010; Morere, this volume). But, given that, prior to intervention, children with severe-profound deafness tend to have poor auditory functioning along with reasonably typical visual functioning, any auditory-based intervention is designed to strengthen children's use of residual hearing, whether electronic or acoustic. Indeed, as a result of auditory-based intervention, children who have learned how to listen and understand what is heard can then function more like typical children with five senses.

Auditory-Verbal Practice as Evidence-Based Intervention

Reviews of research findings pertaining to AV practice (Eriks-Brophy, 2004; Rhoades, 2006, 2010a) show outcome data to be largely positive in that many children attained typical language growth rates, achieving levels of spoken language considered equivalent to their typically hearing peers. Given this corpus of outcome data that includes surveys, interviews, a series of replicated randomized controlled trials, and matched group repeated measures design, AV intervention can no longer be considered controversial. However, the children included in these studies tend to have highly motivated parents, and the families were overwhelmingly affluent Caucasians (Dornan, Hickson, Murdoch, & Houston, 2007, 2010; Easterbrooks, O'Rourke, & Todd, 2000; Hogan, Stokes, White, Tyszkiewicz, & Woolgar, 2008; Neuss, 2006; Rhoades, 2001; Rhoades & Chisolm, 2001; Wu & Brown, 2004). Some parents reported feeling overwhelmed with how they were instructed to implement AV practice (Neuss, 2006; Wu & Brown, 2004). More recent data show that typical spoken language outcomes can also be attained by children from low-income families benefitting from AV intervention (Hogan, Stoke, & Weller, 2010).

For some families and their children with severe-profound deafness, AV practices represent effective intervention, provided conversational levels of sound are afforded each child. In studies focusing on child outcomes, effective intervention means that children showed reasonably good progress in their attainment of spoken language skills; that is, the children evidenced an average of 12 months progress over each 12-month period. Attainment of this benchmark for rate of progress in spoken language, first demonstrated in the Rhoades and Chisolm study (2001), was corroborated by the Dornan et al. (2008, 2010) and Hogan et al. (2008, 2010) studies. Indeed, many of the children in these studies attained communicative skills equivalent to their typically hearing peers. However, only a few of these studies included a significant minority of children with atypicalities in addition to deafness (Hogan et al., 2008, 2010; Rhoades, 2001).

Although mainstreaming the young language learning child during AV intervention is not a required requisite of AV intervention, it is a doable goal that enables literacy and reasonable academic achievement for many children who become linguistically competent in the majority spoken language prior to their formal schooling, particularly in somewhat controlled academic environments (Duquette et al., 2002; Easterbrooks et al., 2000; Eriks-Brophy et al., 2006; Goldberg & Flexer, 2001; Robertson & Flexer, 1993; Wray, Flexer, & Vaccaro, 1999). As noted by Leigh (2008), there is accumulating evidence that strongly associates auditory-based early intervention with improved spoken language and literacy outcomes. However, full inclusion is not always a realistic goal for children first initiating any auditory-based intervention during grade school. Considerably more evidence is needed to ascertain the viability of full inclusion and assimilation on many levels, including psychosocial health and academic achievement (Bat-Chava & Deignan, 2001).

Among the research studies published in the first decade of the 21st century, some characteristic commonalities of AV intervention are noted. These include the following:

1. Parents are proactive in their informed choice of the AV option for their children, as they want their children to develop listening skills and to actively speak the family's anchor language.
2. Parents receiving AV intervention services become knowledgeable about their children's performance and goals relative to those of typically hearing peers.
3. AV practice, sometimes referred to as AV therapy, or AVT, tends to involve hourly or weekly individualized therapy sessions in which practitioners coach parents while demonstrating select strategies with each child.
4. Primary caretakers are responsible for implementing those select strategies at home on a daily basis.
5. Strategies employed on a daily basis are designed to enhance listening skills and the spoken language directed to each child.
6. AV practices include the routine use of spoken language assessment instruments normed on typically hearing peers.
7. Caregivers become knowledgeable about the need for optimizing environmental acoustic conditions.
8. Assertive programming of cochlear implant processors occurs frequently and consistently.

However, AV intervention does not effectively serve all children with severe-profound deafness. Outcomes are variable, so some children benefit more from this intervention model than others. Common sense dictates that many intervention strategies are needed as some are more appropriate for some children and their families than others. There is a continuum of listening and spoken language skills attained by children, if for no other reason than that children and their families represent diverse situations and needs, some more complex than others.

Unfortunately, the educational landscape for children with severe-profound deafness has long been riddled with passionate controversy and oppositional stances (Myers & Fernandes, 2010). Research findings and position statements involving cochlear implants sometimes exacerbate what was formerly referred to as the "oral-manual controversy" (e.g., Connor, Hieber, Arts, & Zwolan, 2006; Sparrow, 2010; Tobey, Rekart, Buckley, & Geers, 2004). Children with severe-profound deafness represent an incredibly diverse group that should be neither categorized nor stereotyped. A somewhat unfortunate product of this polarity has been the label of severe-profound deafness assigned to children, since their respective hearing statuses are considerably varied in degree and type. Each child's neurobiological capacities, experiential histories, family culture, psychosocial status, and quality of intervention services differentially affect intervention outcomes.

Trends

Controversial Histories

During the early 1940s, less than a handful of practitioners working with children with severe-profound deafness advocated capitalizing on usable residual hearing along with the use of high-powered wearable transistorized hearing aids (Beebe, 1953; Fiedler, 1952; Huizing & Pollack, 1951). By the mid-1970s, when increasingly more practitioners joined this movement to develop spoken language primarily through the auditory channel, AV practice became an established, albeit highly controversial intervention model in a few North American cities (Pollack, 1970). Some practitioners advocating the auditory-oral communication option, particularly those who worked in special school settings, did not welcome AV practitioner perspectives, even as recently as the mid-1990s (J. Moog, personal communication, June 1994).

During the 1960s, American Sign Language became recognized as a legitimate language system in its own right (Stokoe, 1965). Shortly thereafter, by the mid-1970s, the intervention model of total communication (TC) was introduced (Lowenbraun, Appelman, & Callahan, 1980). This promoted the concept that fingerspelling, conceptually accurate signs, spoken language, speechreading, and use of residual hearing via hearing devices should be simultaneously employed to reproduce spoken language. TC is intended to morphosyntactically mirror the spoken language so children can optimally use all their senses in the quest to become linguistically and academically competent. However, shortly thereafter, a forceful argument was made for the existence of a Deaf culture and the importance of American Sign Language (Padden & Humphries, 1988).

Current Evolutionary Practices

By the onset of the 21st century, the confluence of three primary factors changed the general attitude of many practitioners and parents toward the viability of hearing as a means to learning spoken language. Those three factors were (1) outcome data emanating from intervention studies involving children with cochlear implants; (2) universal newborn hearing screenings, resulting in many deaf children acquiring spoken language with relative ease, providing they had access to soft conversational sound during infancy; and (3) the Internet, which enabled parents easy access to a current and greater knowledge base pertaining to deafness and intervention models. Indeed, age seems to be the most critical variable affecting auditory and spoken language outcomes (Loy, Warner-Czyz, Tong, Tobey, & Roland, 2010; Niparko et al., 2010; Schramm, Bohnert, & Keilmann, 2009; Sharma, Dorman, & Kral, 2005).

Outcome data are effecting change within the community of practitioners who facilitate listening and spoken language for children with severe-profound deafness, with or without the inclusion of signed language (Easterbrooks & Estes, 2007; Kirk, Miyamoto, Ying, Perdew, & Zuganelis, 2000; Watson, Hardie, Archbold, & Wheeler, 2008). Like the AV model, the TC model has evolved to become a more viable intervention option for increasingly more families. Indeed, AV practices, in particular its strategies and select activities, are being implemented across many communication options (Jiménez, Pino, & Herruzo, 2009; Tobey et al., 2004; Watson, Archbold, & Nikolopoulos, 2006).

Any intervention model that purports to best serve *all* children and their families should be considered controversial (McWilliam, 1999). The practitioners of all communication options and intervention models should become aware of their own prejudices and recognize how their personal beliefs and stereotypes affect their philosophy (Dunham, Baron, & Benaji, 2006). Stereotypes *can* be inhibited (Moskowitz & Li, 2011) and tolerance facilitated by knowledge and self-awareness. If practitioners are to embrace a more inclusive, nonhierarchical perspective, they must consciously strive toward neutrality. Neutral stances lend themselves to "informed choice"—a critical and complex construct that involves many underlying issues warranting practitioner attention (Young et al., 2005).

Bilingualism: Unimodal and Bimodal

A mother tongue is a culturally based language reflective of the communication system typically used in the home (Genesee, Paradis, & Crago, 2004). This language serves as the anchor for family cohesion while facilitating children's linguistic competency (Macrory, 2006). Abandoning the heritage language can have extensive personal, familial, religious, cultural, and academic implications that establish unfavorable conditions for children. As such, the home language should be each child's anchor language (Kohnert, Yim, Nett, Fong Kan, & Duran, 2005).

"Bilingualism," defined here to mean proficient conversational fluency in at least two languages, is an asset that should be treasured on many levels (Rhoades, 2008). Learning two languages during the first 3 years of life is referred to as "simultaneous bilingualism" or "first language acquisition" (Genesee & Nicoladis, 2006), and both languages may be considered native to a child. The notion that linguistic confusion or language delays occur when young children simultaneously learn two languages is a myth (Pearson, 2008). On the other hand, "sequential bilingualism" typically occurs when the first learned language is a child's anchor or native language, and the second language is learned after age 3. Also known as "successive bilingualism," this has implications for different neurobiological and linguistic outcomes (Abutalebi & Green, 2007; Hernandez, 2009).

Knowing and using two spoken languages is referred to as "unimodal bilingualism." Unimodal bilinguals are assumed to perceive both languages via the auditory sense and, given that each person has one vocal tract, they cannot simultaneously produce two spoken words or linguistic units (Emmorey, Borinstein, Thompson, & Gollan, 2008). Specific to spoken language, early exposure to the anchor language is widely considered critical for the development of speech perception (Dietrich, Swingley, & Werker, 2007). Particularly for young language learning children engaged in the process of simultaneous unimodal bilingualism, there is typically some rule-governed language mixing that eventually stabilizes into code-switching, which more often than not involves nouns (Holowka, Brosseau-Lapré, & Petitto, 2002). This can serve social and discourse functions that include the signaling of topic changes, establishing linguistic proficiency, and creating identity or emphasis (Zentella, 1997). However, code-switching seems to diminish with maturation among unimodal bilinguals (Cantone & Muller, 2005).

There are data showing that children with cochlear implants can become unimodally bilingual like their typically hearing peers (Francis & Ho, 2003; Guiberson, 2005; Rhoades, 2009a; Rhoades, Perusse, Douglas, & Zarate, 2008; Thomas, El-Kashlan, & Zwolan, 2008; Waltzman, Robbins, Green, & Cohen, 2003). Current data on unimodal bilingualism indicate that it is particularly important for children to learn at least one language system well, as that can provide a template for another language, and that learning a spoken language system at an early age facilitates literacy in that same language system (Archbold et al., 2008).

Children who sign one language and speak another are representative of a less explored form of bilingualism. Many children, particularly those with typical hearing born to deaf parents, have two native languages, both spoken and signed.

In addition to being bilingual, they are also bicultural in that they affiliate with Deaf/minority and hearing/majority communities. "Bimodal bilinguals," those who know both a signed and a spoken language, are a unique group because each language system differentially influences the brain's neural organization (Emmorey & McCullough, 2009; Kovelman et al., 2009). Instead of code-switching, bimodal bilingual children typically produce code-blends (i.e., simultaneously produced spoken and signed words; Bogaerde & Baker, 2006; Emmorey et al., 2008; Petitto et al., 2001). Code-blending seems to occur more often with verbs than nouns, which tend to differ in combinatorial structure (Emmorey et al., 2008). Neither code-mixing nor code-blending are random or atypical among bilinguals, since they occur for sociolinguistic reasons (Bogaerde & Baker, 2006). However, some code-blending may persist more frequently into adulthood (Bishop & Hicks, 2005).

Although the corpus of data pertaining to bimodal bilingualism is significantly smaller than that pertaining to unimodal bilingualism, some findings are emerging. For example, bimodal bilingualism is also strongly associated with neurobiological advantages manifested in such improved executive capacities as cognitive flexibility (Kushalnagar, Hannay, & Hernandez, 2010). However, there are equivocal data indicating that bimodal bilinguals may or may not perform as well in spoken language as do children relying exclusively on spoken language (Jiménez et al., 2009), particularly if cochlear implantation occurs after the first few years of life (Kos, Deriaz, Guyot, & Pelizzone, 2009). There are insufficient data pertaining to languageless children simultaneously learning two languages after age 3 and then becoming conversationally fluent in both, regardless of whether the languages are signed or spoken. Despite universal newborn hearing screening, cochlear implants, and early intervention programs, many children with severe-profound deafness continue to enter the primary grades without having acquired any language system with any degree of proficiency. These children present highly complex learning needs in very diverse situations (Mayer, 2009).

Subsequent to cochlear implantation, many children change their communication style from exclusively signed to primarily spoken language (Watson et al., 2006). Many of these children and their parents consider the ongoing use of signs and fingerspelling to be a pragmatic resource (Wheeler, Archbold, Gregory, & Skipp, 2007). This may be important because, although cochlear implants can afford people with access to soft conversational sound, the fact remains that their newfound hearing is atypical.

Adding to the array of complexities are data showing that bimodal bilingualism has not yet afforded many deaf children a level of literacy commensurate with hearing peers (Marschark & Spencer, 2005; Mayer & Akamatsu, 2003). Unlike unimodal bilinguals, bimodal bilinguals cannot be biliterate simply because there is no written form of a signed language. For those children who do become literate, their exclusive use of signed language necessitates bimodal bilingualism during

foreordain long-term effectiveness of implantation nor affect implantation decision (Harrison et al., 2005; Fitzpatrick, Séguin, & Schramm, 2004; Kos et al., 2009; Rhoades, 2001). In other words, the notion of "critical period" does not seem to apply, as the window of opportunity for learning spoken language does not close at any particular time. There are clear data indicating that neuronal growth occurs throughout adolescence and thus is subject to reorganization (Giedd, 2008). Indeed, it seems that an older child's state of mind and motivation should be far more critical factors in any decision on implantation or interventions to facilitate spoken language.

Expectation Levels and the Self-Fulfilling Prophecy

Persons involved in the process of enabling a child to develop spoken language typically include at least a practitioner, one of the child's primary caregivers, and the child. Given that expectations drive behaviors, including assessment, decision making, and intervention outcomes (Dunham et al., 2006; Morgan, 2007; Ysseldyke, 2001), it is imperative that all involved persons embrace a positive outlook involving high, albeit realistic expectation levels for the development of spoken language and listening skills. The pessimistic explanatory style, as reflected in the statement, "I/she can't because I'm/she's deaf," is denied. For example, parents selecting AV intervention programs for their children typically have high expectations for their children, and those expectations are encouraged by AV practitioners (Wu & Brown, 2004). Those high expectation levels were shown to serve as predictors of children's comprehension of spoken language (Wu & Brown, 1999).

The self-fulfilling prophecy is an uncontested powerful force; it is a situation in which a person's belief or expectation of an event can cause the actual occurrence of that event (Jones, 1977; Rosenthal, 2002). A literature review (Rhoades, 2010b) indicates that low expectations can create poor performance in learning spoken language via audition. Negative self-fulfilling prophecies may be more powerful than positive ones (Madon, Guyll, & Spoth, 2004). It is therefore important that involved parties understand some essential factors contributing to the success of an intervention program designed to facilitate a communication system among children with hearing loss that differs from their existing system.

Optimism, Motivation, and Sense of Autonomy

Mental state affects learning and mental health (Au, Watkins, Hattie, & Alexander, 2009; Lai, 2009), influencing the development of listening and spoken language skills in children with hearing loss. Regardless of communication history, some children with hearing loss enter preadolescence with a sense of learned helplessness or hopelessness (Marschark & Spencer, 2005; McCrone, 2006). Such deficit-based attitudes are associated with prior academic failures, low self-esteem, poor learning strategies, and ineffective interpersonal skills (Au, Watkins, & Hattie, 2010). As a result of "giving up," some children become disengaged from school and/or peers, erroneously attributing their alienation and academic problems to their hearing loss (Burkley & Blanton, 2008), which may or may not be an indirect result of others' projected perceptions.

In contrast, children who highly value schooling tend to see their achievement as a function of their own efforts and learning competencies. Optimistic children are positive about their future (Peters, Flink, Boersma, & Linton, 2010; Ylvisaker & Feeney, 2002). Practitioners should focus on competency enhancement rather than on existing deficits. Close enduring relationships between children and their supportive parents and mentors can facilitate optimism and positive developmental changes (Rhodes & DuBois, 2008). These relationships should be flexible, involve mutual trust and empathy, and facilitate both identity development and competent autonomy (Deci & Ryan, 2008).

For children with negative perspectives based on past experiences, it is imperative that those adults in their home, extracurricular, and school environments forcefully collaborate to facilitate engagement and "learned optimism" in the child (Kelley, 2004). Negative beliefs maintained by the child need to be ameliorated while developing specific skills; a sense of hope should be established and carefully nurtured. Positive feedback and acquisition of effective learning strategies are among those factors that can reverse a downward self-fulfilling spiral (Hattie, 2009). The nurturance of hope and new learning skills can initiate an ongoing cycle of motivation accompanied by a gradual increase in self-esteem and cognitive capacities (Taylor et al., 2004). A positive mental state encouraged by adults may shield children from interim adversities in the process of learning effective spoken language skills (Massey, Gebhardt, & Garnefski, 2008).

This may necessitate repetitive and varied motivational interventions, one being the persistent use of constructive feedback, reframing, and expressions reflective of positive psychology (Dweck, 2006; Gable & Haidt, 2005; Roberts, Walton, & Viechtbauer, 2006). For auditory-based strategies to be implemented and effect substantive outcomes, it is critical that both adults and children have a positive mind-set toward the development of listening to the language spoken in their familial and academic communities.

Intrinsic motivation, associated with a sense of connectedness and belongingness, comes from within (Juvonen, 2007). However, children's intrinsic motivational levels are largely shaped by those adults in their immediate environments. Informational or positive performance feedback can enhance intrinsic motivation. Common sense dictates that developing a sense of ownership regarding their own hearing loss can facilitate intrinsic motivation (Royal College of Physicians, 2007). This, in turn, can help foster self-confidence in learning (Ryan & Deci, 2003). In short, high motivation and high expectation levels are critical individually learned dispositions that contribute to a positive state of mind.

There are some central components requisite to developing a sense of autonomy. When children feel controlled, judged, rewarded, or pressured due to their communication skills, their drive to learn can be negatively affected. It is important that children feel they have choices in any intervention designed to nonjudgmentally facilitate their listening and spoken language skills. Ultimately, optimism coupled with intrinsic motivation lead toward the need for competency and self-determination (Deci & Ryan, 2008). Convergence of these dispositions can enable children and adolescents with hearing loss with late access to soft conversational sound to persist in their acquisition of listening skills and spoken language.

Management of the Cochlear Implant Processor

More so for older children or adolescents whose primary mode of communication is a signed language, cochlear implants imply significant change on several levels. Intervention occurs on psychosocial, neurobiological, auditory perceptual, and linguistic levels. Aside from communication issues, older children and adolescents agree to surgery and related medical treatment as well as frequent trips to audiologists who provide ongoing optimal programming of processors. Each child or youth, in agreeing to wear a processor, should also agree to accept the responsibilities needed for effective care of the external apparatus. A maximum number of active electrodes and better programmed processors are associated with improved intervention outcomes (Geers et al., 2002). Moreover, all children should understand the necessity of wearing their processors during all waking hours in the home, social, and academic environments.

With older children, it is suggested that practitioners intellectualize the learning process as often as possible. For example, each child can learn some basic information about decibels and frequencies—enough to realize that access to the average level of soft conversational sound of about 30–35 dB HL is needed (Boothroyd, 2008), that understanding what is heard becomes problematic at distances of greater than 5 feet, and that teachers should be heard at 15–30 dB above the level of classroom noise (American Speech-Language-Hearing Association, 2005; Ling & Ling, 1978). While continually stressing the positive, each child's initial goals should be realistic throughout the intervention process—from cochlear implant decision making to spoken language outcomes. Short-term goals may need to be tempered from time to time.

Common sense dictates that family attitudes toward cochlear implants shape family behaviors (Marom, Cohen, & Naon, 2007). Therefore, it is important that hearing devices not be stigmatized; that is, regardless of self-identity, the equipment should be embraced for its potential and possibilities. Children who previously relied on a visual communication system can incorporate the processor into a renegotiated self-identity whereby the individual trumps the group (Crawford, 2007).

Assessment of Communication Skills

Appropriate and efficient planning for intervention is based on varied assessment outcomes. Assessment of communication skills should include the use of instruments standardized on typically hearing children, particularly to determine the functional level of each child's morphosyntactic skills (Rhoades, 2003). Whether the use of signed language should be incorporated into these assessments will vary from situation to situation. In general, if children are not yet in grade school, the exclusion of signed language from the process of assessing receptive and expressive spoken language may be recommended. In any case, a note on the inclusion of signed language should accompany all assessment outcome data as deemed appropriate.

Although there are varied assessment instruments that yield functional information on performance levels of children's perceptual and spoken language skills, practitioners often develop their own informal tools to ascertain at least the following information: (1) child's preferred mode of communication; (2) child's speech parameters pertaining to voice, rhythm, fluency, intonation, and intensity; (3) child's telephone skills, if any; (4) child's interpersonal skills and sense of loneliness or satisfaction with self; (5) child's motivations and expectations of self and cochlear implant; (6) child's communication repair strategies; (7) child's attitudes toward the use of listening and spoken language. Although much of this information can be gleaned from questions asked of such involved adults as family members and teachers, most of it should be obtained directly from each child.

It is also important to secure a baseline, however informal, of each child's auditory discrimination skills. This baseline, if at all possible, should be secured preimplant and preintervention. Discrimination skills include whether each child can differentiate between (1) high and low pitch speech, ranging from voice gender to suprasegmental variations that include statements, queries, and exclamations; (2) loud and soft sounds as well as long and short sounds, ranging from the subtle to the obvious; (3) emotional content in voice, including angry, happy, and sad; (4) discrete number of sounds, ranging from long and short sentences to the number of syllables in a word; (5) high- and low-frequency phonemes, including those consonants that vary in fewer dimensions, for example, /s/ and /f/, which vary only on the dimension of placement (Ling, 1976). It should also be determined if each child can engage in auditory tracking and the extent to which nonauditory cues are needed for ease in tracking.

IMPLEMENTATION OF INDIVIDUALIZED AUDITORY-VERBAL PRACTICE

Knowledge Base

Practitioners understand that language acquisition occurs spirally, with each level building on preceding levels. Language learners must be initially exposed to spoken language for a period of time before language can be understood. During this period of becoming familiar with the spoken language, several processes occur: first, children must find the spoken language and then, to find it, children must block out the noise (Yang, 2006). As this process occurs, they begin attending to speech and they realize that there are certain linguistic patterns. In the process of finding these patterns, children figure out the grammatical rules of spoken language (Tomasello, 2003). Indeed, early receptive language skills, not expressive language, were found to be good predictors of later language performance (Hay-McCutcheon, Kirk, Henning, Gao, & Qi, 2008).

However, this knowledge is sometimes neglected when children are learning a second language or when practitioners operate under the assumption that they must "teach" language to young children. Ancient Hindu linguists recognized that ethics and language are "caught, not taught" (e.g., Handford, 1937). Thus, it may not be wise to inadvertently apply subtle pressure on children to imitate spoken language shortly after they have their processor mapped. Regardless of age or degree of hearing loss, children should not be held differentially accountable for language learning. Ideally, the process of learning any spoken language should be auditory based, enjoyable, meaningful, cognitively oriented, and discoverable (Conway, Bauernschmidt, Huang, & Pisoni, 2010; Tomasello, 2003).

Toward that end, practitioners initially focus on "knowing" rather than "using." This means that newly implanted children engage in activities that involve visual- and movement-based activities while practitioners are providing spoken language. Beyond infancy, this permits intersensory redundancy that naturally confirms what is being heard by the child (Bahrick, Lickliter, & Flom, 2006). When spoken language is synchronized with the repetitive action-oriented activity, children can develop cross-modal integration that may facilitate pattern recognition of the acoustic event.

Over time, "hearing the language" evolves into "understanding the language." Auditory awareness and attention develop so that auditory perception evolves. Production should not be expected until each child is comfortable with listening to spoken language. At this point, language acquisition should focus on morphosyntactical and phonological awareness rather than on building a lexicon (Tomasello, 2003). Because nouns do not provide the perceptual glue of language, nouns as content, concrete entities should not be the focus of language-based activities (Arunachalam & Waxman, 2010; Golinkoff & Hirsh-Patek, 2008; Kedar, Casasola, & Lust, 2006). In short, children of all ages who are just beginning to hear the spoken language must be accorded the same respect as typically hearing first language learner—they are permitted time to listen and develop an appreciation for the multisensory convergence of information.

Finally, "hearing age," a construct essential to AV practice (Pollack, 1964), is considered integral to the ongoing assessment and intervention process. This age dates from the time a child first has access to conversational levels of spoken language and hence is a benchmark for expectations and the typical developmental trajectory of language growth in both knowledge and use. As an example, a child with a chronological age of 3 years but a hearing age of 6 months might be expected to engage in vocal play or babbling while developing both recognitory and true/referential comprehension (Oviatt, 1980; Stager & Werker, 1998).

Critical Operational Strategies to Facilitate Listening

From the outset, it is important to help each child develop some confidence in hearing. Although electronic sounds may initially seem garbled and static-like to many children, practitioners provide continual reassurance that those sensations are temporary and to be expected for some time. Strategies used by practitioners are designed to transition each child from being visually based to auditory based, in short, to optimize each child's use of newfound hearing.

Among the many auditory-based strategies embraced by practitioners with language learners is that of "infant- or child-directed speech" (Matychuk, 2005; Smith & Trainor, 2008). Sometimes known as "motherese" (Durkin, Rutter, & Tucker, 1982) or prosodic bootstrapping (Jusczyk, 1997), this means incorporating slight exaggerations of certain acoustic cues, such as inflection, in spoken language directed to children. This language input should clearly reflect rhythmic, melodic, naturally fluent speech at soft conversational levels in relatively quiet environments. Regardless of each child's age, such acoustic cues in spoken language facilitate the spoken language learning process.

Speaking within earshot is a critical strategy used across the intervention process for the purpose of providing children with the clearest auditory signal (Ling & Ling, 1978). Within earshot is the distance over which speech sounds are intelligible to listeners and, for optimal listening conditions in a quiet room at soft conversational level, this is within 3 to 6 inches from each child's processor microphone. Like whispering into each child's ear or microphone, this enhances speech audibility for children engaged in the listening process. Related to this is the tacit assumption that practitioners sit and speak on the better hearing side of each child during therapy sessions. Typically, AV practitioners do not talk directly in front of children or make any effort to get in children's visual space.

Acoustic highlighting, sometimes referred to as "consonant" and/or "envelope enhancement" (Smith & Levitt, 1999), is a more general strategy used to enhance speech audibility. Acoustic highlighting renders perceptual salience to important sounds and words considered key to facilitating comprehension or production at any particular level to meet each child's linguistic needs. Such aspects may include a specific phoneme, a morphological marker, or a syntactical element. This is similar to syntactic bootstrapping, whereby grammatical parts of sentence streams are exaggerated to facilitate language comprehension for language learners (Bedore & Leonard, 1995).

The "auditory sandwich" is still another highly effective strategy that can be particularly effective for children transitioning from a visually based to auditory-based language system (Koch, 1999). According to all AV pioneering practitioners, listening is the first and last step in any activity. When needed, the visual component in the form of print, picture, sign, subtle gesture, cue, or speech reading is sandwiched between the initial and ending spoken language. In short, for those times when listening is isolated and a child does not understand, this is followed by the visual information redundant to what was heard and then followed by auditory-only input once more. Listen first, then look, then listen again.

Related to this is the strategy of talking before acting. When practitioners discuss what will be seen or done prior to actual activities, children are set up to listen first, thus meaning, relevance, imitation, outcome, and anticipation can be facilitated (Southgate, Chevallier, & Csibra, 2009). For example, before bringing a book to the child's visual attention, a practitioner first informs the child that a book will soon be brought to the table and that a story will then be read.

Although practitioners are encouraged to talk frequently in meaningful contexts to children, silence is another important strategy. Silence can promote (1) listening by bracketing meaningful language, and (2) the processing of linguistic units. Silence can give children time to compensate for an incomplete linguistic signal by "filling in the missing pieces" with what makes sense, thereby understanding the speaker's intended meaning. Silence can also give children time to formulate linguistic responses (Arco & McCluskey, 1981; Halle, Marshall, & Spradlin, 1979).

The interturn or expectant pause is a type of silence or prosodic cue that tends to follow certain inflectional patterns such as a rise at the end of a question or certain statements. This tends to involve eye contact, serving as an additional cue for turn taking by subtly encouraging children to vocalize or formulate appropriate responses (Carey-Sargeant & Brown, 2003).

Still another type of silence is wait time—the length of time that practitioners wait for a response after asking a question (Rowe, 1974). This period of uninterrupted silence should be 3 to 5 seconds for typical hearing children, so it is often recommended that practitioners increase this wait time to 10 to 20 seconds for children with severe-profound deafness. Oftentimes, these children need a bit more time to understand what was heard since the entire linguistic signal may not have been heard; this guessing process based on linguistic redundancy may take a few seconds prior to each child engaging in "speculative thinking" (Tobin, 1987). Evidence shows this wait time results in longer and more confident child responses, reduces child failure to respond, improves child participation, enhances critical and creative thinking, and fosters higher practitioner expectations with fewer but more appropriate practitioner questions (Rowe, 1978, 1987). Moreover, waiting for children to respond rather than being quick to repeat questions demonstrates respect and value for each child's opinion (Black, Harrison, Lee, Marshall, & William, 2003).

"Tell me what you heard" is another strategy that may encourage listening. Rather than automatically repeating what was said because a child did not seem to hear or understand, practitioners ask the child to state what he or she thought he or she heard. Even if the child did not understand everything, repeating what was heard may help "fill in those missing pieces." Because some children are too quick to ask for repetitions, this strategy may help them auditorily process the spoken language.

Related to this is the strategy of rephrasing rather than repeating. Particularly for children who already have some language, poor communication repair strategies need to be replaced with more effective ones. This means the "what" question should be replaced with more meaningful ones such as Can you please rephrase that? What was the name of the —? Where did you say she went? What was the last word said? It is important that practitioners ensure children understand the need for specificity when asking for clarification of what was heard. With linguistic maturation, children should demonstrate increasingly larger repertoires of effective conversational repair strategies (Brinton, Fujiki, Loeb, & Winkler, 1986).

Closing Comments

Each child has a unique history of multitudinous variables that must be considered in a unique family system. Although some practitioners may seek to fully assimilate all children with severe-profound deafness into a typical hearing environment, academically and socially this is likely neither possible nor appropriate. There are myriad educational and social options that must be considered as well. One child may transition from a visually based system to as much of an auditory-based system as possible with very different time lines. Interim steps may reflect dramatically different goals, expectations, and necessary modifications from child to child and family to family. Educational, psychosocial, and linguistic challenges may at times seem insurmountable but with creative collaboration can be successfully met.

Cochlear implants can provide children with severe-profound deafness reasonably good access to soft conversational sound in relatively quiet environments. However, that sound is somewhat limited or distorted, particularly when accessed at ages later than the first few years of life. Regardless, cochlear implants do provide reasonably good acoustic input that can enable children to understand spoken language. The goal of AV intervention is to ultimately invest this limited acoustic input with spoken language significance. Particularly for older children, it is not necessarily an easy task and, without a dedicated commitment to its realization, it will not occur (Ross, 1994). Therefore, it is imperative that all peers and adults, including practitioners and caregivers, collaborate to support children by facilitating the process of spoken language acquisition.

References

Abutalebi, J., & Green, D. (2007). Bilingual language production: The neurocognition of language representation and control. *Journal of Neurolinguistics, 20,* 242–275.

Abutalebi, J., Tettamanti, M., & Perani, D. (2009). The bilingual brain: Linguistic and non-linguistic skills. *Brain & Language, 109*(2–3), 51–54.

American Speech-Language-Hearing Association. (2005). *Acoustics in educational settings: Technical report.* Rockville, MD: Author.

Archbold, S., Harris, M., O'Donoghue, G., Nikolopoulos, T., White, A., & Richmond, H. L. (2008). Reading abilities after cochlear implantation: The effect of age at implantation on outcomes at 5 and 7 years after implantation. *International Journal of Pediatric Otorhinolaryngology, 72,* 1471–1478.

Arco, C. M., & McCluskey, K. A. (1981). "A change of pace": An investigation of the salience of maternal temporal style in mother-infant play. *Child Development, 52,* 941–949.

Arunachalam, S., & Waxman, S. R. (2010). Meaning from syntax: Evidence from 2-year-olds. *Cognition, 114,* 442–446.

Au, R. C. P., Watkins, D. A., & Hattie, J. A. C. (2010). Academic risk factors and deficits of learned helplessness: A longitudinal study of Hong Kong secondary school students. *Educational Psychology, 30*(2), 125–138.

Au, R. C. P., Watkins, D., Hattie, J., & Alexander, P. (2009). Reformulating the depression model of learned helplessness for academic outcomes. *Educational Research Review, 4,* 103–117.

Bahrick, L. E., Lickliter, R., Castellanos, I., & Vaillant-Molina, M. (2010). Increasing task difficulty enhances effects of intersensory redundancy: Testing a new prediction of the intersensory redundancy hypothesis. *Developmental Science, 13*(5), 731–737.

Bahrick, L. E., Lickliter, R., & Flom, R. (2006). Up versus down: The role of intersensory redundancy in the development of infants' sensitivity to the orientation of moving objects. *Infancy, 9*(1), 73–96.

Baker, C. (1995). *A parents' and teachers' guide to bilingualism.* Clevedon, UK: Multilingual Matters.

Barker, D. H., Quittner, A. L., Fink, N. E., Eisenberg, L. S., Tobey, E. A., Niparko, J. K., et al. (2009). Predicting behavior problems in deaf and hearing children: The influences of language, attention, and parent-child communication. *Development and Psychopathology, 21,* 373–392.

Bat-Chava, Y., & Deignan, E. (2001). Peer relationships of children with cochlear implants. *Journal of Deaf Studies and Deaf Education, 6,* 186–199.

Bat-Chava, Y., Martin, D., & Kosciw, J. (2005). Longitudinal improvements in communication and socialization of deaf children with cochlear implants and hearing aids: Evidence from parental reports. *Journal of Child Psychology and Psychiatry, 46*(12), 1287–1296.

Bedore, L. M., & Leonard, L. B. (1995). Prosodic and syntactic bootstrapping and their clinical applications: A tutorial. *American Journal of Speech-Language Pathology, 4*(1), 66–72.

Beebe, H. H. (1953). *A guide to help the severely hard of hearing child*. Basel, Switzerland: S. Karger.

Bishop, M., & Hicks, S. (2005). Orange eyes: Bimodal bilingualism in hearing adults from Deaf families. *Sign Language Studies, 5*(2), 188–230.

Black, P., Harrison, C., Lee, C., Marshall, B., & William, D. (2003). *Working inside the black box: Assessment for learning in the classroom*. London: King's College.

Bogaerde, B. van den, & Baker, A. E. (2006). Code mixing in mother-child interaction in deaf families. *Sign Language and Linguistics, 8*(1–2), 155–178.

Boothroyd, A. (2008). The acoustic speech signal. In J. R. Madell & C. Flexer (Eds.), *Pediatric audiology: Diagnosis, technology, and management* (pp. 159–167). New York: Thieme.

Brinton, B., Fujiki, M., Loeb, D. F., & Winkler, E. (1986). Development of conversational repair strategies in response to requests for clarification. *Journal of Speech and Hearing Research, 29*, 75–81.

Burkley, M., & Blanton, H. (2008). Endorsing a negative in-group stereotype as a self-protective strategy: Sacrificing the group to save the self. *Journal of Experimental Social Psychology, 44*, 37–49.

Cantone, K. F., & Muller, N. (2005). Codeswitching at the interface of language-specific lexicons and the computational system. *International Journal of Bilingualism, 9*(2), 205–225.

Carey-Sargeant, C. L., & Brown, P. M. (2003). Pausing during interactions between deaf toddlers and their hearing mothers. *Deafness and Education International, 5*(1), 39–58.

Ciaramitaro, V. M., Buracas, G. T., & Boynton, G. M. (2007). Spatial and cross-modal attention alter responses to unattended sensory information in early visual and auditory human cortex. *Journal of Neurophysiology, 98*, 2399–2413.

Connor, C. M., Hieber, S., Arts, H. A., & Zwolan, T. A. (2006). Speech, vocabulary, and the education of children using cochlear implants: Oral or total communication? *Journal of Speech, Language, and Hearing Research, 43*(5), 1185–1204.

Conti-Ramsden, G. (2010). Summing up problems in bilingual specific language impairment: Why multiple influences may not be additive. *Applied Psycholinguistics, 31*, 270–273.

Conway, C. M., Bauernschmidt, A., Huang, S. S., & Pisoni, D. B. (2010). Implicit statistical learning in language processing: Word predictability is the key. *Cognition, 114*, 356–371.

Crawford, M. T. (2007). The renegotiation of social identities in response to a threat to self-evaluation maintenance. *Journal of Experimental Social Psychology, 43*, 39–47.

Deci, E. L., & Ryan, R. M. (2008). Facilitating optimal motivation and psychological well-being across life's domains. *Canadian Psychology, 49*(1), 14–23.

Dick, A. S., Solodkin, A., & Small, S. L. (2010). Neural development of networks for audiovisual speech comprehension. *Brain & Language, 114*(2), 101–114.

Dietrich, C., Swingley, D., & Werker, J. F. (2007). Native language governs interpretation of salient speech sound differences at 18 months. *Proceedings of the National Association of Sciences, 104*(41), 16027–16031.

Dornan, D., Hickson, L., Murdoch, B., & Houston, D. (2010). Longitudinal study of speech perception, speech, and language for children with hearing loss in an auditory-verbal therapy program. *The Volta Review, 109*(2–3), 61–86.

Dornan, D., Hickson, L., Murdoch, B., & Houston, T. (2007). Outcomes of an auditory-verbal program for children with hearing loss: A comparative study with a matched group of children with normal hearing. *The Volta Review, 107*(1), 37–54.

Dunham, Y., Baron, A. S., & Banaji, M. R. (2006). From American city to Japanese village: A cross-cultural investigation of implicit race attitudes. *Child Development, 77*(5), 1268–1281.

Duquette, C., Durieux-Smith, A., Olds, J., Fitzpatrick, E., Eriks-Brophy, A., & Whittingham, J. (2002). Parents' perspectives on their roles in facilitating the inclusion of their children with hearing impairment. *Exceptionality Education Canada, 12*(1), 19–36.

Durkin, K., Rutter, D. R., & Tucker, H. (1982). Social interaction and language acquisition: Motherese help you. *First Language, 3*(8), 107–120.

Dweck, C. S. (2006). *Mindset: The new psychology of success.* New York: Random House.

Easterbrooks, S., & Estes, E. (Eds.). (2007). *Helping children who are deaf and hard of hearing learn spoken language.* Thousand Oaks, CA: Corwin Press.

Easterbrooks, S. R., O'Rourke, C. M., & Todd, N. W. (2000). Child and family factors associated with children's success in auditory verbal therapy. *The American Journal of Otology, 21*, 341–344.

Edwards, L. C. (2007). Children with cochlear implants and complex needs: A review of outcome research and psychological practice. *Journal of Deaf Studies and Deaf Education, 12*(3), 258–268.

Edwards, L., & Crocker, S. (2008). *Psychological processes in deaf children with complex needs.* London: Jessica Kingsley.

Emmorey, K. (2002). *Language, cognition, and the brain: Insights from sign language research.* Mahwah, NJ: Erlbaum.

Emmorey, K., Borinstein, H. B., Thompson, R., & Gollan, T. H. (2008). Bimodal bilingualism. *Bilingualism: Language and Cognition, 11*(1), 43–61.

Emmorey, K., & McCullough, S. (2009). The bimodal bilingual brain: Effects of sign language experience. *Brain and Language, 109*(2–3), 124–132.

Eriks-Brophy, A. (2004). Outcomes of auditory-verbal therapy: A review of the evidence and a call for action. *The Volta Review, 104*(1), 21–35.

Eriks-Brophy, A., Durieux-Smith, A., Olds, J., Fitzpatrick, E. F., Duquette, C., & Whittingham, J. (2006). Facilitators and barriers to the inclusion of orally educated children and youth with hearing loss in schools: Promoting partnerships to support inclusion. *The Volta Review, 106*(1), 53–88.

Fiedler, M. (1952). *Deaf children in a hearing world.* New York: Ronald Press.

Fisher, C., & Tokura, H. (1996). Acoustic cues to grammatical structure in infant-directed speech: Cross-linguistic evidence. *Child Development, 67,* 3192–3218.

Fitzpatrick, E., Séguin, C., & Schramm, D. (2004). Cochlear implantation in adolescents and adults with prelinguistic deafness: Outcomes and candidacy issues. *International Congress Series, 1273,* 269–272.

Flexer, C. (1999). *Facilitating hearing and listening in young children.* San Diego, CA: Singular.

Floor, P., & Akhtar, N. (2006). Can 18-month-old infants learn words by listening in on conversations? *Infancy, 9*(3), 327–339.

Francis, A. L., & Ho, D. W. L. (2003). Case report: Acquisition of three spoken languages by a child with a cochlear implant. *Cochlear Implant International, 4*(1), 31–44.

Gable, S. L., & Haidt, J. (2005). What (and why) is positive psychology? *Review of General Psychology, 9*(2), 103–110.

Geers, A., Brenner, C., Nicholas, J., Uchanski, R., Tye-Murray, N., & Tobey, E. (2002). Rehabilitation factors contributing to implant benefit in children. *The Annals of Otology, Rhinology & Laryngology, 111*(5), 127–130.

Geers, A., Tobey, E., Moog, J., & Brenner, C. (2008). Long-term outcomes of cochlear implantation in the preschool tears: From elementary grades to high school. *International Journal of Audiology, 47*(Suppl. 20), S21–S30.

Genesee, F., & Nicoladis, E. (2006). Bilingual first language acquisition. In E. Hoff & M. Shatz (Eds.), *Blackwell handbook of language development* (pp. 324–341). Oxford, UK: Blackwell.

Genesee, F., Paradis, J., & Crago, M. B. (2004). *Dual language development and disorders.* Baltimore, MD: Paul H. Brookes.

Giedd, J. N. (2008). The teen brain: Insights from neuroimaging. *Journal of Adolescent Health, 42,* 335–343.

Goldberg, D. M., & Flexer, C. (2001). Auditory-verbal graduates: Outcome survey of clinical efficacy. *Journal of the American Academy of Audiology, 12,* 406–414.

Golinkoff, R. M., & Hirsh-Patek, K. (2008). How toddlers begin to learn verbs. *Trends in Cognitive Sciences, 12*(10), 397–403.

Grosjean, F. (2010). Bilingualism, biculturalism, and deafness. *International Journal of Bilingual Education and Bilingualism, 13*(2), 133–145.

Guiberson, M. M. (2005). Children with cochlear implants from bilingual families: Considerations for intervention and a case study. *The Volta Review, 105*(1), 29–40.

Halle, J. W., Marshall, A. M., & Spradlin, J. E. (1979). Time delay: A technique to increase language use and facilitate generalization in retarded children. *Journal of Applied Behavioral Analysis, 12,* 431–439.

Handford, B. W. T. (1937). "Revolutionizing" our New Testament teaching. *Religion in Education, 4*(2), 88–94.

Harrison, R. V., Gordon, K. A., & Mount, R. J. (2005). Is there a critical period for cochlear implantation in congenitally deaf children? Analyses of hearing and speech perception performance after implantation. *Developmental Psychobiology, 46*, 252–261.

Hattie, J. A. C. (2009). *Visible learning: A synthesis of 800 meta-analyses on achievement.* Oxford: Routledge.

Hawker, K., Ramirez-Inscoe, J., Bishop, D., Twomey, T., O'Donaghue, G., & Moore, D. (2008). Disproportionate language impairment in children using cochlear implants. *Ear and Hearing, 29*(3), 467–471.

Hay-McCutcheon, M. J., Kirk, K. I., Henning, S. C., Gao, S., & Qi, R. (2008). Using early language outcomes to predict later language in children with cochlear implants. *Audiology & Neuro-Otology, 13*(6), 370–378.

Hayes, H., Geers, A. E., Treiman, R., & Moog, J. S. (2009). Receptive vocabulary development in deaf children with cochlear implants: Achievement in an intensive auditory-oral educational setting. *Ear and Hearing, 30*(1), 128–135.

Hernandez, A. E. (2009). Language switching in the bilingual brain: What's next? *Brain & Language, 109*(2–3), 133–140.

Hogan, S., Stokes, J., & Weller, I. (2010). Language outcomes for children of low-income families enrolled in auditory verbal therapy. *Deafness & Education International, 12*(4), 204–216.

Hogan, S., Stokes, J., White, C., Tyszkiewicz, E., & Woolgar, A. (2008). An evaluation of auditory verbal therapy using the rate of early language development as an outcome measure. *Deafness and Education International, 10*(3), 143–167.

Holowka, S., Brosseau-Lapré, F., & Petitto, L. A. (2002). Semantic and conceptual knowledge underlying bilingual babies' first signs and words. *Language Learning, 52*, 205–262.

Huizing, H. C., & Pollack, D. (1951). Effects of limited hearing on the development of speech in children under three years of age. *Pediatrics, 8*(1), 53–59.

International Congress on Education of the Deaf. (2010). *Statement of principle and accord for the future.* Retrieved March 10, 2011, from http://www.milan1880.com/Resources/iced2010statement.pdf

James, D., Brinton, J., Rajput, K., & Goswami, U. (2007). Phonological awareness, vocabulary, and word reading in children who use cochlear implants: Does age of implantation explain individual variability in performance outcomes and growth? *Journal of Deaf Studies and Deaf Education, 13*(1), 117–137.

Jiménez, M. S., Pino, M. J., & Herruzo, J. (2009). A comparative study of speech development between deaf children with cochlear implants who have been educated with spoken or spoken + sign language. *International Journal of Pediatric Otorhinolaryngology, 73*, 109–114.

Jones, R. A. (1977). *Self-fulfilling prophecies: Social, psychological, and physiological effects of expectancies.* Hillsdale, NJ: Erlbaum.

Jusczyk, P. (1997). *The discovery of spoken language.* Cambridge: Massachusetts Institute of Technology Press.

Juvonen, J. (2007). Reforming middle schools: Focus on continuity, social connectedness, and engagement. *Educational Psychologist, 42*(4), 197–208.

Kedar, Y., Casasola, M., & Lust, B. (2006). Getting there faster: 18- and 24-month-old infants' use of function words to determine reference. *Child Development, 77*(2), 325–338.

Kelley, T. M. (2004). Positive psychology and adolescent mental health: False promise or true breakthrough? *Adolescence, 39*(154), 257–278.

Kirk, K. I., Miyamoto, R. T., Ying, E. A., Perdew, A. E., & Zuganelis, H. (2000). Cochlear implantation in young children: Effects of age at implantation and communication mode. *The Volta Review, 102*(4), 127–144.

Koch, M. E. (1999). *Bringing sound to life: Principles and practices of cochlear implant rehabilitation.* Timonium, MD: York.

Kohnert, K. (2010). Bilingual children with primary language impairment: Issues, evidence and implications for clinical actions. *Journal of Communication Disorders, 43*(6), 456–473.

Kohnert, K., Yim, D., Nett, K., Fong Kan, P., & Duran, L. (2005). Intervention with linguistically diverse preschool children. *Language, Speech, and Hearing Services in Schools, 36,* 251–263.

Kolb, B., Gibb, R., & Robinson, T. E. (2003). Brain plasticity and behavior. *Current Directions in Psychological Science, 12*(1), 1–5.

Kos, M.-I., Deriaz, M., Guyot, J.-P., & Pelizzone, M. (2009). What can be expected from a late cochlear implantation? *International Journal of Pediatric Otorhinolaryngology, 73,* 189–193.

Kovelman, I., Shalinsky, M. H., Whites, K. S., Schmitt, S. N., Berens, M. S., Paymer, N., et al. (2009). Dual language use in sign-speech bimodal bilinguals: fNIRS brain-imaging evidence. *Brain & Language, 109*(2–3), 112–123.

Kushalnagar, P., Hannay, H. J., & Hernandez, A. E. (2010). Bilingualism and attention: A study of unbalanced bilingual deaf users of American Sign Language and English. *Journal of Deaf Studies and Deaf Education, 15*(3), 263–273.

Lai, J. C. L. (2009). Dispositional optimism buffers the impact of daily hassles on mental health in Chinese adolescents. *Personality and Individual Differences, 47,* 247–249.

Leigh, G. (2008). Changing parameters in deafness and deaf education: Greater opportunity but continuing diversity. In M. Marschark & P. Hauser (Eds.), *Deaf cognition: Foundations and outcomes* (pp. 24–51). New York: Oxford University Press.

Ling, D. (1976). *Speech and the hearing-impaired child: Theory and practice.* Washington, DC: AG Bell Association.

Ling, D., & Ling, A. H. (1978). *Aural habilitation: The foundations of verbal learning in hearing-impaired children.* Washington, DC: AG Bell Association.

Lowenbraun, S., Appelman, K., & Callahan, J. (1980). *Teaching the hearing impaired through total communication.* Columbus, OH: Charles E. Merrill.

Loy, B., Warner-Czyz, A. D., Tong, L., Tobey, E. A., & Roland, P. S. (2010). The children speak: An examination of the quality of life of pediatric cochlear implant users. *Otolaryngology—Head and Neck Surgery, 142*(2), 247–253.

Macrory, G. (2006). Bilingual language development: What do early years practitioners need to know? *Early Years, 26*(2), 159–169.

Madon, S., Guyll, M., & Spoth, R. L. (2004). The self-fulfilling prophecy as an intrafamily dynamic. *Journal of Family Psychology, 18*(3), 459–469.

Marom, M., Cohen, D., & Naon, D. (2007). Changing disability-related attitudes and self-efficacy of Israeli children via the Partners to Inclusion Programme. *International Journal of Disability, Development and Education, 54*(1), 113–127.

Marschark, M. (2001). *Language development in children who are deaf: A research synthesis.* Alexandria, VA: National Association of State Directors of Special Education.

Marschark, M., & Spencer, P. E. (2005). *Oxford handbook of deaf studies, language, and education.* New York: Oxford University Press.

Massey, E. K., Gebhardt, W. A., & Garnefski, N. (2008). Adolescent goal content and pursuit: A review of the literature from the past 16 years. *Developmental Review, 28*, 421–460.

Mastropavlou, M. (2010). Morphophonological salience as a compensatory means for deficits in the acquisition of past tense in SLI. *Journal of Communication Disorders, 43*(3), 175–198.

Matychuk, P. (2005). The role of child-directed speech in language acquisition: A case study. *Language Sciences, 27*, 301–379.

Mayer, C. (2009). Issues in second language literacy education with learners who are deaf. *International Journal of Bilingual Education and Bilingualism, 12*(3), 325–334.

Mayer, C., & Akamatsu, C. T. (2003). Bilingualism and literacy. In M. Marschark & P. Spencer (Eds.), *Oxford handbook of deaf studies, language, and education* (pp. 136–147). New York: Oxford University Press.

Mayer, C., & Leigh, G. (2010). The changing context for sign bilingual education programs: Issues in language and the development of literacy. *International Journal of Bilingual Education and Bilingualism, 13*(2), 175–186.

McCrone, W. P. (2006). Learned helplessness and level of underachievement among deaf adolescents. *Psychology in the Schools, 16*(3), 430–434.

McWilliam, R. A. (1999). Controversial practices: The need for a reacculturation of early intervention fields. *Teaching Early Childhood Special Education, 19*(3), 177–188.

Mitchell, R. E., & Karchmer, M. A. (2004). Chasing the mythical ten percent: Parental hearing status of deaf and hard of hearing students in the United States. *Sign Language Studies, 4*(2), 138–163.

Mitchell, R. E., & Karchmer, M. A. (2005). Parental hearing status and signing among deaf and hard of hearing students. *Sign Language Studies, 5*(2), 231–244.

Morgan, S. L. (2007). Expectations and aspirations. In G. Ritzer (Ed.), *The Blackwell encyclopedia of sociology* (pp. 1528–1531). Oxford: Wiley.

Moskowitz, G. B., & Li, P. (2011). Egalitarian goals trigger stereotype inhibition: A proactive form of stereotype control. *Journal of Experimental Social Psychology, 47*(1), 103–116.

Musselman, C., & Kircaali-Iftar, G. (1996). The development of spoken language in deaf children: Explaining the unexplained variance. *Journal of Deaf Studies and Deaf Education, 1*(2), 108–121.

Myers, S. S., & Fernandes, J. K. (2010). Deaf studies: A critique of the predominant U.S. theoretical direction. *Journal of Deaf Studies and Deaf Education, 15*(1), 30–49.

Neuss, D. (2006). The ecological transition to auditory-verbal therapy: Experiences of parents whose children use cochlear implants. *The Volta Review, 106*(2), 195–222.

Nicholas, J. (2008). Expected test scores for preschoolers with a cochlear implant who use spoken language. *American Journal of Speech-Language Pathology, 17*, 121–138.

Nicholas, J. G., & Geers, A. E. (2006). Effects of early auditory experience on the spoken language of deaf children at 3 years of age. *Ear and Hearing, 27*(3), 286–298.

Niparko, J. K., Tobey, E. A., Thal, D. J., Eisenberg, L. S., Wang, N.-Y., Quittner, A. L., et al. (2010). Spoken language development in children following cochlear implantation. *Journal of American Medical Association, 303*(15), 1498–1506.

Ormel, E. A., Gijsel, M. A. R., Hermans, D., Bosman, A. M. T., Knoors, H., & Verhoeven, L. (2010). Semantic categorization: A comparison between deaf and hearing children. *Journal of Communication Disorders, 43*(5), 347–360.

Oviatt, S. L. (1980). The emerging ability to comprehend language: An experimental approach. *Child Development, 51*, 97–106.

Padden, C., & Humphries, T. (1988). *Deaf in America: Voices from a culture.* Cambridge, MA: Harvard University Press.

Pearson, B. Z. (2008). *Raising a bilingual child.* New York: Random House.

Peters, M. L., Flink, I. K., Boersma, K., & Linton, S. J. (2010). Manipulating optimism: Can imagining a best possible self be used to increase positive future expectancies? *The Journal of Positive Psychology, 5*(3), 204–211.

Petitto, L., Katerelos, M., Levy, B., Gauna, K., Tetrault, K., & Ferraro, V. (2001). Bilingual signed and spoken language acquisition from birth: Implications for the mechanisms underlying early bilingual language acquisition. *Journal of Child Language, 8*, 453–496.

Pollack, D. (1964). Acoupedics: A unisensory approach to auditory training. *The Volta Review, 66*, 400–409.

Pollack, D. (1970). *Educational audiology for the limited-hearing infant.* Springfield, IL: Charles C Thomas.

Rhoades, E .A. (2001). Language progress with an auditory-verbal approach for young children with hearing loss. *International Pediatrics, 16*(1), 1–7.

Rhoades, E. A. (2003). Lexical-semantic and morpho-syntactic language assessment in auditory-verbal intervention: A position paper. *The Volta Review, 103*(3), 169–184.

Rhoades, E. A. (2006). Research outcomes of auditory-verbal intervention: Is the approach justified? *Deafness and Education International, 8*(3), 125–143.

Rhoades, E. A. (2008). Working with multicultural and multilingual families of young children. In J. R. Madell & C. Flexer (Eds.), *Pediatric audiology: Diagnosis, technology, and management* (pp. 262–268). New York: Thieme.

Rhoades, E. A. (2009a). Learning a second language: Potentials & diverse possibilities. *Hearing Loss, 30*(2), 20–22.

Rhoades, E. A. (2009b). What the neurosciences tell us about adolescence. *Volta Voices, 16*(1), 16–21.

Rhoades, E. A. (2010a). Evidence-based auditory-verbal practice. In E. A. Rhoades & J. Duncan (Eds.), *Auditory-verbal practice: Toward a family-centered approach* (pp. 23–51). Springfield, IL: Charles C Thomas.

Rhoades, E. A. (2010b). Revisiting labels: 'Hearing' or not? *The Volta Review, 110*(1), 55–67.

Rhoades, E. A., & Chisolm, T. H. (2001). Global language progress with an auditory-verbal approach for children who are deaf or hard of hearing. *The Volta Review, 102*(1), 5–25.

Rhoades, E. A., Perusse, M., Douglas, W. M., & Zarate, C. (2008). Auditory-based bilingual children in North America: Differences and choices. *Volta Voices, 15*(5), 20–22.

Rhoades, E. A., Price, F., & Perigoe, C. B. (2004). The changing American family and ethnically diverse children with multiple needs. *The Volta Review, 104*(4), 285–305.

Rhodes, J. E., & DuBois, D. L. (2008). Mentoring relationships and programs for youth. *Current Directions in Psychological Science, 17*(4), 254–258.

Roberts, B. W., Walton, K. E., & Viechtbauer, W. (2006). Patterns of mean-level change in personality traits across the life course: A meta-analysis of longitudinal studies. *Psychological Bulletin, 132*(1), 1–25.

Robertson, L., & Flexer, C. (1993). Reading development: A parent survey of children with hearing loss who developed speech and language through the auditory-verbal method. *The Volta Review, 95*(3), 253–261.

Rosenthal, R. (2002). Covert communication in classrooms, clinics, courtrooms, and cubicles. *American Psychologist, 57*(11), 839–849.

Ross, M. (1994). Letter to the editor. *American Journal of Audiology, 3*(2), 6.

Rowe, M. B. (1974). Wait time and rewards as instructional variables, their influence in language, logic, and fate control. Part 1: Wait time. *Journal of Research in Science Teaching, 11*, 81–94.

Rowe, M. B. (1978). Wait wait wait . . . *School Science and Mathematics, 78*, 207–216.

Rowe, M. B. (1987). Wait time: Slowing down may be a way of speeding things up. *American Educator, 11*(1), 38–43, 47.

Royal College of Physicians. (2007). *Hearing and balance disorders: Achieving excellence in diagnosis and management. Report of a working party.* London: Lavenham.

Ryan, R. M., & Deci, E. L. (2003). On assimilating identities to the self: A self-determination theory perspective on internalization and integrity within cultures. In M. R. Leary & J. P. Tangney (Eds.), *Handbook of self and identity* (pp. 253–272). New York: Guilford Press.

Schramm, B., Bohnert, A., & Keilmann, A. (2009). The prelexical development in children implanted by 16 months compared with normal hearing children. *International Journal of Pediatric Otorhinolaryngology, 73*, 1673–1681.

Schramm, B., Bohnert, A., & Keilmann, A. (2010). Auditory, speech, and language development in young children with cochlear implants compared with children with normal hearing. *International Journal of Pediatric Otorhinolaryngology, 74*(7), 812–819.

Sharma, A., Dorman, M. F., & Kral, A. (2005). The influence of a sensitive period on central auditory development in children with unilateral and bilateral cochlear implants. *Hearing Research, 203*(1–2), 134–143.

Shaywitz, S. E., Morris, R., & Shaywitz, B. A. (2008). The education of dyslexic children from childhood to young adulthood. *Annual Review of Psychology, 59*, 451–475.

Smith, L. Z., & Levitt, H. (1999). Consonant enhancement effects on speech recognition of hearing-impaired children. *Journal of American Academy of Audiology, 10*, 411–421.

Smith, N. A., & Trainor, L. J. (2008). Infant-directed speech is modulated by infant feedback. *Infancy, 13*(4), 410–420.

Southgate, V., Chevallier, C., & Csibra, G. (2009). Sensitivity to communicative relevance tells young children what to imitate. *Developmental Science, 12*(6), 1013–1019.

Sparrow, R. (2010). Implants and ethnocide: Learning from the cochlear implant controversy. *Disability & Society, 25*(4), 455–466.

Stacey, P. C., Fortnum, H. M., Barton, G. R., & Summerfield, A. Q. (2006). Hearing-impaired children in the United Kingdom, I. Auditory performance, communication skills, educational achievements, quality of life and cochlear implantation. *Ear and Hearing, 27*, 161–186.

Stager, C. L., & Werker, J. F. (1998). Methodological issues in studying the link between speech-perception and word learning. In C. Rovee-Collier,

L. P. Lipsitt, & H. Hayne (Eds.), *Advances in infancy research* (Vol. 12, pp. 237–256). Stamford, CT: Ablex.

Stevenson, J., McCann, D., Watkin, P., Worsfold, S., Kennedy, C., & Hearing Outcomes Study Team. (2010). The relationship between language development and behaviour problems in children with hearing loss. *Journal of Child Psychology and Psychiatry, 51*(1), 77–83.

Stokoe, W. C. (1965). *A dictionary of American Sign Language on linguistic principles.* Washington, DC: Linstock.

Surian, L. (2010). Sensitivity to conversational maxims in deaf and hearing children. *Journal of Child Language, 37*(4), 929–943.

Svirsky, M. A., Teoh, S.-W., & Neuburger, H. (2004). Development of language and speech perception in congenitally, profoundly deaf children as a function of age at cochlear implantation. *Audiology & Neuro-Otology, 9*, 224–233.

Swanwick, R. (2010). Policy and practice in sign bilingual education: Development, challenges and directions. *International Journal of Bilingual Education and Bilingualism, 13*(2), 147–158.

Taylor, S. F., Welsh, R. C., Wager, T. D., Phan, K. L., Fitzgerald, K. D., & Gehring, W. J. (2004). A functional neuroimaging study of motivation and executive function. *NeuroImage, 21*, 1045–1054.

Thomas, E., El-Kashlan, H., & Zwolan, T. A. (2008). Children with cochlear implants who live in monolingual and bilingual homes. *Otology & Neurotology, 29*, 230–234.

Tobey, E. A., Rekart, D., Buckley, K., & Geers, A. E. (2004). Mode of communication and classroom placement impact on speech intelligibility. *Archives of Otolaryngology—Head & Neck Surgery, 130*(5), 639–643.

Tobin, K. (1987). The role of wait time in higher cognitive level learning. *Review of Educational Research, 57*(1), 69–95.

Tomasello, M. (2003). *Constructing a language: A usage-based theory of language acquisition.* Cambridge, MA: Harvard University Press.

Waltzman, S. B., Robbins, A. M., Green, J. E., & Cohen, N. L. (2003). Second oral language capabilities in children with cochlear implants. *Otology & Neurology, 24*(5), 757–763.

Watson, L. M., Archbold, S. M., & Nikolopoulos, T. P. (2006). Children's communication mode five years after cochlear implantation: Changes over time according to age at implant. *Cochlear Implants International, 7*(2), 77–91.

Watson, L. M., Hardie, T., Archbold, S. M., & Wheeler, A. (2008). Parents' views on changing communication after cochlear implantation. *Journal of Deaf Studies and Deaf Education, 13*(1), 104–116.

Wauters, L. N., Tellings, A. E. J. M., van Bon, W. H. J., & Mak, W. M. (2007). Mode of acquisition as a factor in deaf children's reading comprehension. *Journal of Deaf Studies and Deaf Education, 13*(2), 175–192.

Wheeler, A., Archbold, S., Gregory, S., & Skipp, A. (2007). Cochlear implants: The young people's perspective. *Journal of Deaf Studies and Deaf Education, 12*(3), 303–316.

Woolfe, T., Herman, R., Roy, P., & Woll, B. (2010). Early vocabulary development in deaf native signers: A British Sign Language adaptation of the communicative development inventories. *Journal of Child Psychology and Psychiatry, 51*(3), 322–331.

Wray, D., Flexer, C., & Vaccaro, V. (1999). Classroom performance of children who are deaf or hard of hearing and who learned through the auditory-verbal approach: An evaluation of treatment efficacy. *The Volta Review, 99*(2), 107–119.

Wu, C. D., & Brown, P. M. (2004). Parents' and teachers' expectations of auditory-verbal therapy. *The Volta Review, 104*(1), 5–20.

Yang, C. D. (2006). *The infinite gift: How children learn and unlearn the languages of the world*. New York: Scribner.

Ylvisaker, M., & Feeney, T. (2002). Executive functions, self-regulations, optimism in paediatric rehabilitation and implications for intervention. *Pediatric Rehabilitation, 5*(2), 51–70.

Young, A., Hunt, R., Carr, G., Hall, A.-M., McCracken, W., Skipp, A., et al. (2005). Informed choice, deaf children and families—underpinning ideas and project development. *Electronic Journal of Research in Educational Psychology, 3*(3), 253–273.

Ysseldyke, J. (2001). Reflections on a research career: Generalizations from 25 years of research on assessment and instructional decision making. *Exceptional Children, 67*, 295–309.

Zentella, A. C. (1997). *Growing up bilingual: Puerto Rican children in New York*. Oxford: Blackwell.

PART III

Educational Approaches

9

THE COCHLEAR IMPLANT EDUCATION CENTER: PERSPECTIVES ON EFFECTIVE EDUCATIONAL PRACTICES

Debra Berlin Nussbaum and Susanne M. Scott

The number of children using cochlear implant technology is growing.[1] With this growth has emerged a population of children who are similar in the technology they are using, yet disparate in their demographic characteristics and spoken language communication outcomes (Belzner & Seal, 2009). Although the demographics of children using cochlear implant technology are wide ranging, professional recommendations surrounding language and communication approaches for these children often do not reflect their diversity. As a cochlear implant is an "auditory technology," recommendations often lean toward language and communication methodologies that focus on development and use of only spoken language. Although these auditory/oral approaches appear appropriate for a percentage of children with a cochlear implant, they do not appear to meet the comprehensive linguistic, cognitive, communicative, and social needs for many others.

Given this reality, the Laurent Clerc National Deaf Education Center (Clerc Center) at Gallaudet University established the Cochlear Implant Education Center (CIEC) in 2000. The CIEC was established to examine practices including both spoken and signed languages for the heterogeneous children who were obtaining cochlear implants and assimilating into educational programs. Since 2000, the CIEC has annually developed and implemented education, habilitation, and support service programs and services for approximately 20 to 30 students with cochlear implants enrolled at the Clerc Center demonstration schools (Kendall Demonstration Elementary School and the Model Secondary School for

1. According to the U.S. Food and Drug Administration, as of December 2010, approximately 219,000 people worldwide have received implants. In the United States, roughly 42,600 adults and 28,400 children have received them. Most children who receive implants are between 2 and 6 years old (National Institute on Deafness and Other Communication Disorders, 2011).

the Deaf).[2] The CIEC staff has also had the unique opportunity to interact with more than 10,000 professionals and families throughout the United States to network and share information about the common challenges and successes that many experience in their journey to meet the needs of children with cochlear implants. From these experiences, there is a clear message to share. That message is that no single approach fits the characteristics and needs of all children with a cochlear implant. All children with a cochlear implant are unique and should not be defined by the technology they are using. What the CIEC has observed and said many times in interactions with professionals and families is "If you have met one child with a cochlear implant, you have met *one* child with a cochlear implant."

So, if there is not one "right" approach, what does this signify for professionals and families seeking guidance in addressing the comprehensive needs of children with cochlear implants? It suggests the importance of considering whether pursuing solely an oral approach may put a child at risk cognitively, linguistically, and socially (Grosjean, 2008) as well as the need to examine broader recommendations that include both spoken and signed languages. In its journey to define "effective practices" for children with cochlear implants, the CIEC has learned the following:

- Multiple factors affect spoken language performance outcomes with a cochlear implant.
- Children with cochlear implants *can* benefit from the use of a signed language (e.g., American Sign Language [ASL]) and signs used to support spoken English.
- The key to facilitating successful linguistic, communicative, cognitive, and social-emotional development is purposeful language and communication planning.

Factors That Affect Spoken Language Performance Outcomes

Although it appears that most children with a cochlear implant can detect individual speech sounds, this does not automatically guarantee they will develop the necessary skills to comprehend spoken language for learning. All children with a cochlear implant will attain their own level of auditory functioning depending on a variety of characteristics intrinsic to each child (e.g., etiology of loss, additional

2. Kendall Demonstration Elementary School serves students from birth through 8th grade from the Washington, DC, metropolitan area. The Model Secondary School for the Deaf is a residential high school program.

disabilities) and extrinsic to the child (i.e., habilitation history, educational environment, family support, etc). With time and training, some children will develop auditory skill proficiency to a level in which they can "listen to learn" whereas others may not be able to effectively do so. The latter group nonetheless may benefit from the implant for support and access to sound in other areas of life (e.g., music enjoyment, enhancement of speechreading, phonemic awareness, environmental sound awareness). Even though children will not all achieve the same level of auditory functioning and spoken language ability with their cochlear implant, the majority will develop skills beyond those they might have developed while using hearing aids (Eisenberg, Kirk, Martinez, Ying, & Miyamoto, 2004).

There are many complex and interactive factors that will affect a child's spoken language outcomes with his or her cochlear implant (Geers, 2003, 2004; Geers, Tobey, Moog, & Brenner, 2008; Nussbaum, 2003; Spencer & Marschark, 2003, 2006). It is critical that each of these factors be considered in the process of language, communication, and educational planning.

Factors Related to the Child

Age of implantation. Research and observation suggest that spoken language performance outcomes are best for children who are implanted during the early months of life (generally before 18 to 24 months) when language is typically developing. As children are implanted at progressively later ages, outcomes and rates of development vary (Dettman, Pinder, Briggs, Dowell, & Leigh, 2007; Geers, 2002; Geers, Nicholas, & Sedey, 2003; Holt & Svirsky, 2008; McConkey Robbins, Burton Koch, Osberger, Zimmerman-Phillips, & Kishon-Rabin, 2004; Sharma, Dorman, & Kral, 2005; Sommers & Lim, 2006; Spencer, Barker, & Tomblin, 2003; Svirsky, Teoh, & Neuburger, 2004; Waltzman & Roland, 2005; Zwolan et al., 2004). For later implanted children who did not have access to sound during the early years of their lives, observation and research suggest that although there is greater benefit from a cochlear implant compared with traditional hearing aids, existing auditory delays at the time of implantation present continued educational and rehabilitation challenges that oftentimes cannot be overcome (Nicholas & Geers, 2007). It is therefore critical to counsel families regarding these limited outcomes.

Preimplant duration of hearing loss. The shorter the time from the identification of deafness to the time of cochlear implantation, the easier it tends to be for a child to develop spoken language (Hammes et al., 2002). Research suggests that the less time the auditory channels remain dormant and unused, the greater the chance for these pathways to demonstrate the plasticity to accept the new incoming information available through the cochlear implant. It is therefore necessary to understand the importance of stimulating auditory neural pathways via hearing aids as early as possible to prepare for implantation (Sharma et al., 2005; Sharma, Dorman, & Spahr, 2002; Sharma et al., 2004).

Language competence at time of implantation. When parents and children communicate effectively with each other from the time the child is identified with a hearing loss, a foundation for language acquisition (both spoken and signed languages) is established, and language delays may be prevented or minimized (Yoshinaga-Itano, 2003). This also applies to children who obtain cochlear implants. It appears that children who have a strong language foundation (whether signed or spoken) before getting a cochlear implant have an easier time developing spoken language using their implant (Magnuson, 2000; Tait, Lutman, & Robinson; 2000). It has been demonstrated that children with early language foundations via ASL before implantation can transition well to spoken language following implantation. This early exposure prevents delay in establishing language foundations and can then be used to provide a "piggyback" to the development of spoken language (Yoshinaga-Itano, 2006).

Previous listening experience. Children who experience adventitious hearing loss, as well as children who have had meaningful auditory experiences with a hearing aid before implantation, typically achieve high levels of spoken language outcomes with a cochlear implant (Nicholas & Geers, 2006). This relates to past imprinting or memory for this information. Children implanted beyond the early language learning years who have had limited listening experiences before implantation, however, typically require more time and structured approaches to facilitating spoken language development and often do not achieve similar levels of receptive or expressive spoken language skills (Waltzman & Cohen, 2000).

Cause of hearing loss. Some of the associated secondary conditions arising from varying causes of hearing loss may influence the degree of benefit a child actualizes from a cochlear implant. For example, some children with hearing loss from cytomegalovirus have been observed to demonstrate auditory processing problems. Although a cochlear implant provides access to sound, it will not eliminate auditory processing problems related to interpretation of sound in the brain. Also, causes of hearing loss that affect the anatomy of the cochlea may present an obstacle to the insertion of all electrodes available through the cochlear implant, which may then limit outcomes (Pyman, Blamey, Lacy, Clark, & Dowell, 2000). For children with auditory neuropathy or auditory dys-synchrony (Starr, Picton, Sininger, Hood, & Berlin, 1996),[3] there appears to be varied benefit from a cochlear implant, depending on where the dysfunction occurs in the auditory system. It is important that a complete battery of diagnostic evaluations be completed before proceeding with a cochlear implant so that families are clear on the appropriateness of a cochlear implant and varied outcomes for children with this condition (Gardner-Berry, Gibson, & Sanli, 2005).

---

3. "Auditory neuropathy," also known as "auditory dys-synchrony," is a hearing disorder in which sound successfully reaches the inner ear, but for one or more reasons, the signals are not successfully transmitted from the inner ear to the brain.

Additional challenges. Increasing numbers of children with additional challenges are getting cochlear implants and demonstrating a range of outcomes. The type of additional challenge children demonstrate influences the outcomes they may obtain with their implants. For example, children with physical challenges may still demonstrate similar auditory development as their non–physically challenged peers with cochlear implants (Garber & Nevins, 2007). However, if a child demonstrates other complex cognitive, language processing, or social communication challenges, these will affect outcomes related to the rate of spoken language development and the level of spoken language competence achieved (Edwards, 2007; Goldberg & Perigo, 2006). It is important that families and professionals do not expect that obtaining a cochlear implant will resolve these other challenges (Pyman et al., 2000).

Although some children obtain their implants with known additional challenges, other children obtain their implants at young ages before other additional challenges become apparent (e.g., autistic spectrum disorder, learning disabilities). As it is not possible to predict when additional challenges may emerge that can directly affect performance outcomes, it is critical to closely monitor each child for possible complicating issues and make necessary revisions and accommodations to approaches and strategies used as needed.

Learning styles. Some children are auditory learners; others are visual learners. Visual learners may benefit from visual context for learning through the use of visual reinforcement, for example, through books, videos, or diagrams. Auditory learners may benefit from strategies that provide auditory reinforcement, such as repetition of messages, listening to audiotapes, and repeating information aloud. A child's learning style may affect implant outcomes as well as the choice of strategies used to achieve optimal outcomes. Some children may demonstrate more "auditory inclination" than others, with some readily learning auditory information without much guidance and others struggling for similar competence (Chute & Nevins, 2006).

Personality. All children have a unique personality that may influence how they function with their cochlear implant. A child's assertiveness, positive attitude, resiliency, and ability to tolerate frustration are all integral to what outcomes may be actualized (Leigh & Christiansen, 2009). If a child is shy and not willing to participate in activities to support auditory and speech development, this may affect spoken language and communication growth. If the child demonstrates resistant behaviors and is not willing to use the implant consistently, this will also affect optimal outcomes. Successful outcomes will be tied to a child's motivation to use the implant and participate in activities to support auditory, speech, and spoken language development.

Factors Related to Family Characteristics

Family support. Children demonstrating the best outcomes with a cochlear implant (regardless of the other factors discussed) have strong family involvement and support (Moeller, 2000; Spencer, 2004). As expected, families who are integrally involved in providing a rich listening and language learning environment and helping a child to receive all of the necessary supports to maximize benefit from his or her implant will have a positive impact on outcomes.

Language use in the home. There are children with cochlear implants from homes that are multilingual and multicultural. Some families speak English and another language fluently, some are learning English as a new language,[4] and some use a visual language such as ASL. Multilingual/multicultural factors will have an impact on the spoken language outcomes of a child with a cochlear implant. For children in this situation, it is necessary to identify and apply strategies and techniques in bilingual language learning based on which will be most effective for each child in relation to how language is used in the home (American Speech-Language-Hearing Association, 2004; Thordardottir, 2006). The factors that predict the best outcomes for bilingual spoken language development for a child with a cochlear implant are (1) two spoken languages used in the home, (2) early age of implantation (before age 2), (3) strong speech perception skills, (4) absence of additional disabilities, (5) intact language learning ability for the language of the home, (6) parent involvement, (7) motivation for bilingual learning, and (8) opportunities to use both languages in meaningful contexts with native users (McConkey Robbins, 2007). For children who come from families in which ASL is the language used in the home, strong language foundations in ASL coupled with ongoing implementation of strategies to address the development and use of spoken English will positively affect spoken language outcomes (Cummins, 2006; Grosjean, 2008; Yoshinaga-Itano, 2006).

Factors Related to Cochlear Implant Technology

Performance outcomes may vary depending on issues specific to the technology. Children implanted with more current technology appear to demonstrate increased potential in comparison with children implanted with earlier technologies with less sophisticated speech processing capabilities. Outcomes will also be affected by the continued appropriateness of the "MAP" (individualized speech processing settings) of a child's speech processor (Zwolan et al., 2004). It is imperative that the continued appropriateness of a child's MAP be closely monitored to ensure optimal benefit. This requires daily close monitoring of the implant at home and at school and support by the hospital implant center. In addition, increasing numbers of children are obtaining bilateral cochlear implants that can positively affect performance outcomes in relation to enhanced ease of listening and sound localization (Litovsky et al., 2006).

4. "English as a new language" pertains to parents who are just learning to speak English or may have no English proficiency; another language is spoken in the home, and the child typically learns English at school.

In Conclusion

Based on the documented differences in performance outcomes for children with cochlear implants, it would seem logical that strategies and approaches endorsed for children using this technology would be equally diverse. However, we have not found this to be the case. Through our interactions with families and professionals in our demonstration schools, as well as schools for the deaf and mainstream programs nationally, we encounter ongoing reports of medical and educational professionals making recommendations to families to use oral education approaches alone regardless of child characteristics. In consideration of broader practices for children with cochlear implants, the CIEC has focused on examining services and strategies that include sign spoken language, which are described throughout the chapter.

CHILDREN WITH COCHLEAR IMPLANTS CAN BENEFIT FROM THE USE OF SIGN

When considering the use of sign to support the language, communication, educational, and social-emotional development of children with cochlear implants, it is first necessary to address two issues: the definition of "sign" as its use is envisioned by professionals and families, and the controversy of using sign (regardless of how sign is defined) for children with cochlear implants. Without attention to these two issues, it is difficult to continue the discussion regarding recommendations for its use.

Defining "Sign"

Webster's New World College Dictionary (2005) defines sign language as "a system of signs and gestures used as a language." This definition implies that "sign language" encompasses a full language, as is the case with ASL, which is a complete visual language with all of the components of any language with its own vocabulary and grammar (Malloy, 2003). Use of "sign language" to mean ASL is different from using "sign language" when referring to signed representations of English such as Manually Coded English (MCE), Conceptually Accurate Signed English (CASE), Simultaneous Communication, (SimCom), or Sign Supported Speech (SSS), which are English-based sign systems employing sign as a support to English (Moores, 2001). These sign systems are not true languages.

As sign is discussed in professional circles and in research, however, it is often not defined. Consequently, it is important to detail exactly how it should be included. Our experience suggests that when methodologies that include sign are being recommended for children with cochlear implants, these recommendations typically imply the use of sign to support English, not ASL, as a full language.

Professionals do not typically explain this distinction. This also is not generally understood by many families choosing to include sign. In addition, educational programs using both sign and spoken language for children with cochlear implants often do not clearly address how sign is used in their programs. We have found that lack of a clear definition of sign affects research validity when discussing performance outcomes, family decision making regarding its use, and appropriate planning for how sign and spoken language can be jointly addressed in educational approaches for children with cochlear implants.

Addressing the Controversy of Sign Use for Children With Cochlear Implants

The second critical issue that is important to address is the pervasive fear that sign (either a sign system or ASL) may interfere with spoken language development. Although there are many documented factors (many cited earlier in this chapter) that potentially affect outcomes, use of sign often is singled out as the primary factor limiting a child's spoken language progress. This prevents many families from choosing methodologies including sign for their child.

A review of research related to sign use, however, does *not* demonstrate that signing in and of itself impedes the development of spoken language on average across children. Instead, the quality and intensity of the spoken language used with a child has been found to have the most impact on the development of spoken language (Geers, 2006; Moeller, 2006; Moog & Geers, 2003; Spencer & Bass-Ringdahl, 2004; Yoshinaga-Itano, 2006).[5] It is critical to document, research, and share how spoken language can be actively developed, valued, and used in approaches that include sign, so these approaches will be more readily considered as a first choice option for children with implants to effectively meet their comprehensive linguistic, cognitive, communicative, and social needs.

Although there may be debate regarding use of sign for children following implantation, the benefit of providing visual access to language via sign before implantation to prevent linguistic, cognitive, and communicative deprivation appears to be clearly documented (Schick, de Villiers, de Villiers, & Hoffmeister, 2002; Snoddon, 2008). The lack of age appropriate language development can negatively affect a child's cognitive and social development, which in turn interferes with success in school and in later life (Marge & Marge, 2005). Even in the best-case scenario regarding early implantation, children will typically miss approximately 14 to 15 months of prime language learning opportunities before gaining access to sound as they await eligibility for implantation, undergo surgery

5. Patricia Spencer (2009) summarized research findings addressing the use of sign for children with cochlear implants during her presentation titled "Research to Practice" at the CIEC conference, Cochlear Implants and Sign Language: Building Foundations for Effective Educational Practices.

and the initial fitting of the externally worn speech processor, and learn listening skills. If spoken language access during these formative months is inadequate to promote linguistic competence, this alone is a strong justification to use ASL, a full visual language (while also stimulating auditory development through hearing aids and associated auditory/speech habilitation), at least to establish early language foundations and as a bridge to spoken language development (Malloy, 2003; Snoddon, 2008; Yoshinaga-Itano, 2006).

Although direct comparisons cannot be made between how deaf children with cochlear implants and hearing children learn language, it is interesting to observe the popularity of teaching sign to young hearing children. As sign is shown to jump-start cognitive development, reduce communication frustration, enhance early communication confidence, and support speech development for hearing children (Goodwyn, Acredolo, & Brown, 2000), it seems unreasonable to object to the use sign for children who are deaf and could gain similar if not more benefit.

At the Kendall Demonstration Elementary School, we have observed students as they develop spoken language in our ASL/English bimodal–bilingual program, which actively incorporates both ASL and spoken English. Although we have not yet had the opportunity to formally research outcomes, we have documented student progress in both ASL and spoken English for educational planning purposes. The variable spoken English outcomes appear more strongly related to the many other factors that may affect performance rather than the use of ASL. Since 2000, many of our students with cochlear implants have developed spoken English skills at a level to effectively transition to educational settings using primarily spoken English and/or mainstream environments with an interpreter. We have also observed diverse students (e.g., children who are more visually inclined, children from Deaf families, children with additional language processing challenges, children implanted at a later age, children from hearing families interested in a bilingual education for their children) who demonstrate continued growth in their spoken English development but remain in our program as they continue to benefit from and value the development and use of ASL and English for the learning and communication afforded them in a bilingual environment.

Approaches to Sign Use for Children With Cochlear Implants

We have observed the following approaches that include sign (based on Moeller, 2006) in various educational programs throughout the United States:

- *Use of sign vocabulary to facilitate early language development before obtaining a cochlear implant.* Children are exposed to sign vocabulary (conceptually accurate ASL signs or an English-based sign system) to jump-start language development before cochlear implantation. Signing is discontinued immediately upon implantation.

- *Use of sign as a bridge or transition to proficiency in spoken English.* Sign (ASL or an English-based sign system) is used with the child before implantation and as a bridge to transitioning to the use of spoken English following implantation. Sign is slowly diminished as the child demonstrates increased proficiency in spoken English.
- *Continued use of sign as a support to spoken English.* An English-based sign system is used in conjunction with spoken English (either via simultaneous communication, sequentially as a support to English, or via an interpreter).
- *Bilingual development.* ASL and spoken English are each developed and addressed as independent languages. Spoken English is facilitated for both social and academic purposes based on the individual characteristics and goals of each child.
- *Primary use of ASL.* ASL is the child's primary language. Listening through the cochlear implant provides some linguistic support.

It has been our observation that medical and educational professional recommendations often lean toward use of English-based sign systems rather than bilingual approaches that include ASL and spoken English. The inclination to recommend English-based sign systems appears connected to desired long-term aspirations for proficiency in spoken English. Consequently, many professionals and families considering sign will gravitate toward use of an English-based sign system to promote this goal. ASL as a visual language, with a grammatical system separate from English and without a spoken component, is often not favorably viewed nor understood as a choice for children with cochlear implants, as the relationship between ASL as a visual language and English as a spoken and written language is often difficult for many professionals and families to envision. However, as stated earlier, there is research that clearly supports the use of ASL for children with cochlear implants in establishing early language foundations. In addition, there is strong support for the brain's capacity to readily accomplish both sign and spoken language acquisition without detriment to the development of language through either modality (Kovelman et al., 2009; Petitto et al., 2001; Petitto & Kovelman, 2003). Although the rate of developing speech perception/production skills may be slower for some children using both sign language and spoken language, the benefit of using approaches that include sign to safeguard linguistic, cognitive, and literacy development have been documented (Connor, Hieber, Arts, & Zwolen, 2000; Connor & Zwolan, 2004; Courtin, 2000; Fagen, Pisoni, Horn, & Dillon, 2007; Marschark & Hauser, 2008; Marschark, Rhoten, & Fabich, 2007; Mayberry, Lock, & Kazmi, 2002; Petitto et al., 2001).

If ASL/English bilingual programs are to be considered a favorable option for children with cochlear implants, it is important that the benefit of developing and using ASL and English as separate languages be clearly explained to families; strategies demonstrating how ASL can successfully link to and promote development of English be shared; and educational programs explicitly delineate their philosophies, beliefs, and strategies regarding how spoken language can be effectively addressed in this approach. Rationales for why an English-based sign system may or may not be an appropriate recommendation for a child need to be reviewed by professionals as they plan effective programs and discuss these with families.

Sign Language, Cochlear Implants, and the Deaf Community

During the early years of cochlear implantation, there was speculation regarding whether individuals with cochlear implants would choose to be a part of the Deaf community (Christiansen & Leigh, 2002, 2004).[6] This issue emerged from the expectation that these individuals would function as "hearing" and no longer have an interest or need to associate with the larger Deaf community. Our interactions with cochlear implant users and their families in our demonstration school programs suggest that many individuals choose to use cochlear implant technology and maintain associations with the Deaf community. This includes Deaf adults obtaining a cochlear implant for themselves as well as both hearing and Deaf families choosing a cochlear implant for their children.

A connection with the Deaf community can be beneficial for children with cochlear implants in a variety of ways. This community can provide an essential resource for accessing native, proficient ASL language models for children and families who are learning and using ASL. Regardless of the families' language and communication choices, the Deaf community can provide a network for socialization and support. Some of the strategies that may facilitate involvement with the Deaf community are the following:

- Educational placements that include Deaf teachers, support professionals, and paraprofessionals
- Opportunities to participate in summer camps and weekend activities that include deaf children and Deaf adults, especially if children do not have opportunities for interaction with other Deaf individuals through their educational placement
- Availability of support groups for children with cochlear implants with activities to address identity

6. *Deaf* with a capital D, refers to individuals who share the use of ASL and other common values, rules for behavior, traditions, and views of themselves (Padden & Humphries, 1988). The *Deaf community* refers to a cultural group sharing common experiences, concerns, and language (Ladd, 2003).

- Opportunities for families of children with cochlear implants to learn about the Deaf community and interact with Deaf adults and other parents of deaf children (e.g., social gatherings, parent support groups).
- Interaction with organizations that support association with the Deaf community such as the American Society for Deaf Children[7] and the National Association for the Deaf[8]

Considerations for Effective Language and Communication Planning

The CIEC has observed that an important factor in designing effective educational practices for children with cochlear implants is purposeful language and communication planning at both the *schoolwide level* and at the *individual student level.*

Schoolwide Planning

At the schoolwide level, it is important that any program enrolling children with cochlear implants first prepare by clearly articulating the school/program's vision, establishing language use practices, providing access to a range of support services, and promoting professional competence.

A Clearly Articulated Vision on the Use of Spoken and Signed Language

In developing a vision that considers the overall linguistic and cognitive needs of children in conjunction with auditory, speech, and spoken language development, it is helpful for schools to develop philosophy and belief statements to exemplify how the school program values and supports the education of children with cochlear implants (as well as other students who have access to sound through hearing aids). Philosophy and belief statements should reflect the importance of looking at the language, communication, cognitive, linguistic, and social-emotional development of the child. It is critical that this vision be applied to designing and implementing program practices that reflect a balance between development and

7. The American Society for Deaf Children supports and educates families of deaf and hard of hearing children and advocates high-quality educational programs and services. For more information, see http://www.deafchildren.org

8. The National Association for the Deaf is an advocacy organization of, for, and by deaf and hard of hearing individuals. In 2000, the National Association for the Deaf developed a position statement on cochlear implants that supports families in their right to make informed choices regarding language preference and use, educational placement and training opportunities, psychological and social development, and the use of cochlear implants and other assistive devices. For more information, see http://www.nad.org

use of auditory, speech, and spoken language skills and provision of an accessible learning environment through the development and use of sign.

Establishment of Language Use Practices

As educational programs establish practices that include both spoken language and sign, several types of sign-inclusive approaches may be considered. The approach chosen should best fit the needs of each individual child. The effectiveness of the approach should be evaluated regularly to determine whether it provides the child with sufficient opportunities to facilitate and use spoken language.

1. *Sign as a support to spoken English.* Children with a cochlear implant are presumed to have the potential to access, develop, and use spoken English for learning. It is therefore reasoned that if sign is included, it should be used to clarify or support concepts spoken in English. If this approach is chosen, it is important for the child to have the ability to use his or her listening ability to access English as a full language for academic learning as well as for social interactions (see section on diverse outcomes). When determining classroom placement for children based primarily on their auditory, speech, and spoken language goals, it is important to think about how grouping students in this manner will affect planning and implementation of the child's academic program.
2. *Bilingual development of ASL and spoken English.* An ASL/English bimodal–bilingual approach promotes language foundations and access to learning through both modalities (auditory and visual) and both languages (ASL and English). Both ASL and spoken English are addressed as independent languages. Strategies to develop and use spoken English are implemented to match the characteristics and goals of each child. ASL can serve an integral role in promoting linguistic and cognitive competence in varied ways—preimplantation as a child transitions to spoken English learning, and postimplantation as a child continues to develop spoken English (Swanwick & Tsverik, 2007).
3. *Interpreters in the mainstream.* An educational interpreter can provide access to communication and learning in a mainstream environment for children with cochlear implants who do not demonstrate the auditory, speech, and spoken language competency to fully access the curriculum and communicate with their peers without the use of a signed language or sign system. Interpreting services should be evaluated on an ongoing basis to determine how best to support the comprehensive needs of the child in the educational setting.

- As children demonstrate increasing proficiency in understanding complex, fast-paced spoken language, it may become appropriate to transition from ASL to a sign system that supports or clarifies English. This decision should be closely scrutinized and monitored. If interpreting is provided via an English-based sign system, consideration should be given to the use of conceptually accurate signing rather than the use of other MCE systems that do not necessarily convey concepts visually and are typically based on how a word sounds.

- The interpreter's role may be expanded to provide support in areas such as preteaching concepts, clarifying information upon request, clarifying multiple meanings of words (e.g., present, park, run), clarifying words that sound the same but are spelled differently (e.g., bear/bare), and cueing the student during fast-paced discussions. If the interpreter is to take on multiple responsibilities in conjunction with interpreting, it is critical that the interpreter, educational program professionals, and the child's family agree on these services as a component of the planning/Individualized Education Program (IEP) process and that the interpreter be qualified to take on these added responsibilities.
- Interpreters can incorporate strategies that offer students the opportunity (as appropriate) to rely on their spoken language ability. These include allowing a child to listen to the teacher or other students before immediately providing interpretation, allowing the child to first listen to the message and then signing words and concepts for clarification as needed, and assisting the child in making links between sign and spoken language (e.g., say it–sign it or sign it–say it).

Provide a Range of Support Services

Support services are integral to successfully meeting the needs of children with cochlear implants. Regardless of the educational setting, consideration of the following supports can be incorporated into planning and provided by the school or outside professionals.

Auditory and speech training. Effective programs for children with cochlear implants should include opportunities to address development of individualized spoken language skills as well as opportunities for spoken language to be used and valued in the child's daily learning environment. There is extensive discussion in the field regarding who is qualified to provide auditory habilitation, how it should be provided (i.e., incorporated in natural environments or in therapy settings), and how often a child should be seen for services. Our experience suggests that (1) there is no uniform recommendation for all children, (2) there may be professionals with varied credentials and backgrounds qualified to provide auditory and speech habilitation services, and (3) more is not always better. Based on our experience, we recommend that the following issues be taken into consideration as decisions are made regarding spoken language habilitation practices:

- All children with cochlear implants should receive some type of auditory and speech habilitation services following implantation either through their hospital implant center, their school program, or a private professional. A habilitation program should continue as long as the child is progressing in his or her development of spoken language skills.
- Auditory habilitation services should be provided by knowledgeable professionals with cross-disciplinary skills in three primary areas: audiology,

speech-language pathology, and education of the deaf. The professionals should have training and experience with the development of auditory, speech, and language skills for children with hearing loss and demonstrate proficiency in the communication mode that the child uses (American Speech-Language-Hearing Association & Council on Education of the Deaf, 2004). Increasing numbers of training/certification programs are preparing professionals to facilitate spoken language for children with cochlear implants.[9] However, experienced specialists who do not have formal certification may be qualified to provide the necessary services. It is important to explore the qualifications of the professional who will be providing services to each child to assure he or she has the necessary training and experience.

- Development of spoken language skills may effectively be addressed in individualized therapeutic sessions, integrated into the child's natural environments (home or classroom), or a combination of both. Some children may learn best in a therapy setting, whereas others may readily develop skills in more natural settings.
- Recommendations regarding the frequency of habilitation services should be specific to each child. Immediately after implantation, the child may require more frequent and focused attention on skill development. As spoken language foundations are established, the frequency of individualized training should be revisited.

Collaborative planning. Ongoing collaboration between hospital implant centers and educational settings (i.e., observations between centers/schools, workshops, teaming, attendance at Individualized Family Service Plan (IFSP)/IEP meetings) is integral to promoting effective language and communication planning and educational program implementation for children with cochlear implants. It is important that hospital implant centers understand the full range of issues involved in educational placement and language/communication planning, and that the school understand the clinical and medical side of implantation. This collaboration is vital to facilitating unified and cohesive recommendations to the family regarding educational placement and language use as well as habilitation practices.

Equipment troubleshooting. A child's success with an implant depends on the device's consistent functioning. Although it is not common, the internal

---

9. The AG Bell Academy for Listening and Spoken Language offers certification for listening and spoken language specialists (LSLS) as either auditory-verbal therapists (LSLS Cert. AVT) or auditory-verbal educators (LSLS Cert. AVEd). Another training program, the Professional Preparation in Cochlear Implants (PPCI), represents a multicenter collaboration to address both the medical and educational aspects of pediatric cochlear implantation. PPCI is specifically designed for teachers of deaf children, speech-language pathologists, and educational audiologists to provide training and experience in providing (re)habilitation services to children with implants.

component of the implant device can fail (Hughes & Pensak, 2006). More common are issues related to the functioning of the implant's external speech processor. To assure optimal functioning, it is critical that professionals working with the child are comfortable with the device, know the personal device settings for each child, and can check the device on a daily basis. School professionals needing support in this area will benefit from access to an educational audiologist in their school system and/or an audiologist from the hospital implant center. Information about how to troubleshoot implant devices can be found on each manufacturer's Web site. To ensure that children are functioning as expected with their implant, it is recommended that in addition to checking the integrity of the equipment itself (speech processor, cords, batteries, settings, etc.) on a daily basis, someone in the child's environment also complete a daily functional check of the equipment while it is on the child using the Ling Six-Sound Check.[10]

Frequency modulation systems. As more and more children are obtaining cochlear implants, the use of frequency modulation (FM) systems to enhance listening is being evaluated (Schafer, 2008). Although FM systems provide significant benefit in noisy environments and when listening from a distance, questions about the most effective use of these devices for children with implants remain (Thibodeau, 2006). There are questions about whether to use direct audio input (an FM device coupled directly to a child's cochlear implant) or a sound field device (an FM system using speakers placed strategically in the classroom). When FM equipment is used for children in ASL/English bilingual classrooms where spoken English is at times directed to only some children in the classroom, a direct audio input system rather than a sound field system may be better suited to not distract students who are not involved in that communication interaction.

Student support groups. If an educational program has several students with cochlear implants, it is beneficial to set up support groups. Support groups provide students with the opportunity to discuss issues specific to their personal experiences with a cochlear implant. Older students can be role models for younger implanted students.

Family education and support. It is critical that school professionals partner with families who are in the process of considering implantation. It is helpful to identify teachers or staff members who are knowledgeable about cochlear implants and can collaboratively provide the family with information about the technology

10. The Ling Six-Sound Check is a tool used to evaluate children's functioning with their cochlear implant using six sounds representative of varied English phonemes across the frequencies integral to understanding speech (ah, ee, oo, sh, s, mm). A child is asked to produce a conditioned response to sound (put a block in a can, raise hand, etc.) to indicate that they are aware of each of these sounds at a quiet listening level. After a baseline is obtained, a change in the child's responses indicates a red flag for further troubleshooting of the child's cochlear implant. For further information about how to do the Ling Six-Sound Check, see http://www.advancedbionics.com/UserFiles/File/Ling_Six_Sound_Check-6.pdf

itself, the medical and audiological evaluations involved in the implant process, and expected performance outcomes for their child (Chute & Nevins, 2002). The school may consider hosting family education workshops on this topic and providing individual counseling to families. It is also beneficial to identify a professional in the school program to act as a liaison between the school and the hospital implant center and assist families in networking with other families who have already gone through the implant process.

Promote Professional Competence

As increasing numbers of professionals in signing settings work with children who have cochlear implants, school programs need to ensure that these professionals are comfortable with cochlear implant technology, understand the varied outcomes for children with cochlear implants, and are competent in incorporating strategies to support not only signs/ASL but also auditory and speech development, academic learning, and social-emotional growth. There are numerous professional training opportunities and educational training guides available through the three cochlear implant manufacturers as well as agencies and organizations with the mission of promoting oral education. There are currently limited training opportunities available to address strategies and techniques for addressing both sign and spoken languages for children with cochlear implants.

Presently, teachers trained in educational philosophies that include sign often do not have the background and experience in facilitating spoken English skill development, and teachers trained in spoken language methodologies often do not have the sign skills necessary to work with students who may benefit from its use. The CIEC has therefore focused attention on offering professional training opportunities throughout the United States to educate professionals about considerations for establishing bimodal educational programs (use of both sign and spoken languages) for children with cochlear implants. To further address this topic, the CIEC has hosted two conferences[11] to encourage national discussion on how to work collaboratively to identify, research, and share evidence-based practices for the growing diverse population of children with cochlear implants who could benefit from bimodal approaches. In addition, the CIEC has worked collaboratively with the Center for ASL/English Bilingual Education and Research[12] at Gallaudet

11. Cochlear Implants and Sign: Putting It All Together (April 2002) http://clerccenter.gallaudet.edu/Documents/Clerc/CIandSL.pdf and Cochlear Implants and Sign: Building Foundations for Effective Educational Practices (April 2009) http://clerccenter.gallaudet.edu/Clerc_Center/Information_and_Resources/Cochlear_Implant_Education_Center/Cochlear_Implants_and_Sign_Language_Building_Foundations_for_Effective_Educational_Practices.html

12. The Center for ASL/English Bilingual Education and Research is housed at Gallaudet University. Its mission is to foster educational leadership and collaborative opportunities for educators implementing ASL/English bilingual programs in their schools.

University in sharing strategies to address spoken English development and use in an ASL/English bilingual framework. This framework is shared with professionals through the Center for ASL/English Bilingual Education and Research's ASL/English Bilingual Professional Development, which is designed for teachers and staff who work in schools for the deaf that follow an ASL/English bilingual philosophy (Nover, Andrews, Baker, Everhart, & Bradford, 2002).

As school programs that use both sign and spoken languages include children with cochlear implants, it is important that teachers and staff be prepared to work with this population of students. It is important to address the following issues in professional training:

- How teachers, audiologists, speech-language pathologists, sign language specialists, counselors, teaching assistants, and interpreters (if in the mainstream) can work as a team to meet a child's language and communication needs. Ideally, teams should consist of deaf and hearing professionals and paraprofessionals. It is important that all teachers and staff understand their role in relation to working with students with cochlear implants.
- The need to establish guidelines for interpreters working with students who have cochlear implants (i.e., use of ASL or English-based sign systems, interpreting strategies for students with varying levels of auditory and speech competence, the possible expanded role of interpreters for students with cochlear implants).
- The importance of understanding each child's auditory functioning level—the level at which a child is functioning on a hierarchy of auditory development (i.e., detection, discrimination, identification, or comprehension; Erber, 1977). A child's auditory functioning level will determine how spoken language and sign will each be used to facilitate language development and use in communication interactions throughout the day.
- Strategies associated with how to promote a child's access to auditory information by modifying the challenge of a listening situation. Professionals and families can incorporate varying strategies related to managing either the content or presentation of a message to make spoken language information either more accessible or more challenging.[13]
- Strategies related to how and when to include (or not include) visual clarification (sign and/or speechreading) to support spoken English in signing environments so appropriate opportunities are available to promote auditory develop-

13. Mary E. Koch, *Bringing Sound to Life: Principles and Practices of Cochlear Implant Rehabilitation* (available through Advanced Bionics Corporation) is a training program for professionals and parents that offers a systematic approach to learning how to listen and understand the connection between a sound and its meaning. This program includes strategies on how to facilitate a child's auditory learning through modification of "challenge factors" related to the content and presentation of a message.

ment and use. Note: although cued speech[14] is a visual strategy considered for use in supporting the English development of children with cochlear implants, the CIEC has not been involved with using and evaluating cued speech.

- Effective strategies to help children make connections between signed and spoken languages. For example, if a child has established vocabulary and language concepts in sign, professionals (and families) can implement strategies to assist children in making links from their known signs to the correlating spoken vocabulary and concepts.

Individualized Planning

Individualized planning for each child is the second part of the language and communication planning process integral to effective educational programming for children with a cochlear implant. Whether a child is in a school for the deaf, a self-contained classroom, a mainstream program, or a typical classroom, an effective program is a program designed to match a child's individual needs related to language use and necessary support services.

To promote individualized planning, it is helpful to develop an individualized language and communication plan. This plan should include documentation of the following:

- A student profile summarizing integral background information and a description of a child's spoken and sign competence.
- Support service recommendations to promote the development of both spoken and sign skills (e.g., auditory habilitation services, sign language classes/services, family sign language classes).
- Recommendations for spoken language and sign language use throughout the school program to support learning.

Although the framework used to document a child's individualized plan may be unique to each school program, the important issue is to have some type of planning process to guide systematic decision making and program monitoring of classroom characteristics and services for each child. This plan can be incorporated into the IFSP/IEP process or used in other ways to share information with families as decisions are made about appropriate programs and services to meet a child's needs.

14. As defined by the National Cued Speech Association, cued speech is a visual communication system that uses eight handshapes in four different placements near the face in combination with the mouth movements of speech to make the sounds of spoken language look different from each other.

Regardless of the format used, it is recommended that the development of an individualized language and communication plan be facilitated by a team of professionals working with the student including the child's teacher(s), speech-language specialist, audiologist, family members, sign language specialists (when available), interpreters, and the student (when appropriate). If auditory habilitation specialists outside of the school are involved with the child, information sharing to facilitate the development of this plan would be beneficial.

Developing a student profile. When developing student profiles at Kendall Demonstration Elementary School, we have found it beneficial to document and discuss a child's functioning along the following two continuums:[15] a receptive continuum for how a child accesses language (visually, auditorily, or somewhere in between) and an expressive continuum for how a child expresses language (sign, spoken, or somewhere in between) (Nussbaum, Scott, Waddy-Smith, & Koch, 2004). Documenting a child's functioning on each continuum has been valuable in providing a baseline for each child to support decision making regarding language and communication practices to best match his or her unique characteristics.

Children's placement on the receptive continuum (see Figure 1) is based on how they generally tend to access information for communication and learning. When children do not have access to auditory information, they would be described as a **big V** learner, indicating that they best access information for learning visually

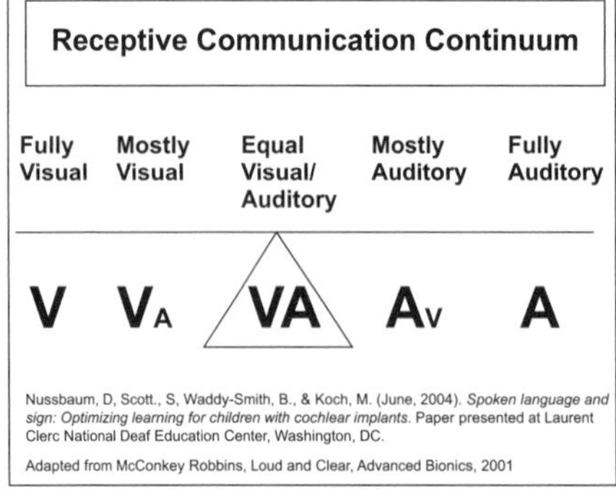

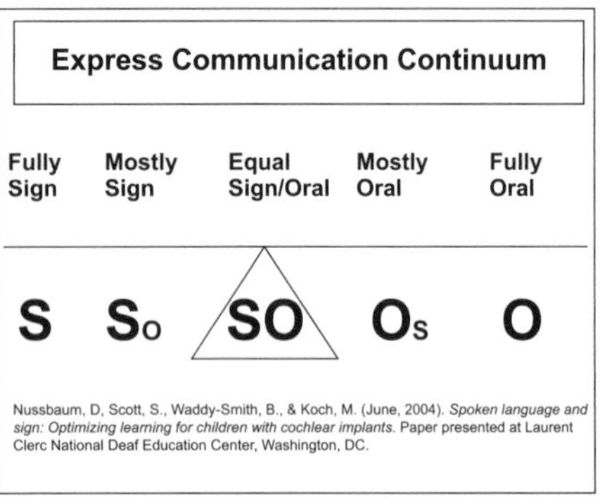

Figure 1: Tool used at the Laurent Clerc National Deaf Education Center to document a child's receptive and expressive communication as part of the individualized language planning process.

15. The receptive continuum was adapted from McConkey Robbins (2001). Both continuums have been included in Clerc Center national professional training workshops provided by the CIEC titled "Spoken language and sign: Optimizing learning for children with cochlear implants" as well as other professional training activities. These continuums are incorporated into the individualized planning process at Kendall Demonstration Elementary School.

through sign. As the child first receives a hearing aid and/or cochlear implant and begins to access auditory information, he or she may move to becoming a **big V, little a** learner, indicating that although primary learning still occurs visually via sign, some learning is beginning to occur through the slowly developing sense of audition. At the **VA** stage of the continuum, the child is able to access information equally through either visual or auditory channels. At the **big A, little v** point in the continuum, the child is able to access auditory information for learning; however, he or she may still benefit from visual information through sign or other visual clarifiers (e.g., pictures, cues, objects). When the child can readily access auditory learning without use of visual information through sign or other visual clarifiers, he or she is described as a **big A** learner. How the child best accesses information either visually or through listening may depend on the characteristics of the listening situation.

It should be noted that even when children have the characteristics to function as **big A** learners they may still demonstrate challenges in listening that affect learning, such as difficulty understanding in background noise and at a distance; difficulty following and understanding the responses and answers of classmates; difficulty understanding the fast rate and complexity of language used in the classroom; difficulty following group discussions, the need for increased processing time to respond; and extra effort listening, which may cause fatigue and loss of focus or attention (Med El Corporation, 2008, p. 31). It is important to consider all of these issues, unique to children with cochlear implants in comparison with their hearing peers, when planning.

It is equally important to describe how children function expressively in their ability to communicate information (see Figure 1). From the expressive perspective, children may be considered a **big S** communicator, indicating that they may most comfortably and readily express themselves through sign. As the child demonstrates beginning development of spoken communication, they may move on the continuum to becoming a **big S, little o** communicator. At this stage, the child primarily uses sign to communicate and oral communication skills are emerging. Children are considered **SO** communicators when they demonstrate the potential to communicate information comfortably through either sign or spoken language. At a **Big O, little s** placement on the continuum, the child primarily uses spoken language with sign used for clarification. When children can comfortably and intelligibly communicate age appropriate language information through spoken language without the use of sign, they may be described as a **Big O** communicator.

As these continuums are incorporated into developing a student profile and an individual language and communication plan, we have found it important to emphasize the following:

- How far each child with a cochlear implant will move along the receptive continuum toward auditory learning and along the expressive continuum toward spoken language competence is not guaranteed. The rate of movement along each continuum will also vary for each child.
- Although a child may have the *potential* to become a **big A** learner or **big O** communicator, school placement and language use decisions should look beyond potential and take into consideration where a child is functioning at the time the plan is developed.
- How a child functions on either continuum may differ in varied settings (e.g., social setting, large classroom, small group or one-on-one communication, noisy environment, complicated fast-paced language use). Language use decisions should reflect a child's needs in these varied settings.
- How a child functions in receptive spoken language understanding may differ from how she or he functions in expressive spoken language use. For example, a child may be able to readily understand spoken language. However, there may be other complicating factors (e.g., oral motor issues) unique to the child that may limit effective use of speech.
- Where a child falls on either continuum will affect recommendations not only in language and communication development but also in all education and social-emotional development areas.

Use of these continuums should be viewed as only one component of individualized planning. It is important to also take into consideration the multitude of other factors affecting a child's development that should be actively addressed in making decisions on school placement and language use (e.g., psychosocial factors, additional learning challenges, language use in the home, the family's and/or child's desire to be in an environment that includes sign language, the child's comfort level and confidence in using either speech or sign). As mentioned earlier, when children have other complex needs in addition to developing listening, speech, and spoken language through their implant (e.g., learning disabilities, second language used in the home, generalized language delays), it cannot be emphasized enough how important it is to also concentrate on these issues in educational planning and family counseling (Edwards, 2007).

Monitoring Progress

It is important to monitor the progress of children with cochlear implants in all areas of development, including spoken language growth. As spoken language skill development in sign-inclusive environments is monitored, it is recommended that available auditory, speech, and spoken language checklists and assessment tools be incorporated to document a child's progress.[16] Any potential red flags

---

16. There is a variety of checklists available to document expected auditory, speech, and spoken language progress for children with cochlear implants. It is important to

should be noted and considered in developing continued recommendations for a child. Decisions regarding educational placement and language use should reflect children's current auditory/speech functioning in relation to their ability to best access learning as well as future aspirations for their spoken language use. Our recommendation is that decisions regarding communication methodology and educational placement be based on comprehensive assessment and monitoring of a child's needs in all areas of development and not solely on the development of spoken language.

If the transition from a signing environment to a speaking environment is under consideration, this process should involve purposeful planning and a systematic approach to evaluating the appropriateness of this transition for the child. As transitioning is considered, keep in mind that even if a child demonstrates spoken language levels to readily access and use spoken language, the appropriateness of an oral mainstream environment should not automatically be assumed. All areas of a child's development should be considered when deciding whether a mainstream oral environment or a setting that includes sign is a more appropriate placement, even if he or she is demonstrating increasing competence as an auditory learner. If transitioning from a sign-based environment to an oral mainstream environment is under consideration, we recommend using *Children with cochlear implants who sign: Guidelines for transitioning to oral education or a mainstream setting* (Boston Center for Deaf and Hard of Hearing Children, Children's Hospital Boston, 2009) as a tool to assist in this process. These guidelines may also be helpful in monitoring children already placed in spoken language settings to ensure that they are appropriately placed or perhaps would be more appropriately served in an environment that includes sign.

Putting it all Together

Although considerations in planning for children with cochlear implants have typically lean toward to oral education approaches, we are optimistic that the field of deaf education is reaching a *tipping point* in viewing language and communication approaches that include both signed and spoken languages for children with cochlear implants. A "tipping point" is a social phenomenon achieved when small numbers of people start behaving differently, that behavior then ripples outward, a critical mass is reached and then large change occurs (Gladwell, 2000). As more children obtain cochlear implants and the obvious diversity in the characteristics and needs of these children and families becomes increasingly apparent, it is hoped

---

chart a child's progress using these guideposts. Checklists include *Tracking Auditory Progress in CI Kids* (McConkey Robbins, 2005), Med El handbook for educators: *Teaching Children who Listen With a Cochlear Implant* (Med El Corporation, 2008, pp. 16–20), and *Benchmarks of Performance for Children With Cochlear Implants* (Nevins & Garber, 2005).

that systemic changes will occur in professional training and educational program development to reflect the considerations discussed in this chapter. We hope that practices that promote linguistic, cognitive, academic, and social competence that include both spoken and sign languages as well as continued connection with the Deaf community will then ripple outward until a critical mass is reached in viewing these practices as accepted and valued recommendations for children with cochlear implants. The CIEC at the Clerc Center looks forward to being a part of this positive change.

REFERENCES

American Speech-Language-Hearing Association. (2004). Knowledge and skills needed by speech-language pathologists and audiologist to provide culturally and linguistically appropriate services. *ASHA Supplement, 24,* 152–158.

Boston Center for Deaf and Hard of Hearing Children, Children's Hospital Boston. (2009). *Children with cochlear implants who sign: Guidelines for transitioning to oral education or a mainstream setting.* Retrieved March 9, 2011, from http://www.childrenshospital.org/clinicalservices/Site2003/Documents/transition.pdf

American Speech-Language-Hearing Association & Council on Education of the Deaf. (2004). *Roles of speech-language pathologists and teachers of children who are deaf and hard of hearing in the development of communicative and linguistic competence* (Position statement). Retrieved March 9, 2011, from http://www.asha.org/docs/html/PS2004-00232.html

Belzner, K. A., & Seal, B. C. (2009). Children with cochlear implants: A review of demographics and communication outcomes. *American Annals of the Deaf, 154*(3), 311–333.

Christiansen, J., & Leigh, I. (2002). *Cochlear implants in children: Ethics and choices.* Washington, DC: Gallaudet University Press.

Christiansen, J., & Leigh, I. (2004). Children with cochlear implants: Changing parent and Deaf community perspectives. *Archives of Otolaryngology, 130*(5), 673–677.

Chute, P., & Nevins, M. E. (2002). *The parents' guide to cochlear implants.* Washington, DC: Gallaudet University Press.

Chute, P., & Nevins, M. E. (2006). *School professionals working with children with cochlear implants.* San Diego, CA: Plural Publishing.

Connor, C., & Zwolan, T. (2004). Examining multiple sources of influence on the reading comprehension skills of children who use cochlear implants. *Journal of Speech, Language, and Hearing Research, 47,* 509–526.

Connor, C. M., Hieber, S., Arts, H. A., & Zwolan, T. A. (2000). Speech, vocabulary, and the education of children using cochlear implants: Oral or total communication? *Journal of Speech, Language, and Hearing Research, 43,* 1185–1204.

Courtin, C. (2000). The impact of sign language on the cognitive development of deaf children: The case of theories of mind. *Journal of Deaf Studies and Deaf Education, 5*(3), 266.

Cummins, J. (2006). *The relationship between American Sign Language proficiency and English academic development: A review of the research.* Retrieved March 11, 2011, from http://aslthinktank.com/files/CumminsASL-Eng.pdf

Dettman, S., Pinder, D., Briggs, R., Dowell, R., & Leigh, J. (2007). Communication development in children who receive the cochlear implant younger than 12 months: Risks versus benefit. *Ear and Hearing, 28*(2), 11S–18S.

Edwards, L. (2007). Children with cochlear implants and complex needs: A review of outcome research and psychological practice. *Journal of Deaf Studies and Deaf Education, 12*(3), 258–268.

Eisenberg, L., Kirk, K., Martinez, A., Ying, E., & Miyamoto, R. (2004). Communication abilities of children with aided residual hearing: Comparison with cochlear implant users. *Archives of Otolaryngology—Head & Neck Surgery, 130*(5), 563–569.

Erber, N. (1977). Evaluating speech perception ability in hearing impaired children. In F. H. Bess (Ed.), *Childhood deafness: Causation, assessment, and management.* New York: Grune & Stratton.

Fagen, M., Pisoni, D., Horn, D., & Dillon, C. (2007). Neuropsychological correlates of vocabulary, reading, and working memory in deaf children with cochlear implants. *Journal of Deaf Studies and Deaf Education, 12*(4), 461–471.

Garber, A., & Nevins, M. E. (2007, July). *Cochlear implants and special populations.* HOPE Note. Retrieved March 9, 2011, from http://www.cochlearamericas.com/PDFs/HOPE_special_populations.pdf

Gardner-Berry, K., Gibson, W., & Sanli, H. (2005, November). Pre-operative testing of patients with neuropathy or dys-synchrony. Emerging trends in cochlear implants. *The Hearing Journal, 11,* 24–25, 28, 30–31.

Geers, A. (2006). Spoken language in children with cochlear implants. In P. Spencer & M. Marschark (Eds.), *Advances in the spoken language development of deaf and hard-of-hearing children* (pp. 244–270). New York: Oxford University Press.

Geers, A. E., Nicholas, J. G., & Sedey, A. L. (2003). Language skills of children with early cochlear implantation. *Ear and Hearing, 24*(1), 46S–58S.

Geers, A., Tobey, E., Moog, J., & Brenner, C. (2008). Long-term outcomes of cochlear implantation in the preschool years: From elementary grades to high school. *International Journal of Audiology, 47*(Suppl. 2), S21–S30.

Geers, A. E. (2002, July). Factors affecting the development of speech, language, and literacy in children with early cochlear implantation. *Language, Speech, and Hearing Services in Schools, 33,* 172–183. Retrieved March 9, 2011, from http://lshss.asha.org/cgi/content/abstract/33/3/172

Geers, A. E. (2003). Predictors of reading skill development in children with early cochlear implantation. *Ear and Hearing, 24*(1), 59S–68S.

Geers, A. E. (2004). Speech, language, and reading skills after early cochlear implantation. *Archives of Otolaryngology—Head & Neck Surgery, 130*(5), 634–638. Retrieved March 9, 2011, from http://archotol.ama-assn.org/cgi/content/abstract/130/5/634

Gladwell, M. (2000). *The tipping point: How little things can make a big difference.* Boston: Little, Brown and Company.

Goldberg, D., & Perigo, C. (2006). *Auditory learning and cochlear implantation for the young child with multiple disabilities.* Audiology Online archived session, HOPE Online Library. Retrieved March 9, 2011, from http://www.audiologyonline.com/ceus/recordedcoursedetails.asp?cp_pid=6&class_id=5253www.cochlear.com/HOPE

Goodwyn, S. W., Acredolo, L. P., & Brown, C. (2000). Impact of symbolic gesturing on early language development. *Journal of Nonverbal Behavior, 24,* 81–103.

Grosjean, F. (2008). *The bilingualism and biculturalism of the Deaf. Studying bilinguals.* Oxford: Oxford University Press.

Hammes, D. M., Novak, M. A., Rotz, L. A., Willis, M., Edmondson, D. M., & Thomas, J. F. (2002). Early identification and cochlear implantation: Critical factors for spoken language development. *The Annals of Otology, Rhinology & Laryngology. Supplement, 189,* 74–78.

Holt, R., & Svirsky, M. (2008). An exploratory look at pediatric cochlear implantation: Is earliest always best? *Ear and Hearing, 29,* 492–511.

Hughes, G. B., & Pensak, M. L. (2006). *Clinical otology.* New York: Thieme Publishers.

Kovelman, I., Shalinsky, M. H., White, K. S., Schmitt, S. N., Berens, M. S., Paymer, N. et al. (2009). Dual language use in sign-speech bimodal bilinguals: fNIRS brain-imaging evidence. *Brain & Language, 109,* 112–123. Retrieved March 9, 2011, from http://www.ncbi.nlm.nih.gov/pmc/articles/PMC2749876

Ladd, P. (2003). *Understanding Deaf culture: In search of Deafhood.* Trowbridge, UK: Cromwell Press.

Leigh, I. W., & Christiansen, J. B. (2009, April). *Psychosocial aspects of cochlear implantation.* Paper presented at Cochlear Implants and Sign Language: Building Foundations for Effective Educational Practices conference, Gallaudet University, Washington, DC.

Litovsky, R. Y., Johnstone, P. M., Godar, S., Agrawal, S., Parkinson, A., Peters, R., et al. (2006). Bilateral cochlear implants in children: Localization acuity measured with minimum audible angle. *Ear Hear, 27*(1), 43–59.

Magnuson, M. (2000). Infants with congenital deafness: On the importance of early sign language acquisition. *American Annals of the Deaf, 145*(1), 6.

Malloy, T. V. (2003, July). *Sign language use for deaf, hard of hearing, and hearing babies: The evidence supports it.* American Society for Deaf Children. Retrieved March 9, 2011, from http://www.deafchildren.org/resources/49_Sign%20Language%20Use.pdf

Marge, D. K., & Marge, M. (2005). *Beyond newborn hearing screening: Meeting the educational and health care needs of infants and young children with hearing loss in America. Report and recommendations of the 2004 National Consensus Conference on Effective Educational and Health Care Interventions for Infants and Young Children with Hearing Loss.* Syracuse, NY: SUNY Upstate Medical University, Department of Physical Medicine and Rehabilitation.

Marschark, M., & Hauser, P. (2008). *Deaf cognition: Foundations and outcomes.* New York: Oxford University Press.

Marschark, M., Rhoten, C., & Fabich, M. (2007, May). Effects of cochlear implants on children's reading and academic achievement. *Journal of Deaf Studies and Deaf Education.* Advance access. Retrieved March 9, 2011, from http://jdsde.oxfordjournals.org/cgi/content/full/enm013v1

Mayberry, R., Lock, E., & Kazmi, H. (2002). Linguistic ability and early language exposure. *Nature, 417,* 38.

McConkey Robbins, A. (2001). Sign of the times: Cochlear implants and total communication. *Loud & Clear!, 4*(2). Retrieved March 9, 2011, from http://www.advancedbionics.com/userfiles/File/Vol4Issue2-Nov2001.pdf

McConkey Robbins, A. (2005). Clinical red flags for slow progress in children with cochlear implants. *Loud & Clear!, 1.* Retrieved March 9, 2011, from http://www.advancedbionics.com/userfiles/File/Issue1-2005.pdf

McConkey Robbins, A. (2007). Clinical management of bilingual families of children with cochlear implants. *Loud & Clear!, 1.* Retrieved March 9, 2011, from http://www.advancedbionics.com/userfiles/File/Loud_and_Clear_107.pdf

McConkey Robbins, A., Burton Koch, D., Osberger, M. J., Zimmerman-Phillips, S., & Kishon-Rabin, L. (2004). Effect of age at cochlear implantation on auditory skill development in infants and toddlers. *Archives of Otolaryngology—Head & Neck Surgery, 130*(5), 570–574.

Med El Corporation. (2008). *Teaching children who listen with a cochlear implant.* Retrieved March 9, 2011, from http://www.cochlearimplants.com/Shared/pdf/en/Handbook_for_Educators.pdf

Moeller, M. P. (2000). Intervention and language development in children who are deaf and hard of hearing. *Pediatrics, 106,* E43.

Moeller, M. P. (2006). Use of sign with children who have cochlear implants: A diverse set of approaches. *Loud & Clear!, 2*(1), 6–12.

Moog, J. S., & Geers, A. E. (2003). Epilogue: Major findings, conclusions and implications for deaf education. *Ear and Hearing, 24*(Suppl. 1): 121S–125S.

Moores, D. (2001). *Educating the deaf: Psychology, principles, and practices* (5th ed.). Boston: Houghton Mifflin.

National Association of the Deaf. (2000, October). *Cochlear implants: NAD position statement.* Retrieved March 9, 2011, from http://www.nad.org/issues/technology/assistive-listening/cochlear-implants

Nevins, M. E., & Garber, A. S. (2005). *Benchmarks of performance for children with cochlear implants.* Audiology Online archived session, HOPE Online Library. Retrieved March 9, 2011, from http://www.audiologyonline.com/ceus/recordedcoursedetails.asp?cp_pid=6&class_id=4774

National Institute on Deafness and Other Communication Disorders. (2011). *Cochlear implants.* Retrieved March 9, 2011, from http://www.nidcd.nih.gov/health/hearing/coch.asp

Nicholas, J., & Geers, A. (2007). Will they catch up? The role of age at cochlear implantation in the spoken language development of children with severe to profound hearing loss. *Journal of Speech, Language, and Hearing Research, 50,* 1048–1062.

Nicholas, J. G., & Geers, A. E. (2006, June). Effects of early auditory experience on the spoken language of deaf children at 3 years of age. *Ear and Hearing, 27*(3), 286–298.

Nover, S. M., Andrews, J. F., Baker, S., Everhart, V. S., & Bradford, M. (2002). *USDLC Star Schools Report No. 5. Staff development in ASL/English instruction for deaf students: Evaluation and impact study.* Santa Fe: New Mexico School for the Deaf.

Nussbaum, D. (2003). *Cochlear implants: Navigating a forest of information . . . one tree at a time.* Washington, DC: Gallaudet University Laurent Clerc National Deaf Education Center. Retrieved March 9, 2011, from http://clerccenter.gallaudet.edu/Clerc_Center/Information_and_Resources/Cochlear_Implant_Education_Center/CI_Navigating_a_Forest.html

Nussbaum, D., Scott, S., Waddy-Smith, B., & Koch, M. (2004, June). *Spoken language and sign: Optimizing learning for children with cochlear implants.* Paper presented at Laurent Clerc National Deaf Education Center, Washington, DC.

Padden, C., & Humphries, T. (1988). *Deaf in America: Voices from a culture.* Cambridge, MA: Harvard University Press.

Petitto, L. A., Katerelos, M., Levy, B., Gauna, K., Tétrault, K., & Ferraro, V. (2001). Bilingual signed and spoken language acquisition from birth: Implications for mechanisms underlying bilingual language acquisition. *Journal of Child Language, 28*(2), 1–44.

Petitto, L. A., & Kovelman, I. (2003). The bilingual paradox: How signing-speaking bilingual children help us to resolve it and teach us about the brain's mechanisms underlying all language acquisition. *Learning Languages, 8(3),* 5–18. Retrieved March 9, 2011, from http://sitemaker.umich.edu/childlanguage/files/petitto___kovelman_2003.pdf

Pyman, B., Blamey, P., Lacy, P., Clark, G., & Dowell, R. (2000). The development of speech perception in children using cochlear implants: Effects of etiologic factors and delayed milestones. *American Journal of Otology, 21,* 57–61.

Schafer, E. (2008, March). Selecting the optimal FM system for children with cochlear implants. *Perspectives on Hearing and Hearing Disorders in Childhood, 18,* 19–24.

Schick, B., de Villiers, J., de Villiers, P., & Hoffmeister, B. (2002, December). Theory of mind: Language and cognition in deaf children. *ASHA Leader, 7,* 6–14.

The ASHA Leader Online, 22. Retrieved March 9, 2011, from http://www.asha.org/Publications/leader/2002/021203/f021203.htm

Sharma, A., Dorman, M., & Kral, A. (2005). The influence of a sensitive period on central auditory development in children with unilateral and bilateral cochlear implants. *Hearing Research, 203,* 134–143.

Sharma, A., Dorman, J., & Spahr, A. (2002). A sensitive period for the development of the central auditory system in children with cochlear implants: Implications for age of implantation. *Ear and Hearing, 23,* 532–539.

Sharma, A., Tobey, E., Dorman, M., Martin, K., Gilley, P., & Kunkel, F. (2004). Central auditory maturation and babbling development in infants with cochlear implants. *Archives of Otolaryngology—Head & Neck Surgery, 130*(5), 511–516.

Snoddon, K. (2008, June). American Sign Language and early intervention. *The Canadian Modern Language Review, 64*(4). Retrieved March 9, 2011, from http://muse.jhu.edu/journals/cml/v064/64.4.snoddon.html

Sommers, R. K., & Lim, S. (2006, July). *How well do young children using cochlear implants succeed in the development of language, speech, and academic skills? What are current research findings telling us?* Retrieved March 9, 2011, from http://www.auditoryoptions.org/research.htm

Spencer, L. J., Barker, B. A., & Tomblin, J. B. (2003). Exploring the language and literacy outcomes of pediatric cochlear implant users. *Ear and Hearing, 24,* 236–247. Retrieved March 9, 2011, from http://www.uiowa.edu/~clrc/pdfs/literacy.pdf

Spencer, L. J., & Bass-Ringdahl, S. (2004). An evolution of communication modalities: Very young cochlear implant users who transitioned from sign to speech during the first years of use. *International Congress Series, 1273,* 352–355. Retrieved March 9, 2011, from http://www.uiowa.edu/~clrc/pdfs/evolution-ci.pdf

Spencer, P. (2004). Individual differences in language performance after cochlear implantation at one to three years of age: Child, family, and linguistic factors. *Journal of Deaf Studies and Deaf Education, 9,* 395–412.

Spencer, P. (2009, April). *Research to practice.* Paper presented at the Cochlear Implants and Sign Language: Building Foundations for Effective Educational Practices conference, Laurent Clerc National Deaf Education Center, Washington, DC. Retrieved March 9, 2011, from http://clerccenter.gallaudet.edu/Clerc_Center/Information_and_Resources/Cochlear_Implant_Education_Center/Cochlear_Implants_and_Sign_Language_Building_Foundations_for_Effective_Educational_Practices/Research_to_Practice.html

Spencer, P., & Marschark, M. (2003). Cochlear implants: Issues and implications. In M. Marschark & P. Spencer (Eds.), *Oxford handbook of deaf studies, language, and education* (pp. 434–450). New York: Oxford University Press.

Spencer, P. E., & Marschark, M. (2006). *Advances in the spoken language development of deaf and hard-of-hearing children.* New York: Oxford University Press.

Starr, A., Picton, T. W., Sininger, Y., Hood, L. J., & Berlin, L. I. (1996). Auditory neuropathy. *Brain, 119,* 741–753. Retrieved March 9, 2011, from http://brain.oxfordjournals.org/cgi/reprint/119/3/741

Svirsky, M. A., Teoh, S. W., & Neuburger, H. (2004). Development of language and speech perception in congenitally, profoundly deaf children as a function of age at cochlear implantation. *Audiology Neurotology, 9*(4), 224–233.

Swanwick, R., & Tsverik, I. (2007). The role of sign language for deaf children with cochlear implants: Good practice in sign bilingual settings. *Deafness and Education International, 9*(4), 214–231.

Tait, M., Lutman, M. E., & Robinson, K. (2000). Pre-implant measures of preverbal communicative behavior as predictors of cochlear implant outcomes in children. *Ear and Hearing, 21*(1), 18–24.

Thibodeau, L. M. (2006, November 28). Five important questions about FM systems and cochlear implants. *The ASHA Leader.* Retrieved March 9, 2011, from http://www.asha.org/Publications/leader/2006/061128/061128e.htm

Thordardottir, E. (2006, August). Language intervention from a bilingual mindset. *The ASHA Leader, 11*(10), 6–7, 20–21.

Waltzman, S., & Cohen, N. (2000). *Cochlear implants.* New York: Thieme.

Waltzman, S., & Roland, T. (2005, October). Cochlear implantation in children younger than 12 months. *Pediatrics, 116*(4), e487–e493. Retrieved March 9, 2011, from http://pediatrics.aappublications.org/cgi/content/full/116/4/e487

Webster's New World College Dictionary. (2005). Cleveland, OH: Wiley.

Yoshinaga-Itano, C. (2003). From screening to early identification and intervention: Discovering predictors to successful outcomes for children with significant hearing loss. *Journal of Deaf Studies and Deaf Education, 8,* 11–30.

Yoshinaga-Itano, C. (2006). Early identification, communication modality, and the development of speech and spoken language skills: Patterns and considerations. In P. Spencer, and M. Marschark (Eds.), *Advances in the spoken language development of deaf and hard-of-hearing children* (pp. 298–327). New York: Oxford University Press.

Zwolan, T. A., Ashbaugh, C. M., Alarfaj, A., Kileny, P. R., Arts, H. A., El-Kashlan, H. K., et al. (2004). Pediatric cochlear implant patient performance as a function of age at implantation. *Otology & Neurotology, 25*(2), 112–120.

Resources

Alexander Graham Bell Academy. http://www.agbellacademy.org

Center for ASL/English Bilingual Education and Research (CAEBER). http://caeber.gallaudet.edu

Children's Hospital Boston. (2003). *Children with cochlear implants who sign: Guidelines for transitioning to oral education or a mainstream setting.* http://www.childrenshospital.org/clinicalservices/Site2003/Documents/transition.pdf

The Children's Hospital of Philadelphia, Cochlear Implant Program. *Professional preparation in cochlear implants.* http://www.chop.edu/consumer/jsp/division/generic.jsp?id=73440

Koch, M. E. (2000). Bringing sound to life. *Loud & Clear!,* 3(1). http://www.advancedbionics.com/printables/archive/v3_1_2000.pdf

National Institute on Deafness and Other Communication Disorders. *Cochlear implants.* http://www.nidcd.nih.gov/health/hearing/coch.asp

10

EDUCATING CHILDREN WITH COCHLEAR IMPLANTS IN AN ASL/ENGLISH BILINGUAL CLASSROOM

Maribel Gárate

The growing number of children receiving cochlear implants and the variability in their speech and language outcomes (Pisoni et al., 2008) has brought increased attention to their educational needs (Leigh, 2008). Within the medical community, emphasis on the exclusive use of spoken language following implantation continues to prevail (Moog, 2007). The use of a signed language with these children is often seen as an obstacle to spoken language development. As a result of this view, educational placements that emphasize speech production and oral communication are considered more beneficial for children with cochlear implants (Geers, 2003). In contrast to these philosophies, an American Sign Language (ASL)/English bilingual approach aims to develop social and academic language proficiency in both languages so that deaf and hard of hearing children benefit from the affective, cognitive, and academic advantages of bilingualism (Nover & Andrews, 1998). In presenting an overview of the current ASL/English bilingual framework for deaf education, this chapter will address the place of spoken English within it and describe the methodologies that provide a space for oral/aural development for children with cochlear implants in these classrooms.

The following ideas frame the information provided in this chapter. First, early language exposure is paramount to language development (Mayberry, 2007; Morford & Mayberry, 2000). Regardless of the degree or type of auditory access, a natural signed language, such as ASL, can provide the linguistic stimulation required for language acquisition (Mayberry, 2007). Second, being bilingual is a desirable quality that results in, but is not limited to, mental flexibility, creative thinking, and concept development (Hamers, 1998). Deaf children *can* and *do* become bilingual in ASL and English in its spoken and/or written form. Lastly, a maintenance model (Baker, 2006) of bilingual education, which will be further discussed in this chapter, is a viable option for deaf children—including children with cochlear implants. Bilingual methodologies within this model allow the development of two languages and each of their receptive and expressive abilities.

HEARING AND DEAF BILINGUALS: SIMILARITIES AND DIFFERENCES

A bilingual person has functional knowledge of two languages. The level of ability in each language may vary depending on the contexts, and the functions and purposes for their use (Baker, 2006). Thus, a bilingual person may have varied levels of fluency in one of his or her languages based on the functions and the various purposes it serves in his or her life. Fluency can also vary over time when a bilingual favors the use of one language over the other. Defined in this manner, communicative competency is viewed in light of the social, cultural, and linguistic demands that different contexts place on a bilingual person (Baker, 2006).

In terms of language use, deaf bilinguals exhibit many of the same characteristics as do hearing bilinguals. However, one significant difference is the variability in the quality and quantity of access deaf children have to a natural language from an early age, be it signed or spoken (Mayberry, 2007). Unlike hearing bilinguals, many deaf children may spend their first years of life unable to access the language of their environment and may receive their first exposure to accessible language via a parent-infant program that introduces the family to ASL. Another group of deaf children is not taught a first language until they enroll in school (Mayberry, 2007). When the child's auditory access is limited, and the language of instruction is an oral language, this process can be arduous. On the other hand, some deaf children may have enough residual hearing to benefit from the use of hearing aids, which allow them to partially access spoken language prior to entering school. This may provide the child with a basis, albeit weak, for continued language acquisition. An additional group consists of deaf children whose auditory access to spoken language may be enhanced by a cochlear implant, creating the possibility for early speech and language development (Ackley & Decker, 2006). In all of these cases, the type of educational placement—and their communication and educational philosophy—will largely determine the levels of fluency a child will attain in one or two languages.

A second important difference between hearing and deaf bilinguals derives from the modality of the two languages deaf bilinguals use—signed and spoken. Notwithstanding this difference, deaf and hearing children who are exposed to both ASL and English acquire linguistic milestones and communicative competencies in a maturational time line equivalent to that of hearing bilinguals who are exposed to two spoken languages (Mayberry, 2007; Morford & Mayberry, 2000; Newport & Meier, 1985; Petitto et al., 2001; Schick, 2003; Spencer, 2004; Volterra & Iverson, 1995). These similarities lend support to the argument in favor of educating deaf children in a bilingual environment and contest concerns about a signed language negatively affecting the development of a spoken language.

language during the pre-school years [as] a prerequisite for subsequent literacy development in English" (p. 7). The data also showed that access to ASL—or other signed languages—provides children with the linguistic input required for concept development. With regard to the second relationship, the research showed a "consistent significant relationship between students' proficiency in ASL and their development of English reading and writing" (p. 11), which offers support for an interdependence between ASL and English much like the one that takes place between two spoken languages. Drawing on these conclusions, Cummins claims that, taken together, these data invalidate the concerns that "acquisition of ASL will inhibit speech or literacy development among children with cochlear implants" (p. 11). Although the bulk of the research reviewed addressed the impact of ASL proficiency on English literacy, not on speech development, Cummins cites a study by Preisler, Tvingstedt, and Ahlström (2002), whose findings suggest a relationship exists between signing proficiency and speech production in children with cochlear implants.

Preisler et al. (2002) reported on a longitudinal study about the communication patterns of 22 Swedish children with cochlear implants, their parents, teachers, and peers. The purpose of the study was to determine factors that contributed to the "positive development of children with cochlear implants, as well as factors being a hindrance to such development" (p. 406). Videotaped interactions and interviews over the course of 2 years were analyzed. The authors identified patterns of interaction, including adult communication style, complexity of dialogue, quality of peer interaction, and the use of sign language, as important factors in the children's individual development. Preisler et al. noted that the 8 children who had worn their implant from 1.5 to 3.5 years and who communicated using Swedish Sign Language were also those with the best spoken language skills.

Cummins's (2006) review also addressed the question "Does the use of ASL as a language of instruction within a bilingual/bicultural program contribute to English academic development?" (p. 11). In response, he noted the paucity of research in program evaluation needed to provide direct evidence for the efficacy of bilingual programs. Nevertheless, he concluded that the evidence provided by the first two relationships described above "supports the overall rationale for bilingual/bicultural programs" (p. 13). Finally, Cummins concluded that, overall, the research consistently showed

- the importance of acquiring a first language as a prerequisite to future literacy development,
- the lack of research evidence to support the claim that ASL will inhibit English acquisition,
- the relationship between ASL proficiency and the development of English reading and writing indicate that bilingual education programs need to focus

on expanding language fluency, conceptual foundation, and intellectual functions in ASL to facilitate the transfer into English literacy skills, and
- the need to establish criteria to evaluate ASL proficiency, articulate effective instructional practices, and develop policy for the teaching of ASL language arts.

Research studies conducted in the United States with deaf children who signed when they received a cochlear implant also support the existence of linguistic interdependence and refute the interference of signing skills with spoken English development (Connor, Hieber, Arts, & Zwolan, 2000). Connor et al. reported that when comparing children who were implanted before the age of 5, there was no significant difference in (1) rates of performance and growth on consonant-production accuracy, (2) receptive spoken vocabulary scores, and (3) rate of improvement over time in spoken vocabulary scores between children with cochlear implants educated in oral program and those educated in total communication programs that used both sign and spoken English. In addition, children who signed and were implanted during preschool or early elementary school demonstrated superior scores and rate of growth over time on their expressive vocabulary (spoken and/or signed). Connor et al. (2000) concluded that the advantage of children who signed may be related to early language stimulation.

Perhaps the most significant findings to date about children who signed preimplantation have come from research studies conducted by Yoshinaga-Itano (2006). The author reported on the knowledge gained from research conducted on deaf children identified via the universal newborn hearing screening program who had also participated in the Colorado Home Intervention Program Colorado between 1994 and 2004. The longitudinal data revealed that of all variables considered, expressive language ability—regardless of modality (spoken or signed) and degree of hearing—influenced spoken language development. That is, children with preimplantation expressive language scores within the normal range, whether spoken or signed, are more likely to develop spoken language skills. Children with milder degrees of hearing loss are also more likely to develop intelligible speech (Yoshinaga-Itano, 2006).

Yoshinaga-Itano (2006) also reported the results from the case studies of 3 profoundly deaf children who had well-established sign language skills and no reported speech perception prior to receiving the implant. Data showed a rapid growth in spoken vocabulary development, reaching near age appropriate production within 12–14 months after implantation. Yoshinaga-Itano concluded that the rapid development may indicate a transfer between the existing lexical foundation present in sign language and the subsequent spoken production. In a presentation about the results from this research at the Conference of Educational Administrators of Schools and Programs, Yoshinaga-Itano, Sedey, and Uhler (2008) reported that, to their knowledge, the success rate for both speech and language for these children is greater compared with children in any other published studies.

Taken together, the literature points to a relationship and a transfer, which supports Cummins's interdependence hypothesis. The children in Yoshinaga-Itano's (2006) study deduced that spoken English was another code for the concepts they already knew in sign. As long as the children continue to develop both languages, they will contribute to and benefit from a shared reservoir of cognitive resources, concepts, subject knowledge, and metalinguistic skills.

Deaf children who receive a cochlear implant need time to become effective implant users, and this process may take up to 5 years (Spencer, 2002). During this time, they still need cognitive stimulation, effective means of communication, unrestricted socializing, and general learning. At the end of this period, outcomes for individual children vary. In many instances, a cochlear implant user functions much like a hard of hearing child (Spencer, 2002; Spencer & Marschark, 2003). Irrespective of the benefits children derive from the implant, when they begin acquiring a signed language prior to implantation and continue signing, cognitive stimulation, communication, socialization, and learning are not interrupted (Preisler et al., 2002). Rather, learning for these children is enhanced.

However, the concern with educating children with cochlear implants in a bilingual environment hinges on the following questions: How will the children's spoken language needs be addressed within a signing environment? Can sufficient access to spoken English be provided? The following section describes the current ASL/English bilingual framework for deaf education to address how spoken English development is planned within the framework.

ASL/English Bilingual: A Framework for Deaf Education

The current ASL/English bilingual education framework adheres to the bilingual maintenance model and emphasizes the development of ASL and English and all their corresponding abilities. English includes two categories, literacy and oracy, and four abilities. Receptive abilities include listening and reading, and expressive abilities include speaking and writing (Baker, 2006). Nover et al. (1998) proposed that ASL/English bilinguals develop receptive signacy skills in ASL, which include the ability to watch or attend to a signed message and the expressive skill of signing. Nover et al. recognize the development of fingerspelling/finger reading, lipreading /mouthing English, and typing as special abilities that incorporate skills from both languages and serve as bridges between the two. The framework does not ignore the development of a child's speaking and listening skills. It does, however, caution that the development should be commensurate with the child's potential for oral/aural development.

To become bilingual, deaf children "need critical opportunities to develop different language abilities in all three categories: signacy, literacy, and oracy" (Nover et al., 1998, p. 67). Signacy entails the child's ability to (1) watch and comprehend signed messages in face-to-face situations, (2) view and comprehend signed messages presented via electronic media, and (3) produce sign messages appropriately in both face-to-face conversations and recorded media. To ensure its development, signacy activities should be integrated throughout content areas; ASL should be used for both social and academic purposes; and opportunities to study ASL and ASL literature should be provided at school (Nover, 2005a, 2005b; Nover et al., 1998). The rationale for signacy development is to provide the child with the linguistic means to both develop and sustain cognitive, conceptual, and communicative competencies, as well as develop overall language fluency that supports literacy development in the second language (Cummins, 2006). Consequently, signacy development should be monitored for all students, but particularly for new signers.

Literacy is defined within the framework as the development of reading and writing via evidence-based instructional strategies, which include reading aloud, shared reading and writing, guided reading and writing, independent reading and writing, writers workshop, interactive writing, and language and word study (Fountas & Pinnell, 2000, 2006). Additionally, literacy instruction should be planned from a sociopsycholinguistic orientation as shown by Freeman and Freeman (1998) in their seven principles for successfully educating English-as-a-second-language and English-as-a-foreign-language students. The principles are (1) learning goes from whole to part, (2) lessons should be learner centered, (3) lessons should have meaning and purpose for learners now, (4) learning takes place in social interactions, (5) lessons should include all four modes,[3] (6) lessons should support students' first languages and cultures, and (7) faith in the learner expands students' potential (pp. xiii–xviii).

Oracy[4] includes listening and speaking skills, and for many deaf children, it also includes lipreading/speechreading and mouthing of English visemes[5] to facilitate communication and comprehension for spoken English. The conceptualization of oracy as an ability that is important for deaf bilingual children departs from the medical model that has long viewed listening and speaking abilities as needing intervention in the form of therapy, rehabilitation, and training. Instead, oracy is seen as an integral part of the educational and life experience of bilingual deaf students at the level that is appropriate for each student's potential.

The development of these three areas, signacy, literacy, and oracy, and their corresponding expressive and receptive abilities hinges on carefully planned instruction and the use of both ASL and English independently. Within the ASL/

3. Freeman and Freeman refer to the four modes of spoken language: listening, speaking, reading, and writing.

4. The term "oracy" was coined by Andrew Wilkinson to bring attention to the oral skills development of hearing students in the United Kingdom (Peate, 1995).

5. A "viseme" is the movement of the face and the lips that occurs alongside the production of a phoneme. Speechreading skills are based on the ability to comprehend visemes during speech production.

English bilingual framework, English and ASL are equal. As such, both languages are languages used for instruction, and both should be given equal attention within the curriculum. The variability in auditory access that deaf children have—with and without amplification—often makes the natural acquisition of English difficult, and this problem has led practitioners to refer to English as the deaf child's second language; and ASL, which uses the more readily available visual channel, has been referred to as the student's first and natural language. However, the ASL/English bilingual framework also considers the needs of deaf children who have initial access to English and learn ASL as a second language as well as the needs of simultaneous bilinguals for whom both languages are acquired from an early age. Deaf children who are exposed to ASL and also receive a cochlear implant at an early age, thereby continuing to develop both languages, are examples of simultaneous bilinguals.

This framework allows us to see deaf children as developing bilinguals and reminds teachers to dedicate time to each of the abilities (signacy, literacy, and oracy) in both languages. By identifying the linguistic abilities children bring to the classroom, the teacher can support their existing abilities, recognize which abilities are in need of remediation, and plan for the introduction and development of any missing or weak skills and abilities. Planning for the development of two languages requires, at a minimum, clear structures and expectations—with models of behavior for the use of both languages in different contexts, for different purposes, and ample opportunities for using each language. As a result, students will learn to recognize what is expected of them when each language is used. The following bilingual methodologies offer teachers options to structure their classrooms based on the linguistic needs of their students and the instructional objectives of their lessons.

Bilingual Methodologies: Description and Application

The bilingual methodologies to be described here have their origin in general bilingual education. The adaptations for the purpose of applying them in an ASL/English setting have resulted from the collaboration between mentors and teachers who have participated in ASL/English Bilingual Professional Development (AEBPD[6]) and the lead mentors and staff from the Center for ASL/English Bilingual Educational Research, who led the training. AEBPD provides in-service K–12

6. AEBPD was formerly known as the STAR schools project. Stephen Nover and colleagues designed the training in 1997 with a grant from the U.S. Department of Education under the United Star Distance Learning Consortium. Nover is the director of the Center for ASL/English Bilingual Education and Research, which continues to provide training to teachers and school administrators interested in implementing bilingual education. For more information visit http://caeber.gallaudet.edu.

teachers of deaf students with information about bilingual theories, principles of English as a second language, theories of first and second language acquisition, and bilingual methodologies that teachers can apply with their students to develop their two languages.

Bilingual methodologies can be grouped into two main categories based on the type of language allocation they fall under: (1) language separation, and (2) integrated or concurrent use of two languages (Baker, 2001; Jacobson & Faltis, 1990). Language separation aims to develop the two languages independently from each other. Presenting the languages in separate contexts and for separate educational purposes, the students are expected to associate each language with specific experiences, contents, and/or settings, thereby developing proficiency in two separate linguistic systems. The two languages can be separated by time, topic/subject, person, place, medium of activity, curriculum materials, function, and student (Baker, 2001; Jacobson & Faltis, 1990). These options can be further classified into those that require program-level decisions for implementation and those that teachers have the autonomy to select and use in their classrooms.

Separation by time, topic/subject, person, and place apply differently depending on decisions made by individual programs. For example, a bilingual program may decide to separate the two languages based on time and design a schedule to use one language in the morning and another in the afternoon. An alternative separation may be to dedicate an entire day to one language and the following day to the other. Similarly, a program that decides to use topic/subject matter as the basis for separation may design a schedule in which social studies is taught in one language and mathematics is taught in the other.

The separation of two languages by person and place can go hand in hand and be applied both at a program level and within individual classrooms. At a program level, a different language is assigned to different classrooms and to specific school personnel. This plan may include, for example, the librarian, computer teacher, and the school secretary, who are "assigned" to use a specific language when interacting with the students. Within the classroom, two teachers (including the classroom aide, volunteer, resource person, and specialist) team up, and each becomes a consistent user of a specific language. The separation by place can also be accomplished within the classroom by designating areas that cue children to use a specific language. A communication center, an activity area, the manipulatives table, the building blocks corner, the media center, and the reading couch are a few examples of places in a classroom that can be assigned to a particular language.

In an ASL/English bilingual classroom, a communication center can be clearly designated for a specific language—one for spoken language use and practice and one for ASL use and practice. Each communication center should be equipped with resources and materials to support the language being used. The spoken English center should have audio CDs, a CD player, and card games and/or computer games that attract students and allow them to use their aural/oral skills.

The ASL center should include ASL videos, DVDs, dictionaries, flashcards, and access to ASL Web sites where students can practice their signacy skills. The speech-language teacher, the classroom teacher, or a language model can also use the centers in a structured manner to hold individual and group sessions. With younger children, it can be an option during free choice time.

Separation by medium of activity, curriculum materials, function, and student are more classroom and language determined than they are programmatic. An example for medium of activity is seen in a classroom where the students' first language is Hmong. The teacher decides to have a group discussion prior to reading a passage. The medium for the discussion would be oral and carried out in Hmong. Once the activity turns to reading, unless there are texts available in Hmong for the specific content, the default language for reading is English. This separation greatly overlaps with curricular materials and their availability or scarcity in each language. Or, as is the case with ASL, the absence of a written form of the language leaves English texts as the sole source of materials for reading purposes.

Separation by medium of activity can still occur in an ASL/English bilingual setting when the medium of the activity is verbal. A selection can be made between the signed or spoken mode (providing such a selection is appropriate for the students in question) for activities that require sharing, discussing, or presenting. Similarly, selected materials in each language such as CDs, DVDs, and computer-based interactive programs and Web sites can be used to allocate time to listening or viewing skills. Technological advances for visual media production make it possible for teachers to assign and evaluate either written or signed homework. Assigning either a blog or a vlog entry is an example of language separation by medium of activity. With multimedia platforms such as VoiceThread™, students can individually create and submit assignments or collaborate using voice via a microphone or phone, text, audio files, or video files via a webcam.

Within the scenarios discussed thus far, there will be moments during which the teacher sees the need to switch the language being used. The reasons may include giving a brief explanation to an individual student, refocusing students to the task, or helping students transition to a new activity. When the teacher initiates this separation, it is labeled a separation of language by function. A separation by student happens when a student wishes to expand on a concept or asks for clarification in his or her more fluent language and initiates the switch.

The ultimate goal of all language separation options is the same: to cue students to the language they should use while providing ample and varied opportunities to use each of the two languages for different purposes. When the decisions are made at the program level, clear expectations and policies are set to ensure everyone is aware of the chosen allocation. Within a classroom, teachers who select and plan for language separation need to spend time modeling and explaining to students the purposes each language serves to help them recognize each language by its characteristics and functions.

The second category of bilingual methodologies is the concurrent,[7] or integrated, use of two languages; this encompasses the following four types: Preview, View, Review; new concurrent approach (NCA); translanguaging; and translation. The concurrent, or integrated, use of two languages aims to promote acquisition of a second language as well as learning curricular content by providing comprehensible input and the use of the students' first language within an activity, a lesson, or a school day.

Freeman and Freeman (2002) proposed the strategy they named "Preview, View, Review" as a way for teachers to structure their lessons so that multilingual learners can access the curriculum regardless of their grade level, English proficiency, or the teacher's proficiency in the students' language (Freeman & Freeman, 2005).[8] The strategy consists of beginning a lesson, activity, or project with a preview of its content in the students' primary language (e.g., ASL). The preview can take several forms such as covering the goals of the lesson, expectations for the activity, reviewing vocabulary, reading a book, previewing a PowerPoint presentation, or watching a slide show. The preview serves to bring forth the students' background knowledge and prepare them for the view portion. During the view portion, the teacher uses English to deliver the lesson in conjunction with strategies that make the language comprehensible: hands-on activities, visual support, demonstrations, paired and group work, role-playing, and graphic organizers, all the while checking students' comprehension. The goal here is to make both the language and the content accessible. When finishing, the teacher and students review the lesson—using the students' primary language again. The review can be a discussion, an oral summary, or a report of the main points, a written summary, a chart, or reading a different book about the same topic. The review can also be a combination of these suggestions when students are preliterate or their literacy skills vary. In an ASL/English classroom, once the teacher has previewed the lesson in ASL, he or she can lead an online discussion within an environment similar to a chat room where students follow along and contribute to the discussion. During the review the group comes together to summarize, discuss, report, or list the main points. The teacher can evaluate and keep a record of the students' comprehension by asking them to videotape their summaries or reports, which is easily achieved on a computer with a webcam. With students who have sufficient auditory access to process content through spoken English, the teacher can substitute the online

7. The term "concurrent" should not be taken to mean "simultaneous." Within the general bilingual education field where this term was first coined, simultaneous use of two spoken languages is not a possibility, nor is "simultaneous communication" an endorsed practice in ASL/English bilingual education.

8. Freeman & Freeman (2005) suggest that a bilingual aide, a tutor, peer, or a parent can preview the lesson with the student(s) when the teacher is not conversant in the first language.

discussion with a lesson or activity in spoken English while applying strategies that make the language comprehensible and checking students' comprehension frequently (Freeman & Freeman, 2005).

The NCA developed by Jacobson (1981, 1990) aims to provide teachers with a systematic way to make decisions about the need to switch between languages within a lesson. During NCA, English is the consistent language of instruction, but the aim is to give the languages equal amounts of time. Grouping considerations for implementing NCA include the students' English proficiency, their socioeconomic status and positive self-identity, the potential need for further first language development, and the teacher's bilingual proficiency (Jacobson & Faltis, 1990).

The decision to switch to the students' language is made by the teacher and regulated by 16 antecedent cues.[9] Jacobson (1981) classified these cues into four main categories: classroom strategies, curriculum, language development, and interpersonal relationships. The teacher becomes attuned to the different cues and responds to them by switching into the students' primary language. For example, the teacher may see the need to switch languages when the purpose is to review, to provide conceptual reinforcement (classroom strategies), or to establish rapport with a student, (interpersonal relationships) or when the type of text or topic (curriculum) warrants the switch. In every instance, language switching should only occur after a complete sentence or idea has been completed. This point is emphasized to ensure students receive complete models of each language. Additionally, the message the teacher provides during a switch should not be an exact translation of what he or she said in English.

The decision to implement NCA for the duration of an activity, a lesson, or the entire school day is heavily dependent on the students' English proficiency. Using NCA during the entire school day with students with beginning level English proficiency or using spoken English all day with deaf children who do not (or not yet—as is the case with newly implanted children) benefit from amplification may not be the most productive choice. A more beneficial approach would be to implement NCA starting with short activities or individual lessons and building to longer periods. Above all, the teacher needs to be attuned to the linguistic and educational needs of the students to support them.

Translanguaging (Baker, 2003) is a methodology that originated in Wales. It consists of providing the input in one language and expecting the output in the other language. For example, during a lesson, the teacher speaks Welsh while giving a presentation, assigns a reading, and provides a handout written in Welsh. The students write notes in English during the lesson, lead a discussion in English based on the reading, and answer the handout in English. This methodology assumes that students have fluency in both languages. The aim with translanguaging is to promote greater fluency, metalinguistic awareness, and deeper understanding

9. For a complete review of the cues and purposes, see Jacobson and Faltis (1990).

of the students' content knowledge in both languages. Baker (2003) suggests that translanguaging is most valuable with science and mathematics because of the cumulative nature of their content. Individual topics within a unit can be taught by alternating languages, thereby allowing students to gradually increase their understanding while using notes, having discussions, and completing assignments in both languages. In an ASL/English bilingual classroom, a lesson (input) can begin with viewing a signed narrative from which the teacher has selected story elements to discuss. The students take notes in English. Once the lesson is over, the teacher asks questions—in sign—and gives students time to answer them in writing (output). Students can also work in pairs or groups and discuss—in English—the questions with each other before writing the group's answer. If students do not have sufficient oracy skills to engage in a spoken conversation, they can work in pairs, and instead of talking or signing their discussion, they can share a computer and coconstruct their answer in writing.

Translating entails expressing a message written or spoken in one language into another. Within the ASL/English bilingual framework a distinction is made between literal and free translations. In literal translation, "the linguistic structure of the source text is followed, but it is normalized according to the rules of the target language" (Nover, 2005b, p. 22). Literal translation is used when the goal is to study the structure of the source language. However, the literal translation of an English text into ASL is not a sign-to-word mapping; rather, syntactic units such as prepositional phrases and dependent clauses within a sentence are translated as a unit using conceptually appropriate signs to maintain their meaning.

In free translation, "the linguistic structure of the source language is ignored and an equivalent is found based on the meaning it conveys" (Nover, 2005b, p. 23). Free translations do not have to adhere to the structure or the organization of the original source. Instead, the structure of the target language is fully used. The purpose is to explore the meaning of the original text via the target language. Therefore, a free translation can also include translation of the implicit meaning conveyed by the word choice and organization of the original text. Teachers can use translation to compare and contrast characteristics of the two languages. For example, teachers can use literal translation to compare a sentence in ASL and its English equivalent to identify the position of adjectives within it or how each language marks adverbs. Free translation from ASL to English can be used to explore the meaning contained in ASL directional verbs or classifier predicates. In each instance, there is a learning objective and an ultimate goal to enhance the students' understanding of language form or meaning. When a teacher routinely translates for the students without a specific goal, this strategy ceases to be effective in developing bilingual skills because students can just wait for the teacher to translate for them when something is too hard to understand (Baker, 2001; Freeman & Freeman, 2005; Jacobson & Faltis, 1990).

Selecting a way to allocate the two languages (separation or integration) and implementing the methodologies within them ensures that intentional planning has taken place and prevents random switching between languages without conscious regard for the clarity of the linguistic message and the content knowledge. Every methodology may not be appropriate for every group of students. Therefore, choices must carefully consider (1) the type of linguistic skills among students—ASL, English, both, neither, or a different language; (2) the levels of fluency in each language—emergent, developing, fluent; (3) the levels of proficiency in each language ability—signacy, literacy, and oracy, and 4) appropriate and diverse resources that support signacy, literacy, and oracy.

Bilingual Instruction: Classroom-Based Examples

Swanwick and Tsverik (2007) investigated the role of sign language for children with cochlear implants within sign bilingual[10] settings and explored whether the goals of sign bilingual education were compatible with the goals of cochlear implantation. Their methodology was to survey school personnel and observe the literacy classes of six programs that operate under the United Kingdom's provisions for sign bilingualism.

Swanwick and Tsverik (2007) focused on three main features within each program: "i) support for spoken language development; ii) the role of sign language; and iii) the attention to the social/emotional and cultural needs of the individual" (p. 216). The practices below come from four schools for the deaf and two mainstream schools identified as sign bilingual programs. The programs served 37 children with cochlear implants between the ages of 5 and 11.

Support for Spoken Language

1. Instruction in small groups in spoken English with British Sign Language (BSL) used to elicit background knowledge, introduce new concepts, and explain terminology[11]
2. Use of spoken English during small group work time
3. Partial or complete lessons taught in spoken English with switches to BSL for support

10. In the United Kingdom, where this study took place, the term "sign bilingual" designates children educated with both British Sign Language and English. It is equivalent to the "ASL/English bilingual" term used throughout this chapter.
11. As described by the authors, this practice resembles a separation of language by person in which a hearing teacher used English and a deaf teacher used BSL during a team teaching situation.

4. Integration of speech and language targets into the curriculum
5. Mainstream classes in spoken English with focused instruction in BSL about curricular content prior to class and with BSL interpreters available for students who need it
6. Continuous collaboration between the bilingual teachers and the speech-language therapist, which includes teaming and planning and training school staff on the needs of students with cochlear implants
7. High expectations for spoken English development and monitoring listening and speaking skills through regular evaluations

The Role of Sign Language

1. To continue development of BSL skills
2. To use with students with cochlear implants at their required level
3. To use as the language of instruction for partial or whole lessons
4. To prepare students for or support students with new curricular information

Social/Emotional and Cultural Needs

1. Deaf adults working with individual students to develop awareness of language and communication choices
2. Deaf adults leading group discussions about culture, identity, and cochlear implants
3. Focusing on students' identity as implant users
4. Viewing deafness positively and respecting students' communication choices

Overall, Swanwick and Tsverik (2007) identified the amount of language flexibility and a strong value for individual identity as important and interrelated factors in sign bilingual environments educating children with cochlear implants. Although not all of the practices were seen in all settings, purposeful language planning and language support for students with cochlear implants were part of each practice observed. The authors caution that these findings cannot be generalized to other programs because different groups of students may require different practices.

The second study evaluated changes in 3 teachers' beliefs and their classroom practices. These 3 teachers were deaf and participated in the AEBPD program. Gárate (2007) interviewed the teachers over 2 years and documented the application of bilingual methodologies via videotaped classroom observations. The teachers were interviewed before, during, and after the AEBPD training. Classroom observations were videotaped for analysis. These observations captured practices that were used to establish the relationship between reported and actual practices. All documents pertaining to their training were collected and reviewed (e.g., assignments, syllabuses, PowerPoint presentations). The interviews and assignments from the training provided the teachers' stated beliefs and reported practices. Finally, to establish whether any changes had occurred as a result of the training, observed instructional practices were compared with the bilingual methodologies (described earlier in this chapter) teachers had learned. The examples of bilingual methodologies shared here come from classroom observations carried out during the fourth and final level[12] of the training.

Language Separation

Medium of activity. ASL/English digital dictionary. The class worked on their entries for the selected list of signs and their translation.

- ASL activities included videotaping the sign, fingerspelling the word, videotaping the sign used in a sentence, and providing feedback to peers on clarity and accuracy of signed entries.
- English activities included typing the words, typing the sentences, and editing peers' sentences.
- ASL/English activities included the teacher using the students' videos and their writing to teach minilessons about the grammatical features of both languages. (The students performed all media-related activities—taping, uploading, cutting, editing, and formatting—after instruction by the media teacher.)

Time

- English only. A set amount of time was designated for students to converse using written English for social purposes. In this classroom, students wrote back and forth about their weekend activities, upcoming games, and video games, among other topics. Learning logs were used for students to reflect about a lesson, a project, or a school day. Their aim was writing for academic purposes.

Place

- Spoken English table. Students could choose to do their assignments, group work, independent reading, or talk to a peer by sitting at a particular table in the classroom.
- ASL corner. Students had access to videos, DVDs, Web-based ASL dictionaries, and Web sites for expressive and receptive fingerspelling practice. The teacher used this space to develop signacy skills.

12. AEBPD training consists of levels I–IV taken over the course of 2 years. Each level is 12-weeks long, and seminars last 2 hours.

Concurrent Use of Language

Preview, View, Review. Science lesson about hurricanes.

- ASL preview. The teacher prepares a PowerPoint presentation, which includes pictures with labels of parts and short videoclips of the formation, stages, and destructive power of hurricanes. With each slide, the teacher either elicits students' contributions or gives a short description/explanation, which often includes the sign and definition of the terms they will learn. The teacher also fingerspells throughout and explains that the students will be asked to identify the parts and at least one of their characteristics.
- English view. The teacher provides students with a copy of the PowerPoint presentation, which contains arrows and spaces for writing terminology and lined areas for notes. The teacher projects the PowerPoint again, and as the labels (i.e., eye, eye wall, rain bands, etc.) appear, the students copy the information onto the designated spaces. The video is shown again, and both audio and captions are added. Another slide shows a text with the description, location, and functions of each of the parts of the hurricane and the instructions "For each part, underline one characteristic (location or function)." The students read the passage on their handout and underline their choice. The teacher walks around the room and helps some students using ASL and checks on others by tracking their text.
- ASL review. Students are asked to find a partner and share their answers. The teacher briefly summarizes the lesson while fingerspelling and pointing to the text. For each part, the teacher asks for a student volunteer to share the characteristic he or she chooses.

In the course of 2 years, all 3 teachers demonstrated increased used of bilingual methodologies and incorporation of specific strategies to bridge ASL and English. Their selection of a methodology was heavily influenced by the linguistic characteristics and needs of the students in the classroom (Gárate, 2007, 2008). For example, the class that worked on the ASL/English digital dictionary consisted of eight students, half of whom had recently arrived in the United States. As such, they were new to both ASL and English and came from non-English speaking homes. In the classroom with the designated spoken English table, five out of six students were functionally hard of hearing; three of them had deaf parents. They were highly adept at switching between languages at designated times and places.

CONCLUSION

Because a cochlear implant provides access to sound and speech perception and as such facilitates spoken language development at levels that were not previously accessible via conventional hearing aids for profoundly deaf children, many people recommend against the use of sign language. Rather, these individuals advocate that children with cochlear implants be educated in oral programs (Geers, 2003; Moog, 2007)—an option that leads to becoming monolingual. This review of research suggests that the attainment of bilingual competencies can result in a range of language skills, communication options, and cognitive benefits applicable across contexts. Children with cochlear implants have the potential to benefit from the acquisition of ASL while still developing their spoken language within a maintenance model, which aims for bilingualism. Given that these children are still deaf, they also have the right to a visual language that is fully accessible and can provide the linguistic basis onto which spoken language development can be mapped.

However, people express concern about the feasibility of the transfer of skills between a signed and a spoken language. Available data suggest a relationship between early ASL fluency and subsequent English academic development (Cummins, 2006). Additional support for the existence of this transfer is emerging from studies on young deaf children who had well-developed signed expressive language prior to implantation (Yoshinaga-Itano, 2006). As a result, their speech and overall language gains postimplantation surpassed the performance of all other results reported to date (Yoshinaga-Itano et al., 2008).

A second concern hinges on the availability of opportunities for children with cochlear implants to develop spoken English within a bilingual program. The ASL/English bilingual framework for deaf education described here views ASL and English as equally important languages in the lives of deaf children. As such, it emphasizes the need for their development by addressing each of the language abilities—signacy, literacy, and oracy—to the degree that is appropriate for each individual learner.

The framework combines knowledge, pedagogy, and methodologies from bilingual education, English as a second language instruction, second language acquisition, and best practices in literacy instruction for second language learners. It guides school personnel and teachers to think about deaf children as bilingual individuals and to plan accordingly. Teachers who attend AEBPD training learn to apply these bilingual methodologies and strategies effectively in the classroom. Within this framework, bilingual methodologies help teachers plan for the allocation of both languages.

Language separation provides students the opportunity to acquire and learn each language by using it, studying it, and learning through it. Language separation also develops fluency in ASL, and in spoken/written English, independently. Teachers select options for separation based on the linguistic levels and educational needs of their students. As these change, teachers implement variations of these options to challenge or support students' growth. Methodologies that emphasize the concurrent use of language aim to support students' language development and access to the curriculum by providing more immediate support for both.

There is little research about the application of bilingual methodologies with deaf children and about the ways bilingual programs can meet the needs of children with cochlear implants. Examples from two sources were shared (Gárate, 2007; Swanwick & Tsverik, 2007). In both instances, provisions were made to allocate language use to support students' signacy, literacy, and oracy, and those decisions were made based on the students' characteristics. Additional research in this area is highly recommended.

References

Ackley, S. R., & Decker, T. N. (2006). Audiological advances and the acquisition of spoken language in deaf children. In P. Spencer & M. Marschark (Eds.), *Advances in the spoken language development of deaf and hard of hearing children* (pp. 298–327). New York: Oxford University Press.

Baker, C. (2001). *Foundations of bilingual education and bilingualism* (3rd ed.). Clevedon, England: Multilingual Matters.

Baker, C. (2003). Biliteracy and transliteracy in Wales: Language planning and the Welsh National Curriculum. In N. H. Hornberger (Ed.), *Continua of biliteracy* (pp. 71–90). Clevedon, England: Multilingual Matters.

Baker, C. (2006). *Foundations of bilingual education and bilingualism* (4th ed.). Clevedon, England: Multilingual Matters.

Connor, M. C., Hieber, S., Arts, A., & Zwolan, T. A. (2000). Speech, vocabulary, and the education of children using cochlear implants. *Journal of Speech, Language, and Hearing Research Communication, 43,* 1185–1204.

Cummins, J. (1981). The role of primary language development in promoting educational success for language minority students. In California State Department of Education (Ed.), *Schooling and language minority students: A theoretical framework* (pp. 3–49). Los Angeles: California State University, Evaluation, Dissemination and Assessment Center.

Cummins, J. (2001). *Negotiating identities: Education for empowerment in a diverse society* (2nd ed.). Los Angeles: Association for Bilingual Education.

Cummins, J. (2006, October). *The relationship between American Sign Language proficiency and English academic development: A review of the research.* Paper presented at the workshop Challenges, Opportunities, and Choices in Educating Minority Group Students, Hamar University College, Norway.

Ferguson, C. A., Houghton, C., & Wells, M. H. (1977). Bilingual education: An international perspective. In B. Spolsky & R. Cooper (Eds.), *Frontiers of bilingual education* (pp. 159–174). Rowley, MA: Newbury House.

Fountas, I. C., & Pinnell, G. S. (2000). *Guiding readers and writers (grades 3–6) teaching comprehension, genre, and content literacy.* Portsmouth, NH: Heinemann.

Fountas, I. C., & Pinnell, G. S. (2006). *Teaching for comprehending and fluency K-8: Thinking, talking, and writing about reading.* Portsmouth, NH: Heinemann.

Freeman, Y. S., & Freeman, D. E. (1998). *ESL/EFL teaching: Principles for success.* Portsmouth, NH: Heinemann.

Freeman, Y. S., & Freeman, D. E. (2002). *Closing the achievement gap: How to reach the limited formal schooling and long-term learners.* Portsmouth, NH: Heinemann.

Freeman, Y. S., & Freeman, D. E. (2005). Preview, view, review: Giving multilingual learners access to the curriculum. In L. Hoyt (Ed.), *Spotlight on comprehension* (pp. 453–457). Portsmouth, NH: Heinemann.

Gárate, M. (2007). *A case study of an in-service professional development model on bilingual deaf education: Changes in teachers' stated beliefs and classroom practices.* Unpublished doctoral dissertation, Gallaudet University, Washington, DC.

Gárate, M. (2008). Bilingual deaf education: Changes in teacher's stated beliefs and classroom practices. *Rivista Di Sicolinguistica Applicata, 3,* 64–73.

Geers, A. E. (2003, May). Cochlear implant and education for the deaf child. *Hearing review.* Retrieved August 7, 2009, from www.hearingreview.com/issues/articles/2003-05_01.asp

Genesee, F., Lindholm-Leary, K., Saunders, W. M., & Christian, D. (2006). *Educating English language learners.* New York: Cambridge University Press.

Grosjean, F. (2001). The right of the deaf child to grow up bilingual. *Sign Language Studies, 1*(2), 110–114.

Hamers, J. (1998). Cognitive and language development of bilingual children. In I. Parasnis (Ed.), *Cultural and language diversity and the deaf experience* (pp. 51–75). New York: Cambridge University Press.

Jacobson, R. (1981). The implementation of a bilingual instructional model: The new concurrent approach. In R. V. Padilla (Ed.), *Ethnoperspectives in bilingual education research. Vol. 3: Bilingual education technology* (pp. 14–29). Ypsilanti: Eastern Michigan University Press.

Jacobson, R. (1990). Allocating two languages as a key feature of a bilingual methodology. In R. Jacobson & C. Faltis (Eds.), *Language distribution issues in bilingual schooling* (pp. 3–17). Clevedon, England: Multilingual Matters.

Jacobson, R., & Faltis, C. (1990). *Language distribution issues in bilingual schooling.* Clevedon, England: Multilingual Matters.

Johnson, R. E., Liddell, S. K., & Erting, C. J. (1989). Unlocking the curriculum: Principles for achieving access in deaf education. *GRI Working Paper Series, No. 89–3.* Washington, DC: Gallaudet Research Institute, Gallaudet University.

Leigh, G. (2008). Changing parameters in deafness and deaf education: Greater opportunities but continuing diversity. In M. Marschark & P. Hauser (Eds.), *Deaf cognition* (pp. 24–51). New York: Oxford University Press.

Mayberry, R. (2007). When timing is everything: Age of first-language acquisition effects on second-language learning. *Applied Psycholinguistics, 28,* 537–549.

Moog, J. S. (2007). The auditory-oral approach: A professional perspective. In S. Schwartz (Ed.), *Choices in deafness: A parents' guide to communication options* (pp. 131–158). Bethesda, MD: Woodbine House.

Morford, J., & Mayberry, R. (2000). A reexamination of 'early exposure' and its implications for language acquisition by eye. In C. Chamberlain, J. Morford, & R. Mayberry (Eds.), *Language acquisition by eye* (pp. 111–127). Mahwah, NJ: Erlbaum.

Newport, E., & Meier, R. (1985). The acquisition of American Sign Language. In D. Slobin (Ed.), *The crosslinguistic study of language acquisition* (Vol. 1, pp. 881–938). Hillsdale, NJ: Erlbaum.

Nover, S. (2005a, March). *Language planning in (deaf) education.* Paper presented at the Center for ASL/English Bilingual Education and Research conference, Washington, DC.

Nover, S. (2005b, July). *Signacy framework.* PowerPoint presentation at Enhancing Deaf Education: Language Planning and Leadership, Washington, DC.

Nover, S., & Andrews, J. (1998). *Critical pedagogy in deaf education: Bilingual methodology and staff development: Year 1 (1997–1998).* Santa Fe: New Mexico School for the Deaf.

Nover, S., Andrews, J., Baker, S., Everhart, V., & Bradford, M. (2002). *Critical pedagogy in deaf education: Bilingual methodology and staff development: Year 5 (2001–2002).* Santa Fe: New Mexico School for the Deaf.

Nover, S., Christensen, K., & Cheng, L. (1998). Development of ASL and English competence for learners who are deaf. *Topics in Language Disorders, 18*(4), 61–72.

Nover, S., & Ruíz, R. (1994). The politics of American Sign Language in deaf education. In B. Schick & M. P. Moeller. (Eds.), *The use of sign language in instructional settings: Current concepts and controversies* (pp. 73–84). Omaha, NE: Boys Town National Research Hospital.

Ovando, C., & Collier, V. (1998). *The politics of multiculturalism and bilingual education: Students and teachers caught in the crossfire.* Boston: McGraw Hill.

Peate, M. P. (1995). Oracy issues in ESL teaching in key stage 2: Using the language master as a bridge between non-standard and standard English. In M. K. Verma, K. P. Corrigan, & S. Firth (Eds.), *Working with bilingual children: Good practice in the primary classroom* (pp. 154–163). Clevedon, England: Multilingual Matters.

Petitto, L., Katerelos, M., Levy, B., Gauna, K., Tétreault, K., & Ferraro, V. (2001). Bilingual signed and spoken language acquisition from birth: Implications for the mechanisms underlying early bilingual language acquisition. *Journal of Child Language, 28*(2), 453–496.

Pisoni, D. B., Conway, C. M., Kronenberger, W. G., Horn, D. L., Karpicke, J., & Henning, S. C. (2008). Efficacy and effectiveness of cochlear implants in deaf children. In M. Marschark & P. Hauser (Eds.), *Deaf cognition* (pp. 52–101). New York: Oxford University Press.

Plaza-Pust, C., & Morales-López, E. (Eds.). (2008). *Sign bilingualism: Language development, interaction, and maintenance in sign language contact situations.* Amsterdam: John Benjamins.

Preisler, G., Tvingstedt, A., & Ahlström, M. (2002). A psychosocial follow-up study of deaf preschool children using cochlear implants. *Child: Care, Health and Development, 28*(5), 403–418.

Ruíz, R. (1984). Orientations in language planning. *NABE Journal, 8*(2), 15–34.

Schick, B. (2003). The development of American Sign Language and manually coded English systems. In M. Marschark & P. E. Spencer (Eds.), *Oxford handbook of deaf studies, language, and education* (pp. 219–231). New York: Oxford University Press.

Spencer, P. (2002). Considerations for the future: Putting it all together. In D. Nussbaum, R. LaPorta, & J. Hinger (Eds.), *Cochlear implants and sign language: Putting it all together (Identifying effective practices for educational settings)* (pp. 23–29). Washington, DC: Laurent Clerc National Deaf Education Center.

Spencer, P. (2004). Language at 12 and 18 months: Characteristics and accessibility of linguistic models. In K. Meadow-Orlans, P. Spencer, & L. Koester (Eds.), *The world of deaf infants: A longitudinal study* (pp. 147–167). New York: Oxford University Press.

Spencer, P., & Marschark, M. (2003). Cochlear implants: Issues and implications. In M. Marschark & P. E. Spencer (Eds.), *Oxford handbook of deaf studies, language, and education* (pp. 434–448). New York: Oxford University Press.

Swanwick, R., & Tsverik, I. (2007). The role of sign language for deaf children with cochlear implants: Good practices in sign bilingual settings. *Deafness and Education International, 9*(4), 214–231.

Volterra, V., & Iverson, J. (1995). When do modality factors affect the course of language acquisition? In K. Emmorey & J. Reilly (Eds.), *Language, gesture and space* (pp. 371–390). Hillsdale, NJ: Erlbaum.

Yoshinaga-Itano, C. (2006). Early identification, communication modality, and the development of speech and spoken language skills: patterns and considerations. In P. Spencer & M. Marschark (Eds.), *Advances in the spoken language development of deaf and hard of hearing children* (pp. 298–327). New York: Oxford University Press.

Yoshinaga-Itano, C., Sedey, A., & Uhler, K. (2008). *Speech piggybacks onto sign: Fast-mapping from sign to speech.* Paper presented at the Conference of Educational Administrators of Schools and Programs, Boulder, CO.

11

APPLICATION OF AUDITORY (RE)HABILITATION TEACHING BEHAVIORS TO A SIGNED COMMUNICATION EDUCATION CONTEXT

Jill Duncan

This chapter focuses explicitly on teaching behaviors that can be used by the teacher of the deaf[1] to facilitate the auditory-based spoken language development of students in a signed communication education environment. It presents potential challenges the teacher of the deaf may face in this special learning context. What this chapter does not do is prescribe when auditory-based spoken language is to be used in this unique education environment. That is a matter for the family, school leaders, and the education team to decide. The reader is encouraged to see Mayer and Leigh (2010) for a review of pertinent issues regarding the changing context of sign bilingual education and the applicability of simultaneous production of signed and spoken codes. This chapter closes with a case study pertinent to the topic.

In addition to the teaching behaviors presented here and as a matter of principle and regardless of communication methodology, teachers of the deaf are encouraged to use an integrated, developmental approach whereby the progression of cognitive and linguistic functioning is accomplished through social interaction. Attention is consistently placed on the development of communication through natural social discourse as well as activities within and outside of the formal learning context. The teacher is encouraged to maintain a process focus at all times so that "how the student is learning" as compared with "what the student is learning" is identified to the students and made explicit throughout all interactions (Duncan, Rhoades, & Fitzpatrick, in press).

Ten core teaching behaviors presented in this chapter are excerpts from the work of Duncan, Kendrick, McGinnis, and Perigoe (2010). Many of the teaching behaviors were identified by Caleffe-Schenck (1983, 1992a, 1992b) and later refined by Perigoe (Auditory-Verbal International, 2004; Auditory-Verbal International,

1. The "teacher of the deaf" is the practitioner who holds an undergraduate qualification in education and a graduate qualification in deaf education.

Certification Council, 2004; Auditory-Verbal International, Professional Education Committee, 1998–1999). All teaching behaviors can be identified in the work of Helen Beebe (1953, 1976, 1982), Beebe, Pearson, and Koch (1984), Doreen Pollack (1964, 1970, 1981, 1984), and Daniel Ling (1964, 1973, 1976, 1984, 1989, 2002).

Due to the origin of the teaching behaviors presented, each is linked to the auditory-verbal methodology (see, for example, Duncan, 2006). In recent times, the term "auditory (re)habilitation" has been used by the author instead of auditory-verbal due to its inclusiveness of all children and students using auditory-based spoken language regardless of age, culture, and language preference (Duncan et al., 2010).

For the purpose of this chapter, 10 key teaching behaviors have been chosen. Many more teaching behaviors can be applied to this pedagogical context; however, these 10 are fundamental to the facilitation of auditory-based spoken communication (Duncan et al., 2010). After the teacher of the deaf becomes confident employing these teaching behaviors, additional behaviors can be incorporated when appropriate.

For children using hearing technology such as cochlear implants or hearing aids, upon enrollment in a class, teachers are expected to engage in a discussion with families regarding the anticipated use and purpose of the student's hearing technology. It is essential that the teacher understand the extent to which the student is expected to use audition in day-to-day communication. Following this family discussion, the teacher is encouraged to have an ongoing open discussion with the whole class and individual students regarding the use of hearing technology in the classroom. Students themselves need to be aware of who is and who is not using hearing technology. Among other things, this facilitates the development of empathy as the students without hearing technology endeavor to help maintain an appropriate acoustic environment. To this end, all class members understand the importance of hearing technology and listening when using auditory-based spoken language to communicate.

In this chapter the teaching behaviors are categorized into cognitive linguistic, auditory, and speech. These teaching behaviors are thought to facilitate listening and spoken language development for students with hearing loss (Duncan et al., 2010). Bear in mind that these teaching behaviors are to be used not in isolation but as part of a repertoire of strategies (Duncan, 2006).

AUDITORY

A critical element of enhancing auditory-based spoken language development is regular access to the speech spectrum. This requires ongoing surveillance of both the acoustic environment and the student's personal hearing technology. If the student does not have access to the speech spectrum then spoken language development will be encumbered. The teacher of the deaf is encouraged to be continuously cognizant of the acoustic environment every time spoken language is used in the classroom. To this end, half of the teaching behaviors presented here focus on the auditory domain.

1. Monitor Hearing Device Function

Appropriate, early, and consistent fitting and programming of all hearing technology is necessary to access auditory-based spoken language. Fundamental to this is the teacher's audiological knowledge and skill and its application to the student's use of the hearing technology. To predict student auditory-based spoken language reception and expression, it is essential that the teacher understand the cochlear implant MAP[2] in general and the individual student's MAP in particular. Teachers must also be aware of each MAP's limitations. In addition to this, the teacher needs to understand the individual student's cochlear implant speech processor settings so that students can be encouraged to change the setting depending on the acoustic environment.

The teacher of the deaf supports the family in scheduling regular audiology appointments so that the MAP is stable and student benefit is maximized. The teacher can encourage the audiologist to complete annual speech perception tests to glean a greater understanding of how the hearing technology is assisting auditory-based spoken language development.

The teacher of the deaf supports the student in becoming an efficient manager of hearing technology by arranging opportunities to understand and practice basic equipment maintenance (Duncan et al., 2010). When a student is able, care of listening technology can become the student's exclusive responsibility; however, the teacher of the deaf continues to monitor the device systematically throughout formal instruction.

2. Provide Spoken Language Input Through Audition

Auditory-based spoken language is a reflection of what is heard (Ling, 2002). Put simply, the student requires the opportunity to hear abundant, unambiguous, clear spoken language so that its acoustic properties, including all segmental and suprasegmental information, can be incorporated into the child's production of spoken language. Regular attention must be drawn by the teacher of the deaf to the auditory signal so that the student learns to identify, discriminate, and comprehend its intended meaning. To this end, the use of a classroom assistive listening

2. The cochlear implant MAP is the specifications of threshold, suprathresholds, and frequency by which the speech processor processes the auditory signal and delivers it in electrical form to the electrode array (Tye-Murray, 2009).

device in which the teacher wears a microphone that transmits the auditory signal directly to the listener may benefit the student by minimizing background noise and improving the quality of spoken language input.

As a matter of principle and to maximize development, the family and school team structure regular opportunities for the student's exposure to auditory-based spoken language and practice of associated skills—in both an informal social discourse context and a formal didactic context. This is best accomplished through precise planning to minimize the risk of insufficient exposure resulting in less than adequate progress.

3. Maximize Audition by Positioning the Student as Close as Practicable to the Speaker

Strategic positioning of students can maximize auditory input (Ling, 1989, 2002). The teacher of the deaf should take care to sit on the side of the student's cochlear implant so the student can hear the auditory signal. A favorable acoustic environment can be created by minimizing background noise (acoustic clutter) and maximizing auditory input to support the student's auditory learning.

Spoken language must be loud enough to hear. Background noise may interfere with the student's ability to hear and process spoken language. For example, a computer, data projector, or air conditioner may create background noise that results in an inferior speech reception opportunity. In addition, the teacher of the deaf must be aware of and endeavor to monitor nonlinguistic student noise in the classroom, as this too may interfere with the auditory signal. Again, the use of a classroom assistive listening device by students with hearing aids and/or cochlear implants may assist in improving the signal to noise ratio within the classroom environment. Regardless, the teacher of the deaf is encouraged to keep the students with hearing technology close to the speaker when auditory-based spoken language is used. In addition, it may be prudent to place the student with hearing technology so that the hearing technology itself is positioned away from the noise source.

4. Use Acoustic Highlighting to Enhance Key Elements of Spoken Language

Acoustic highlighting is the practice of enhancing the audibility of specific elements of auditory-based spoken language to assist the listener by making specific components of the message more salient (Daniel, 1987). Acoustically highlighted words generally have vowels that are elongated and made slightly louder than the rest of the word or phrase. As necessary, teachers of the deaf should acoustically highlight new, unfamiliar vocabulary words while encouraging the student to listen to the new stimulus. As the student becomes skilled in processing information through audition, the teacher of the deaf decreases the amount of acoustic highlighting. Acoustic highlighting techniques also include singing, whispering, and emphasizing specific suprasegmentals and/or segmental features (Duncan et al., 2010).

Acoustic highlighting can also be used by the student when communicating with peers who use auditory-based spoken language. The teacher of the deaf models a stimulus for the student and when appropriate may request that the child imitate the production to encourage carryover into spoken language.

5. Develop and Use the Auditory Feedback System to Facilitate Speech and Spoken Language Production

The "auditory feedback loop" or "speech chain" (Denes & Pinson, 1993) involves the student correcting the production of his or her spoken language based on self-identified errors or feedback from the communication partner indicating an error. To develop and monitor speech intelligibility, it is important for students who use auditory-based spoken language to learn to listen to their own speech. This will require the teacher of the deaf to draw attention to the students' speech and the speech of others.

In the course of daily instruction and when the student is engaging in auditory-based spoken language, the teacher of the deaf chooses speech targets appropriate to the students and consistently monitors the student production as well as speech reception of the target (Duncan et al., 2010). To ensure reasonable expectations, the teacher is encouraged to limit speech corrections to identified targets. The student is not required to meet one speech goal before progressing to the next one. The teacher of the deaf can choose a few goals and cycle through them accordingly. This is not to say that habituation of speech errors is encouraged.

Cognitive Linguistic

The following three teaching behaviors assist in focusing attention on auditory-based spoken language itself.

6. Communicate With the Student in a Manner That Facilitates Natural Social Discourse

The teacher of the deaf monitors the student's spoken language contribution to social discourse and is careful to wait for the student to process the information and reciprocate verbally. During this interaction, it is important for the teacher to demonstrate a high level of support. The teacher draws information from the student using a range of scaffolding strategies including questioning and expanding and directing while taking every opportunity to engage the student in an age appropriate metacognitive and metalinguistic discussion (Duncan et al., 2010). Throughout the auditory-based spoken language interaction, the teacher uses clear and unambiguous language while conversing with the student slightly above his or her cognitive and linguistic levels.

7. Use Wait Time (Expectant Pauses) to Encourage Turn Taking and Auditory Processing

A strategically used pause allows the student time to process the auditory signal while provoking a verbal response (Duncan et al., 2010). It also facilitates the development of turn taking. As the student's skill develops, the teacher of the deaf reduces the scaffolding, which, in this instance, is the length of the pause. The teacher of the deaf is careful to maintain appropriate pacing that allows the student to learn while continuously monitoring the student's responses to check for comprehension and alter pacing, if required (Duncan et al., 2010). Adequate time must be given to the student to process the auditory-based spoken message. The importance of allowing adequate time to process information is explicitly conveyed to parents, teacher's aides, and volunteers so that they too may facilitate auditory-based spoken language with patience.

8. Use Strategies to Stimulate Thinking About Listening and Spoken Language

In all lessons, teachers are encouraged to highlight metacognitive and metalinguistic skills to students. Habitual and explicit use of the vocabulary of thinking (e.g., "forget," "remember," "elaborate," "judge," "reflect," "consider," "imagine") will facilitate a focus on process rather than on product in teaching (Duncan et al., in press). The teacher of the deaf is careful to bring thinking processes to the awareness of students. Strategies for improving auditory skills, in particular, should be highlighted.

SPEECH

9. Model and Facilitate Speech and Spoken Language With Natural Rate, Rhythm, and Prosody

To develop fluent spoken language, the student must hear language that is pragmatically, syntactically, semantically, and phonologically correct (Duncan et al., 2010). Prosodic information is carried primarily in the lower frequency range, which means that the majority of students who use cochlear implants can access this information. The use of prosodic features increases speech intelligibility.

Keep in mind that for students to produce intelligible speech, intelligible speech must be regularly modeled for and heard by the student. Again, explicit exposure to this speech model ought to be scheduled into the student's learning experience.

10. Accept or Facilitate Students' Intelligible Speech Production, Including Effectively Implementing Appropriate Strategies for Development/Remediation

Caution: Speech errors that occur regularly and are not brought to the attention of the speaker may habituate with time. Care is taken to discourage habituating speech errors. In general, speech remediation is far more difficult than facilitation of speech development. It is far better to prevent a speech error from interfering with speech intelligibility than to implement speech remediation to eliminate it from spoken language.

This acquisition of speech patterns can be promoted through rigorous use of audition. The process of facilitating speech development involves extensive knowledge of the principles of both speech perception (acoustics) and speech production, including how speech sounds develop and how they build on previously learned speech patterns (Duncan et al., 2010). Important skills required of the teacher of the deaf who is expected to facilitate auditory-based spoken language development includes the following: the ability to assess which features of speech the student is able to access through hearing, which speech sounds and processes are developmentally appropriate, and which prerequisite skills the student has mastered (Duncan et al., 2010). It is critical that the teacher of the deaf be skilled at using appropriate strategies for both informal and formal speech development and remediation (Ling, 1976, 1989, 2002).

POTENTIAL CHALLENGES

The teacher of the deaf may encounter numerous challenges when endeavoring to facilitate development of both an auditory-based spoken language and a signed language in a singular group of children. Five challenges are highlighted here along with a few possible solutions.

Asynchronous Signed Language and Auditory-Based Spoken Language

Fluent signed language and spoken language cannot occur simultaneously, making communication within one classroom potentially challenging. The timing of auditory-based spoken language and signed language is critical. This requires the teacher of the deaf to be explicit when using both communication systems. A classroom-based teacher's aide who is fluent in both languages may facilitate the availability of abundant linguistic exposure. Alternatively, at strategic times school volunteers may be used to facilitate small group lessons to allow the teacher time to use auditory-based spoken language with individual students.

Nature of the Student

Children with hearing loss who do not use hearing technology and who use signed language to communicate may produce verbal nonlinguistic noises that may interfere with the reception of an auditory-based spoken language. Explicit explanation to all students regarding the need for a quiet listening environment is essential, as is the placement of students who are developing an auditory-based spoken language.

Some students may lack fluency in their first language, which will result in language learning difficulties when a second language is introduced. Students who receive hearing technology "late" may struggle to use audition in developing an auditory-based spoken language. In particular, some students with additional special needs may be introduced to a signed language after lack of success in an auditory-based spoken language program because of the inability to acquire a spoken language. These students and their families may require additional intensive involvement from a school-based speech-language pathologist to maximize spoken language development opportunities.

Nature of the Family

Family members who are introduced to either a signed language or an auditory-based spoken language as a first language may struggle with the introduction and use of a second language. The introduction of a second language may also interfere with the parents' capacity to use both languages within the family context. Parents who learned a signed language may be distracted from using an auditory-based spoken language and vice versa. Again, these families may require supplementary support from a specialist. In addition, parent support groups consisting of families in similar situations may facilitate problem solving related to this specific context.

Nature of the Class

The teacher of the deaf may find it overly demanding to provide appropriate stimuli in two languages. Balancing teaching behaviors in the context of diverse student needs requires extensive expert knowledge and skill. The educational leader must ensure that a number of mechanisms are in place to support the teacher. This can include ongoing professional development in facilitating the development of both languages, additional planning time, and student access to additional support such as a school-based speech-language pathologist. (See also Gárate, this volume, and Nussbaum and Scott, this volume, for additional strategies.)

Congruent Family, Teacher, and School Expectations

This diverse learning context has the potential to result in confused parent-school-teacher assumptions. In this situation, ongoing open communication among parents, the school, and the teacher is essential. Clear unambiguous policies must be in place, with individual classroom teacher's daily lessons reflecting policy implementation.

CASE STUDY

Background

Rafi is a happy 6 year, 8 month old boy with bilateral congenital profound hearing loss, which is genetic in nature.[3] There are two other children in his extended family with similar etiology and hearing loss. Rafi was diagnosed at birth and fit with hearing aids at 6 months. Rafi received a cochlear implant in his left ear at 18 months when it was determined that after intensive intervention, he was making minimal progress in speech and environmental sound detection. Prior to his cochlear implant candidacy, Rafi's family was counseled that the cochlear implant prognosis was "guarded" due to likely congenital central processing difficulties.

Arabic is the family's first language. Rafi's father and three older siblings are fluent in English, but his mother is not. Although all families in the school Rafi attends are enrolled in Auslan classes and have as a minimum basic Auslan skill, Auslan is not used in Rafi's home; however, gestures are used to supplement spoken Arabic and English. Rafi's preferred language is Arabic at home and Auslan at school.

Rafi's teacher reports that he has age appropriate Auslan skills and that his expressive spoken English skills are at the two-word phrase level. His teacher also reports that Rafi's English speech intelligibility is rated 4 out of 5 to the unfamiliar listener—with most of his speech intelligible.

	Rafi	Mother	Father	Siblings
L1	Arabic	Arabic	Arabic	Arabic
L2	Auslan	English	English	English
L3	English			

Auslan was introduced to Rafi's family as a supplemental communication approach when he was approaching 3 years of age because he was making minimal spoken language progress and his behavior was becoming aggressive and

3. "Rafi" is a pseudonym used to ensure family confidentiality.

disruptive. His parents enrolled him in a bilingual-bicultural (Auslan and spoken English) preschool program when he was 3 years of age. Rafi is currently enrolled in a year 1 Auslan class of five students. Rafi and one other student use a cochlear implant, a third student uses hearing aids, and the fourth and fifth students do not use hearing technology.

Auditory (Re)habilitation Teaching Behaviors

Each morning upon entry into the classroom, Rafi's teacher asks him if his cochlear implant is working and if he has worn it at home. Rafi reports that he uses his cochlear implant at home most of the time. The teacher routinely performs a daily listening check of the cochlear implant. The teacher engages Rafi individually and the class as a whole in frequent discussion regarding hearing technology and the associated requirements of all children in the class who use it, such as reduction of auditory clutter.

In all small group work, Rafi sits on the far left of the other students so that his cochlear implant is positioned away from his peers. Auslan is the principal language of Rafi's classroom and indeed the entire school. Rafi uses Auslan exclusively to communicate with his school peers. Occasionally Rafi's teacher will use spoken English in small group work if she deems the vocabulary of significant importance to his spoken language repertoire. When his teacher uses auditory-based spoken language with Rafi, she endeavors to position herself slightly behind Rafi and to his left so that the auditory signal reaches his cochlear implant speech processor within a reasonable distance. She frequently reminds Rafi to listen to the auditory stimulus when she uses spoken language followed by her request for Rafi to repeat the stimulus. The teacher is careful to use exaggerated pauses in her auditory-based spoken communication with Rafi to allow him the opportunity to process the information and to allow him to respond with spoken English.

In one-on-one literacy work with Rafi, his teacher uses auditory-based spoken English exclusively and consistently uses acoustic highlighting to draw attention to unfamiliar vocabulary words. She requires Rafi to read aloud and is careful to incorporate the auditory feedback loop into correcting his speech errors to continuously improve his speech intelligibility. Rafi's teacher is careful to give explicit, age appropriate feedback to Rafi regarding his spoken English.

In addition, Rafi receives weekly individual sessions with a school-based speech-language pathologist, whose role is to assess, facilitate the development of, and remediate spoken English. Goals and objectives of these sessions are chosen with the assistance of Rafi's parents and classroom teacher. The parents, classroom teacher, and speech-language pathologist meet regularly to communicate Rafi's triumphs and challenges and to set new goals if necessary.

Rafi is a well-liked member of his school community and socializes with his Auslan-using peers appropriately for his age. Rafi's socialization outside of school is mainly limited to family and extended family with spoken Arabic the primary language of use. Family members report that he is able to communicate well in spoken Arabic but that gestures are used to supplement expressive and receptive language. At this point, Rafi has very little contact with hearing peers although his school has recently commenced an integration program with the local primary school where he will attend sports and recreation classes with hearing peers. Rafi's teacher reports that he uses gestures to communicate during integration as do his Auslan-using classmates. The teacher is beginning to encourage Rafi to use his voice with his hearing peers.

Rafi is performing above average in all academic work. His family is pleased with his progress and is happy to allow him the opportunity to develop two auditory-based spoken languages and a signed language simultaneously.

Conclusion

This chapter brings to light 10 key teaching behaviors that may assist the teacher of the deaf in facilitating auditory-based spoken language for students using hearing technology in a signed communication learning environment. Teaching behaviors presented here are taken from Duncan et al. (2010) and incorporate teaching behaviors originally identified by Helen Beebe (1953, 1976, 1982), Beebe, Pearson, and Koch (1984), Doreen Pollack (1964, 1970, 1981, 1984), and Daniel Ling (1964, 1973, 1976, 1984, 1989, 2002). They resemble the work originally developed by Caleffe-Schenck (1983, 1992a, 1992b) and later refined by Perigoe (Auditory-Verbal International, 2004; Auditory-Verbal International, Certification Council, 2004; Auditory-Verbal International, Professional Education Committee, 1998–1999). The chapter closes with identification of some potential challenges the teacher of the deaf may encounter. Teachers, school leaders, and families are cautioned to put systems in place to circumvent these potential challenges.

Acknowledgments

The author is grateful to Melina Priem and Laisarn Leong, primary teachers at RIDBC Thomas Pattison School, for the opportunity to observe their teaching and discuss teaching behaviors with them and for their feedback on an earlier draft of this chapter. In addition, the author is indebted to Jan North, RIDBC Director of Children's Services, and Professor Greg Leigh, Director, RIDBC Renwick Centre/Conjoint Professor of Education, University of Newcastle, for the opportunity to engage in forthright and honest discussion of teaching behaviors with this special population.

REFERENCES

Auditory-Verbal International. (2004). *Certification in auditory-verbal intervention: Bulletin of information*. Alexandria, VA: Author.

Auditory-Verbal International, Certification Council. (2004). *Auditory-verbal teaching behaviors*. Alexandria, VA: Author.

Auditory-Verbal International, Professional Education Committee. (1998–1999). *Auditory-verbal teaching behaviors*. Alexandria, VA: Author.

Beebe, H. (1953). *A guide to help the severely hard of hearing child*. New York: Karger.

Beebe, H. (1976). Deaf children can learn to hear. In G. W. Nix (Ed.), *Mainstream education of hearing impaired children and youth* (pp. 239–246). New York: Grune & Stratton.

Beebe, H. (1982). When parents suspect their child is deaf: Where to turn? What to consider? *Hearing Rehabilitation Quarterly, 7*(4), 4–6.

Beebe, H., Pearson, H., & Koch, M. (1984). The Helen Beebe Speech and Hearing Center. In D. Ling (Ed.), *Early intervention for hearing-impaired children: Oral options* (pp. 15–63). San Diego, CA: College-Hill Press.

Caleffe-Schenck, N. (1983). *Children, children, what do you hear?* Handout from the Denver Ear Institute.

Caleffe-Schenck, N. (1992a). The auditory-verbal method: Description of a training program for audiologists, speech language pathologists, and teachers of children with hearing loss. *Volta Review, 94*, 65–68.

Caleffe-Schenck, N. (1992b). *Auditory-verbal training program handbook*. Englewood, CA: The Listen Foundation.

Daniel, L. (1987). *Effects of acoustic exaggeration on the imitation of selected suprasegmental patterns by profoundly hearing-impaired children.* Unpublished thesis, University of Wisconsin, Madison.

Denes, P. B., & Pinson. E. N. (1993). *The speech chain. The physics and biology of spoken language.* New York: W. H. Freeman.

Duncan, J. (2006). Application of the auditory-verbal methodology and pedagogy to school age children. *Journal of Educational Audiology, 13*, 39–49.

Duncan, J., Kendrick, A., McGinnis, M., & Perigoe, C. (2010). Auditory (re)habilitation teaching behavior rating scale. *Journal of the Academy of Rehabilitative Audiology, 43*, 65–86.

Duncan, J., Rhoades, E. A., & Fitzpatrick, E. (in press). *Adolescents with hearing loss: Auditory rehabilitation.* New York: Oxford University Press.

Ling, D. (1964). An auditory approach to the education of deaf children. *Audecibel, 13*, 96–101.

Ling, D. (1973). The auditory approach. *Volta Review, 75*, 354–356.

Ling, D. (1976). *Speech and the hearing impaired child: Theory and practice*. Washington, DC: Alexander Graham Bell Association for the Deaf.

Ling, D. (Ed.). (1984). *Early intervention for hearing impaired children: Oral options*. Boston: College-Hill Press.

Ling, D. (1989). *Foundations of spoken language for hearing-impaired children*. Washington, DC: Alexander Graham Bell Association for the Deaf.

Ling, D. (2002). *Speech and the hearing-impaired child: Theory and practice* (2nd ed.). Washington, DC: Alexander Graham Bell Association for the Deaf.

Mayer, C., & Leigh, G. (2010). The changing context for sign bilingual education programs: Issues in language and the development of literacy. *International Journal of Bilingual Education and Bilingualism, 13*(2), 175–186.

Pollack, D. (1964). Acoupedics: A unisensory approach to auditory training. *Volta Review, 66*, 400–409.

Pollack, D. (1970). *Educational audiology for the limited-hearing infant*. Springfield, IL: Charles C. Thomas.

Pollack, D. (1981). Acoupedics: An approach to early management. In G. T. Mencher & S. E. Gerber (Eds.), *Early management of hearing loss* (pp. 301–318). New York: Grune & Stratton.

Pollack, D. (1984). An acoupedic program. In D. Ling (Ed.), *Early intervention for hearing impaired children: Oral options*. (pp. 181–253). Boston: College-Hill Press.

Tye-Murray, N. (2009). *Foundations of aural rehabilitation: Children, adults, and their family members* (3rd ed.). New York: Delmar.

PART IV

Some Final Thoughts

12

SENSORY POLITICS AND THE COCHLEAR IMPLANT DEBATES

Joseph Michael Valente, Benjamin Bahan, and H-Dirksen L. Bauman

The human brain does not discriminate between the hand or the tongue . . . people do.

—Laura-Ann Petitto (2009)

. . . people of different cultures not only speak different languages, but what is possibly more important, inhabit different sensory worlds.

—Edward T. Hall (1982)

The cochlear implant controversy is frequently portrayed by popular media and framed by stakeholders as a battle between science and technology versus culture. Cochlear implant proponents claim that early childhood is the most critical period of development if implants are to increase spoken language and literacy development. On the other end, members of the Deaf community assert that cochlear implants are an assault on their culture by interfering with deaf children's right to acquire a fully accessible signed language. As they play out in the public media, these arguments pit the well-funded biopower industries against a tiny linguistic minority (Ladd, 2003; Lane, 1992; Bauman, 2008). This imbalanced portrayal of the argument forms the story line of most media coverage of the cochlear implant controversy, for example, the film *Sound and Fury*, in which articulate white-coated doctors espouse the wisdom of early implantation and emotionally charged Deaf community members seem to be Luddites shunning technological advancements. But these familiar narratives do not take into account all the complexities of the issues at the crux of the cochlear implant debates.

This chapter attempts to defamiliarize two familiar yet polarizing narratives, that is, Deaf culture versus hearing culture. Although the Deaf culture side of the argument has been faulted for its embrace of essentialist identity politics and for ignoring ways Deaf culture actually benefits by positioning itself in opposition to biopower institutions (Friedner, 2010), we also recognize how the medical-educational-industrial complex that promotes cochlear implants is equally motivated by a particular cultural orientation favoring its own sensory orientation in the world. This chapter uses the lens of what we refer to as "sensory politics" (Bahan, 2007, 2009, 2010) to explain the political implications of the enforcement of dominant cultural norms of sensory experience. In other words, sensory politics looks at the intersection of biological perception and cultural mediation and interpretation within a field of power. Sensory politics, as will be discussed below, often finds tension in the culturally determined hierarchy that values and devalues sensory experience, especially between visual and auditory perception.

As we unpack the notion of sensory politics as it applies to the cochlear implant debates, we see that the allegedly neutral rhetoric of medicine and science are just as motivated by a cultural orientation as the Deaf cultural argument. This demystification paves the way for more balanced and culturally aware perspectives that provide insights into the implications and orientations involved in decisions of whether to implant.

Prior to any consideration of ethics of cochlear implants, preconceived notions and dominant Western assumptions about the senses must be disentangled and made explicit. Before we can better understand the implications of cochlear implants, we must understand how senses and sensory politics work in complex and diverse ways around the world. To provide insights that come from what has long been thought to be a neutral biological process, sensory perception is now being studied for how it is culturally mediated and interpreted. A growing field of sensory anthropology has inquired into the relation of sensory experience and culture, foregrounding the fact that not all cultures in the world define and describe sensory experience in the same way (Geurts, 2002; Howes, 2005; Hall, 1982). This provocative body of research brings fundamental epistemic questions to the fore. For example, do all cultures claim to possess five senses? How do disparate cultures parse sensory experience in their epistemological framework and linguistic expression? These questions open the way for an understanding of sensory politics that erodes the bedrock foundations of Western epistemology. In short, the natural and biological notion of normative sensory experience is not so natural and normal after all but is, rather, a phenomenon formed through the complex interplay of biological function and cultural and political mediation.

The primary focus of this chapter, then, is to begin discussion of a framework of sensory politics within which debates of cochlear implants and educational choices for deaf children may be realigned.

Making Sense of Senses and Culture

How many senses are there? Without a doubt, five is the most commonly understood answer to this question. Yet, this is not a historically or universally accepted fact. Several other senses are often cited in scientific literature, such as proprioception, awareness of one's body in space; equilibrioception, the sense of balance; and magnetoreception, the sense of direction. Sensory anthropologist Kathryn Geurts provides a genealogy of senses that challenges preconceived ideas of what senses are and can be. Geurts (2002) takes issue with Western notions of senses that attempt to propose that sensory data is both objective and rational, perpetuating a "folk ideology" of senses (p. 228). She also argues that "our taxonomy of senses is organ-based," perpetuating the belief that there is a direct link between discrete organs and their assigned sensory domain: eyes = vision, ears = hearing, skin = touch, nose = smell, tongue = taste (Geurts, 2002, p. 228). This model, however, does not account for the actual work of perception. Smell and taste are deeply related, as anyone with a cold knows; similarly, sound waves are registered not just by the ear but also through skin and muscle. Clearly, organs are deeply tied to sensory experience, but the history of the senses shows us that there has been great variation over the years regarding the relation of sensory perception and knowledge and the hierarchy and relation of the senses to each other.

As Jütte (2005), Geurts (2002), Howes (2005), Jay (1992), and others have explained, our use of the senses coevolved with historical shifts in epistemologies. "The idea that perception or sensation," writes Robert Jütte, "may be localized in certain physical organs has a long tradition. It pervades many cultures, although not all of them set the number of these organs at the sacred or magical figure of five" (p. 20). According to Geurts, Aristotle is most likely responsible for setting in motion a particular hierarchy of the five senses in this order: seeing, hearing, tasting, smelling, and touching. But Aristotle's definition, as Howes (2005) would remind us, was culturally and historically bound and included a different set of understandings of the five senses from what we have today. For instance, Aristotle combined the five senses with "the elements—earth, air, fire, water, and the quintessence" (Geurts, p. 229). As we moved away from such earlier theological and allegorical explanations of the world toward the Enlightenment, the assigned roles of the senses also shifted. The relative value assigned to sensory data as a key element in knowing the world changed dramatically, for example, from Descartes's rationalist position that it was the mind, not the senses that lead to truth to John Locke's epistemology, which asserted that all knowledge was derived from sensory experience. For an updated version, consider also the evolving ability to extend our sensory reach, which includes x-ray vision, infrared vision, and navigational abilities such as homing devices, not to mention the Hubble telescope, which enables us to see back in time and toward the far reaches of the universe.

Although we have seen that interpretation and explanation of sensory experience has been malleable over time, it is also contingent on particular cultural interpretations. As Geurts (2002) shows, the Anlo, a Western African tribe parse their sensory experience along six rather than five categories, adding the sense of "balance" to sensory experience. Howes (2005) also shows that even within a single sense, there is wide cultural variation of the explanation and attributes of perception. In English there are four flavors, this contrasts with the Japanese who have five, Weyewa of Sumba, seven, and Sereer Ndut of Senegal, three. Even within each of these distinct cultures, there are differences in constructions of smell or "odor categories": Sereer Ndut has five odors; Weyewa, three; Japanese, two; and English, definitive descriptors. Owing to these findings, Howes suggests an integrated approach to the study of senses that does not privilege one sense over the other. By providing a historical summary of traps that Western scientists fall into with senses, Howes calls into question how scientists become so ingrained and unquestioned in cultural representations, explaining, "What these facts reflect is rather the extent cultures differ in the intensity with which they attend to a given field of sense at a given moment in their history" (2005, p. 9). How a culture values or devalues a sense tells us more about the culture than the sense itself.

Sensory Politics

We have argued so far that sensory experience is a culturally mediated and understood phenomenon with considerable variation across time and from culture to culture. Once understood in this light, senses gain a political dimension. Sensory politics are invoked when a dominant culture imposes its culturally mediated sensory dispositions onto a minority culture. In cross-cultural situations, what happens when a member of a minority culture violates the sensory norms of a dominant culture? Members of the dominant culture will, by default, make judgments based on sensory data. Arguably in the United States, loud = uncouth and obnoxious; detectible body odor = slob, disgusting; too soft-spoken = insecure. When a member of the dominant culture evaluates different defiant sensorial/behavioral signals then makes judgments, he or she is engaging in an act called "sensory politics." According to Pierre Bourdieu (1995), a French social scientist and philosopher, this is a common occurrence across economic classes.

Sensory Politics and Class Distinctions

Within the realm of senses, there are class distinctions based on dominant cultural ideas of what it is to be sensorially sophisticated or unsophisticated. Senses themselves can belong to a high or low culture. Bourdieu (1995) argues that those in power determine what is considered to be *taste* and that these distinctions work to help us identify who belongs where. Whether we use classes to refer to economic, social, or even, we would argue, sensory classes, the distinct features of each class are not only to define but also to include or exclude based on these distinctions.

Bourdieu (1995) explains how senses drive:

> The socially informed body, with its tastes and distastes, its compulsions and repulsions, with, in a word, all its senses, that is to say, not only the traditional five senses—which never escape the structuring action of social

determinisms—but also the sense of necessity and sense of duty, the sense of direction and the sense of reality, the sense of balance and the sense of beauty, common sense and the sense of the sacred. (p. 124)

According to Geurts (2002), Bourdieu is highlighting the connection between the five senses in relation to 16 sensibilities. For instance, Geurts asks, "Why does Bourdieu want us to consider the similarities between the ability to see and a sensitivity to funny things?" (p. 243). The answer rests in the "isomorphic relationship" meaning "the conditioning of what you consider moral, what you find funny, what is absurd, what is beautiful, and so forth" (p. 243). What it all comes down to is Bourdieu's notions of "tastes," Geurts argues, what connects "mind, body, behavioral practices and cultural background" (p. 243). The idea of taste explains how those in control determine what is aesthetically pleasing. Wacquant (2006) explains how it all works: "Taste is first and foremost the distaste of the tastes of others" (p. 223). By drawing these distinctions, class structures can be more clearly delineated. To this, we would add, taste also uncovers how limited Western notions of the power of senses are in relation to cultures around the world.

When looking at senses across cultures, it becomes evident how much senses are both socially determined and culturally constructed. From the standpoint of social justice and equity, critics from many historically marginalized communities within the United States would argue that senses fall under the purview of white, middle-class, ethnocentric thinking. Take, for example, the violent relationships involved in a colonialist imposition of sensory experience by Native Americans who were sent to boarding schools. Removed from their sensory engagement with the land, sky, and plants, they were subjected instead to an education within a square schoolhouse and cramped dorms that critically undermined their sensory engagement with the world (Zitkala-Sa, 1900/1992).

Disciplining the Senses: On the Control of Sound and Human Voice[1]

We have now argued that sensory experience is culturally mediated and therefore is implicated in unequal power relations in majority-minority relations. At this point, we turn specifically to how sound and the voice are disciplined to fit culturally acceptable norms.

The process of enculturation is largely one of disciplining the senses. Infants are born without awareness of the noises they make. As they grow older, they are taught to learn what noise production is acceptable in which social spaces. The disciplining of noise production permeates nearly every activity, from eating, playing, and learning, to attending religious ceremonies and sporting events.

1. Issues discussed in this section also appeared in Bahan (2010).

All cultures set a range of what is acceptable and what is considered excess for noises like grunting, snorting, hollering, and laughing. As grunts are generally associated with heavy work or physical force, they have become associated with those who perform "mundane" physical labor. When grunts are heard outside the normal space where they are generally produced, such as gyms and construction sites, politically laden interpretations emerge: the grunter's intelligence and social status are questioned. Take, for example, the controversy about the grunting in professional tennis, a sport that has developed in the context of economically elite country clubs. A 9-year-old girl was banned from playing tennis at her local club because she grunted while playing in tennis matches (ESPN.com, 2008). In addition, a 16-year-old player Michelle Larcher de Brito was booed when she walked off the tennis court because she grunted excessively during the 2009 French Open (Flatman, 2009). The noise may be distracting, but deeper down the guttural noise itself carries social meaning that is more at home with wrestling than with the elite sport of tennis.

In another example of national political consequence, take the case of Howard Dean, a former Democratic presidential candidate. In 2004, he came in third in the Iowa caucus. In trying to rouse the crowd during his concession speech, he emitted a primal scream, which became an instant news item played and replayed on national media outlets. The verdict of "the scream" in the court of sensory politics was guilty for having exceeded a norm that was clearly unpresidential. The underlying thought was if he could not keep his voice under control, how could he possibly control the country?

The point here is to become aware of the context of disciplining the senses that takes place for all persons, including the most elite, and to extrapolate that context to appreciate the extreme measures of disciplining sound production that takes place for deaf and hard of hearing individuals. For deaf children, an entire oralist effort has been and continues to be underway in education to teach proper speech and sound production, including now surgical procedures to enhance socially acceptable sound and voice production. Acceptable sights and sounds are grounded in how a culture mediates the meaning attached to visual and auditory ways of knowing and being. The roots of all this uncovers how unquestionably ocularcentric and phonocentric Western society is in its thinking about the senses.

Sensory Politics: Ocularcentrism Versus Phonocentrism

We have argued that senses are a means of identifying class distinctions and exercising power and instilling discipline on bodies (Foucault, 1995). Although this is the case for all citizens, the deaf body is a particularly fraught terrain of sensory politics. The tension between the dominant hearing society and Deaf culture is at the intersection of visual and auditory ways of being. Clearly, all sighted hearing individuals are not exclusively auditory-dominant individuals. Yet, deaf individuals experience a different sensory alignment in which vision assumes a preeminent role.

The tension between the primacy of visual and auditory ways of being is not a new phenomenon. This tension is articulated within critical theory as "ocularcentrism versus phonocentrism." The beginning of the comparative role of the senses can be found in Aristotle's opening paragraphs of *The Metaphysics:*

> ALL men by nature desire to know. An indication of this is the delight we take in our senses; for even apart from their usefulness they are loved for themselves; and above all others the sense of sight. For not only with a view to action, but even when we are not going to do anything, we prefer seeing (one might say) to everything else. The reason is that this, most of all the senses, makes us know and brings to light many differences between things. (p. 243)

Aristotle is unequivocal in ranking the sense of sight the highest, setting in motion a long tradition of what has been called "ocularcentrism." As Aristotle sees it, this fundamental visual grasp on reality literally brings light to the world, making the world available to those who are able to see it. Yet, the following paragraph of *The Metaphysics* introduces the crucial role that hearing plays in gaining deeper knowledge of the world than sight may provide.

> By nature animals are born with the faculty of sensation, and from sensation memory is produced in some of them, though not in others. And therefore the former are more intelligent and apt at learning than those which cannot remember; those which are incapable of hearing sounds are intelligent though they cannot be taught, e.g. the bee, and any other race of animals that may be like it; and those which besides memory have this sense of hearing can be taught. (p. 243)

In this passage, it is unclear here whether Aristotle conflates "man" with "animals," so we may be wary of definitive claims about Aristotle's view on deaf individuals' capacity to be taught. Most important for our purpose, though, is the philosophical alignment that posits hearing as a necessary means of instruction by a teacher. In this way, both senses—sight and hearing—play vital roles in the construction of theories of human intelligence and being, in vastly different ways. On the one hand, sight provides access to the world and the knowledge that is revealed within it, whereas hearing may open up avenues for deeper discourse of instruction beyond the knowledge revealed through sight. For more on the history of the tension of the hierarchy and political alignment of the senses, see Martin Jay (1992), David Howes (2005), Robert Jütte (2005), and Kathryn Geurts (2002).

The point here is that there may be more to the concept of "centrism" than that which occurs with "ocular" or "phono." Each sense has accumulated a historically constructed role and interpretation mapped onto its particular biological functioning. Neither the theory of ocularcentrism nor that of phonocentrism is absolute in all aspects of life and throughout history.

To appreciate the full reach of phonocentrism within the lives of deaf individuals, we must grasp the significance of the human voice.

Phonocentrism: Voice and Identity

The role of human voice as communication apparatus is valued in most cultures and is seen as a stimulus for life force. Anne Karpf (2006) explains, "For some people the very act of using their voice, its kinetic attack, reminds them they are alive" (p. 114). The notion of presence is created as individuals hear themselves speak. "The system of hearing-oneself-speak, through the phonic substance," writes French philosopher Jacques Derrida, "has necessarily dominated the history of the world during an entire epoch and has even produced the idea of the world, the idea of world-origin" (1973, p. 8). Such a wide-ranging claim has been explored elsewhere (Bauman, 2004, 2008). For the purposes of this discussion, though, it is crucial that the production of presence not be underestimated or overlooked in its profoundly influential role in forming ontologies of hearing ways of being. One of the telltale symptoms of phonocentrism is the experience of individuals who experience sudden deafness. Often it is not just the lack of hearing that is disturbing but also the lack of a solid reminder of one's presence through hearing oneself speak. Frequently, these individuals relate that they "feel like a ghost" upon first experiencing the loss of hearing oneself speak. A similar phenomenon happens on a daily basis as portable media player (e.g., iPod or Walkman) users frequently raise their voices when speaking so that they can hear themselves speak. Without the feedback, one feels less present, less confirmed in one's existence.

Each culture generates interpretations for various sounds uttered from the mouth, ranging from grunting and laughing to speaking. The voice as an apparatus plays as a cultural identification card (see, for example, voice printing technology) and broadcasts information about the self. One can often determine the biological status (e.g., age, gender, race), psychological status (e.g., intelligence, educational background), and social status (e.g., occupation, class) by the use of one's voice. Tempos also have cultural dimensions. For instance, Karpf (2006) notes that fast talkers are seen as quick thinkers, intelligent, and knowledgeable, whereas slow talkers are viewed as being less so. Consider also the interpretation that happens when listening to unknown individuals over the phone. Now what happens when a member of a culture with such hearing practices meets someone who does not talk? The mute's identity and personality cannot be extracted. Without the voice, that prime transmitter of one's identity, the mute individual cannot be read. In the void left by the lack of voice, this person becomes stigmatized with cultural interpretations. In general the mute person is not seen as an intelligent and capable person but rather as a caricature of all that society preconceives about those who do not speak.

When a person talks, there are also evaluations of vocal qualities. In American culture, for example, certain voices are found to be irritating to a lot of people, specifically nasal, high-pitched, and loud voices (Karpf, 2006). People with loud voices are seen as being boisterous. The characterizations of deaf speech do not fall far from what is found to be irritating among hearing Americans, in particular nasal resonance distortion, breathy, and tense (Subtelny, 1975). As mentioned earlier, even when a deaf person speaks well, he or she may still have characteristics of deaf speech. Some call it the deaf accent. What is interesting is in the way hearing people would compliment a deaf person who speaks well by saying, "You have good speech!" Hearing people do not go around complimenting each other with, "You have good speech." Rather, they compliment each other on the quality of their voices. What are the underlying assumptions in the discrepant complimentary procedure?

When hearing persons assume that deaf people cannot talk and then find their assumption to be erroneous, the compliment is directed at praising the production rather than the quality.

> It sometimes seems as if we only pay attention to the voice when it goes wrong. There's a whole literature on teachers' voice disorders going back over thirty years, yet the role of the teacher's voice in enthusing a class has been barely researched. (Karpf, 2006, p. 14)

This appears to reflect Western culture's tendency to drive and corral defiant sensory behaviors. The vast industry of speech and hearing sciences in Western culture and their focus on the pathologies of speech and auditory deprivation led to the establishment of the National Institute on Deafness and Other Communication Disorders (NIDCD), the Alexander Graham Bell Association for the Deaf and Hard of Hearing, and hundreds of other rehabilitative organizations and associations. For instance, the NIDCD mission statement explains that it

> conducts and supports research and research training related to disease prevention and health promotion; addresses special biomedical and behavioral problems associated with people who have communication impairments or disorders; and supports efforts to create devices which substitute for lost and impaired sensory and communication function. (NIDCD, 2010)

This overwhelming push toward auditory rehabilitation needs to be placed in the context of biological facts that were revealed in the last half of the twentieth century: There is nothing necessarily "natural" or "essential" about speech as the primary form of human language production. Speech is clearly the majority modality; but the minority modality in this case is *no less human*. Although sign has been studied seriously for only 50 years, its differences signify some of the more remarkable insights into the human capacity to make meaning. As William Stokoe and others have suggested—we, the Deaf, essentially became human as we entered the realm of meaning making through the gestural modality (Stokoe, 1999). Humans have continued to develop gesture into language—a fact evidenced by reports of sign language extending as far back as 7,000 years ago (Woll & Ladd, 2005) and the widespread use of signing among Native Americans (Farnell, 2009) and aboriginals (Kendon, 1998) in addition to hundreds of sign languages of Deaf communities throughout the world (Moores & Miller, 2009). In this light, we see that signed languages provide cognitive, creative, and cultural benefits as opposed to being supplements to and replacements for speech (Bauman & Murray, 2010).

Conclusion: Sensory Politics and Ethical Implications

Given that sensory experience is a social construction, as we have seen, what are the implications for the cochlear implant controversy? The lens of sensory politics allows us to take a few steps back and see that not all of the arguments in favor of implantation are made for biological, scientific reasons. The decision to implant is as culturally mediated as the argument to preserve Deaf culture. Clearly, this does not mean, on the merit of this argument alone, that implants are a form of inherently oppressive mechanism. Few would begrudge adults for receiving an implant. The difference arises with early implantation: sensory politics is only asking that those who implant consider that those who favor implantation are making a medical decision that forces their own sensory orientation in the world on the world of their children. Yet sensory politics has us asking a previously unasked question: Is it inherently better to be hearing than deaf? This paradigm shift in the understanding of human language raises questions of a fundamental nature. Does the difference between being deaf and hearing have an intrinsic negative value? Is it always better to hear than not? There are clearly situations when hearing is not better than its opposite. Hearing can often be a damaging sense. Noise stress has been linked to cognitive functioning difficulties, cardiovascular disease, and mental illness (Arnstein & Goldman-Rakic, 1998; Boer & Schroten, 2007; Stansfeld & Matheson, 2004) and produces stress-related hormones, the effects of which can be very damaging, potentially leading to violent behavior such as infant shaking. In fact, the social costs of traffic noise in the European Union has been estimated at 40 billion per year (Boer & Schroten, 2007). Although many tolerate increased noise production in urban environments, traffic noise alone has reached epidemic proportions. According to the World Health Organization Regional Office for Europe, one in five Europeans is regularly exposed to sound levels at night that could significantly damage health.

The point here is not to play defensive sensory politics but simply to point out that there are many unconsidered angles when assumptions that fixing what may be seen as a medical condition such as deafness does not always result in increased overall health. Suppose emphasis was placed instead on increasing sensory input for deaf children through signed language and a visually rich learning environment. By bringing issues of sensory politics to the fore, we may now see issues around implantation through a new lens.

Clearly there is a ready-made social arrangement that favors being hearing over being deaf. Yet if social structures were the determining factor then it would follow that it is inherently better to be male, White, and economically advantaged. But those positions are made better through social arrangement, not biological being.

Cochlear implants, then, may be seen as a means of ensuring the phonocentric orientation that appears in the form of the belief that speech is the normative means of language, when we now know that the brain is just as capable of functioning with visual as auditory linguistic input (Petitto, 2009). Further, the correlation with the human voice and identity saturates our sense of being and self-identity. To the hearing world, the deaf person without voice appears to lack a sense of presence, identity, and being. Even as there has been a great acceptance of the visual orientation of the Deaf community and their members, the Deaf community is still viewed by larger society as somehow lacking. This association is clearly false and can only be explained as a cultural construction informed by a phonocentric orientation. In this light, we may see the alignment of education and speech as a particular cultural bias against sign language and alternative sensory worlds. Deaf education is the story of this bias, culminating in a medico-pedagogical orientation that drives parents toward surgical procedures and rehabilitation as opposed to letting the human language potential express itself in a modality that is *equally as human, equally a biological norm* as speech.

When parents learn of their children's deafness, they are faced with the existential question: to implant or not to implant? To sign or not to sign? What are the factors involved in this choice? Are the choices that parents make conducted in a politically neutral environment? The argument of sensory politics is to foreground that there is nothing *essentially* better about corralling children to follow the socially dominant sensory order. This argument highlights the fact that decisions are often made with regard to the heavy weight of the social construction of the senses, of the role of voice as presence and the policing of sound and the interpretation of social class that ensues. As the sensory order has become naturalized as the normal state of affairs, it operates as a profoundly influential and unrecognized force. Yet, this argument suggests that we step back or out of our traditionally constructed sensorium and consider that there are other ways of being and that these alternative ways of being are, in fact, intrinsically and extrinsically valid. Decisions are often made before one is able to consider the value in ways of being different from the norm.

Moores, D. F., & Miller, M. S. (2009). *Deaf people around the world: Educational and social perspectives.* Washington, DC: Gallaudet University Press.

National Institute on Deafness and Other Communication Disorders. (2010). Mission statement. Retrieved November 1, 2010, from http://www.nidcd.nih.gov/about/learn/mission.html

Petitto, L. A. (2009, October). *Scientific research on the positive effect of signed language in the human brain.* Effect of Language Delay on Mental Health Conference, Toronto, Canada.

Sandel, M. J. (2007). *The case against perfection: Ethics in the age of genetic engineering.* Cambridge, MA: Belknap Press.

Stansfeld, S. A., & Matheson, M. P. (2003). Noise pollution: Non-auditory effects on health. *British Medical Bulletin, 68,* 243–257.

Subtelny, J. (1975). Speech assessment of the Deaf adult. *Journal of the Academy of Rehabilitative Audiology, 8,* 110–116.

Wacquant, L. (2006). Pierre Bourdieu. In R. Stones (Ed.), *Key contemporary thinkers* (pp. 261–277). London: Macmillan.

Woll, B., & Ladd, P. (2005). Deaf communities. In M. Marschark & P. E. Spencer (Eds.), *Oxford handbook of deaf studies, language, and education.* Oxford: Oxford University Press.

World Health Organization Regional Office for Europe. (2009). *Information for the media.* Retrieved April 13, 2011, from http://www.euro.who.int/en/what-we-publish/information-for-the-media/sections/press-releases/2009/10/one-in-five-europeans-is-regularly-exposed-to-sound-levels-at-night-that-could-significantly-damage-health.

World Health Organization Regional Office for Europe. (2010). *Noise.* Retrieved November 1, 2010, from http://www.euro.who.int/en/what-we-do/health-topics/environmental-health/noise/facts-and-figures.

Zitkala-Sa. (1992). The school days of an Indian girl. In W. L. Andrews (Ed.), *Classic American autobiographies.* New York: Signet Classic. (Original work published 1900).

13

EMBRACING CHANGE: COCHLEAR IMPLANTS AND THE NEW DEAF COMMUNITY PARADIGM

Josh Swiller

The U.S. Deaf community has reached a moment of unprecedented transition. The advent of cochlear implants and other auditory technology, the improvements in medical care and early hearing loss detection, the rise and ubiquity of mainstreaming for deaf students, and the financial uncertainties of the current era are leading the community toward new and unknown realities. The future of the community is impossible to predict save for one thing: it will be different. How it responds to these demographic and technological changes will determine its future character and may even determine, in fact, whether the community continues in a recognizable form. Understandably, these recent developments have created an emotional firestorm.

At the center of this transitional moment is Gallaudet University—the geographic and spiritual center of the Deaf community. Can Gallaudet University effectively evolve? How can it? Need it even do so? These questions are being energetically debated in the university community, and task forces have been formed and consultants hired to work on them.[1]

In the past few decades, the Deaf community has taken substantial strides toward visibility and equality, and in doing so has become a leader in the push for equal rights for one of the last marginalized populations, people with disabilities. Gallaudet itself has had a prominent role throughout this push. The Deaf President Now protests of 1988 and the passage of the Americans With Disabilities Act (ADA) 2 years later are intrinsically related.[2] Gallaudet has taken concrete strides to improve educational standards, and empirical research has verified American Sign

1. There are several examples; the most prominent perhaps is the university's Long Range Strategic Plan task force of 2008–2009 led by Booz Allen Consultants.

2. Soukup (2008) writes, "[Deaf President Now] brought to light in a very public forum the kinds of oppression and discrimination that deaf and hard of hearing people have faced in employment and throughout society. . . . This movement was a catalyst for equal rights, equal opportunity, and equal access for all people with disabilities."

Language's (ASL's) value in the intellectual, linguistic, and emotional maturation of deaf individuals (see, e.g., Gallaudet University, 2008). More broadly, aided by legislative victories, strong leaders, and the shift in general society toward the recognition of the inviolability of the individual human spirit, the Deaf community has trended toward a more open, visible, and equal presence in the global community. But the current technological transitions and demographic and financial pressures make clear that all these gains and efforts, in and outside the university, are not enough to ensure the university's survival.

It seems unfair. It seems to break basic moral doctrines regarding respect for human diversity and individuality. Unfortunately, it is happening whether one likes it or not.

This chapter will place the challenges facing Gallaudet University in a historical perspective that recognizes the magnitude of the current situation and the uniqueness of it but also its parallels to other communities in similar situations. The hope is that doing so will delineate the necessity of action, raise the need and methods to avoid emotional maelstroms, and highlight the enormous potential for positive, empowering transformation that the current situation holds.

The paramount force stressing Gallaudet is one that has threatened and disbanded minority communities throughout recorded human history: the force of economics. Economic forces have never respected moral arguments, and so to put too much weight on and effort into constructing moral arguments for Gallaudet University and the Deaf community would be counterproductive. However, constructing a new philosophical paradigm recognizing the hegemony of economic forces suggests practical steps that could lead to the immediate and long-term security of the university.

Part I: Gallaudet's Coming Demographic Imperative, National and Local Numbers, the Necessity of Action

It is easy and perhaps correct to call hubristic a broad reconnaissance of and broad recommendations for Gallaudet's situation. For that, I apologize in advance. However, a quick survey of the dramatic scale of the demographic shifts taking place in the U.S. deaf and hard of hearing population shows how such a reckoning is necessary.

Over the past 2 decades, new technologies, chief among them cochlear implants, have led to an increasing number of parents choosing spoken language as the primary communication mode for their deaf children. A key moment in this trend was the Food and Drug Administration's decision in 2000 to approve cochlear implant surgery for children as young as 12 months old (National Institute on Deafness and Other Communication Disorders, 2009). Since then the shift toward spoken language as the primary communication modality for deaf children has escalated. Federal funding to compile national data on hearing loss and communication choices is currently pending (Deaf and Hard of Hearing Alliance, 2010), leading to significant gaps in the national numbers. But there are a few stark estimates: an August 2009 *Los Angeles Times* article approximated that in that year about 40% of deaf children under the age of 3 received a cochlear implant, up from 25% just 5 years before (Roan, 2009). And there are compelling figures from the latest Gallaudet Research Institute (2006) national data. Of 36,710 deaf and hard of hearing students in the national school system in the 2007–2008 school year, more than 50% were taught in speech-only settings.

An analysis of state and county trends in deaf education further reveals this trend. In North Carolina, the state department of education has an early intervention program called "Beginnings" that serves infants and toddlers with hearing loss up to the age of 3. In the 1997–1998 school year, 60% of the children in this program were in ASL-focused language programs and 40% in listening and spoken language programs. Just 6 years later, those percentages had shifted to 16% ASL and 84% listening and spoken language (North Carolina Office of Educational Services, 2004). In Bergen County, New Jersey, a similar reshaping took place in the period from 1997 to 2009. In that period, elementary students on a listening and spoken language track went from 16% to 73%, and secondary students went from 0% to 68% (Treni, 2009).

An accelerating factor in these educational shifts is the dire financial condition of national, state, and local governments. In the current fiscal climate, often called the weakest since the Great Depression, drained states are finding it too expensive to sustain the budgets of schools for the deaf. Although there are other possible factors, such as leadership issues and a lack of community support, it is inarguable that financial difficulties have contributed to the list of states that have recently closed or merged the budgets of deaf schools. These states include Nebraska, Pennsylvania, New York, North Carolina, South Dakota, Kansas, Mississippi, and Washington (e.g., Zena, 2009). Only a handful of states have been spared. Cochlear implants are often paired with the decision to educate the implantee in a mainstream setting, as mainstream education is less of a financial strain on the state than education at traditional institutions for the deaf. Although implants do carry a hefty price tag over the short and long terms, the cost is diffused, as it is split among families, insurers, professionals, and local school districts, whereas the cost of educating students in deaf schools is more centralized on the state.

Clearly, more and more parents are choosing spoken language for their deaf children. The ramifications of this trend toward implants and mainstreaming for deaf and hard of hearing children's emotional, psychological, and intellectual development are far reaching and worthy of intensive study—and are currently being studied (Gallaudet University, 2008). These studies may yet reveal that cochlear implants and a strictly spoken language approach in mainstream programs are counterproductive to the development of a child's whole being, although current research has not demonstrated this to be the case (see Leigh & Maxwell-McCaw, this volume, for example). However, it is not the focus of this chapter to discourage or encourage the trend, nor to debate its validity; rather, it is to explore possible ways for Gallaudet to respond pragmatically to the trend.

Part II: Tension in the Deaf Community, Emotional Reactions, Ethical Dead Ends

Understandably, the speed and depth of the demographic changes in communication and educational choices for deaf individuals have produced powerful emotional reactions in all factions of the deaf and hard of hearing world. It is important to note how these reactions and the moral arguments they thrive on and help propagate have been unsuccessful and even counterproductive to Gallaudet University's efforts to secure its future.

The 2006 Gallaudet protest can be read as a manifestation and embodiment of those emotions. When Jane Fernandes was announced as the ninth president of Gallaudet University in spring 2006, a diverse collection of the student body, staff, faculty, and Deaf community orchestrated a protracted but ultimately successful protest to unseat the president-designate. They garnered national media attention. Dr. Dirksen Bauman, a professor in the deaf studies department at Gallaudet, pointed out that the protest's elaborate, complex list of grievances included the following:

> The lack of diversity among the finalists, the Board of Trustees' lack of responsiveness to students of color, the persistence of audism on campus, and the appearance of an unfair search process that led to the appointment of a widely unpopular, internal candidate. (2008, p. 328)

Whether these points were valid or not, it is a jump from them to the scores of arrests and heightened, bitter, discriminatory rhetoric from all sides (and even from the media) that dominated the protests and led to a limited and judgmental portrayal of the Gallaudet community from which it is just now emerging.

Clearly, it is counterproductive to frame the issues facing Gallaudet on moral grounds. And yet those issues continue to be framed just that way by the defenders of both spoken and sign language. Definitive, discriminatory, and inflammatory talk unfortunately remains popular. Some spoken language advocates see parents' informed choice of sign language as the primary communication modality for their deaf children as a choice for isolation and mediocrity (van der Merwe & Clark, 2009). They argue that deaf children should not be exposed to sign language at all. Some in the signing community say a discomfort with the "other" that being deaf and using ASL represents is the main reason hearing parents push for speech over sign. They argue, if parents could only be made comfortable with that "other," with the beauty of signed languages and their community, they would not make the choice for spoken language (Silva, 2005).

The first argument is, among other things, callous in its dismissal of the hundreds of millions of deaf people who do not have access to First World education and technology. The second argument, popular among those who would like to keep Gallaudet focused on signed languages, has a fundamental problem: although the argument for the continuation of the Deaf community on moral grounds is real and true—because at root humans are whole in whatever form they take and do not need to be fixed—it has not proven to be a pragmatically workable one. More and more deaf children swing rapidly toward spoken language regardless of sign language's cultural and linguistic value. Persisting in addressing this shift through moralistic appeals, the Deaf community could very easily win hearts at the expense of losing numbers.

Furthermore, to protect the community by arguing that there is a particularly pernicious bias against deaf individuals and sign language is to ignore overwhelming precedent; in all of history an ethical or moral argument for the survival of minority cultures has rarely, if ever, worked. Morally, Native Americans had the right to their land and their culture; so did African tribes in the slavery era; so do the Amazonian tribes discovered as deforestation and commerce relentlessly push farther into the South American jungle; and so do Aborigines in Australia, Tibetans in China, and Inuit in the Arctic. All had and have the moral right to exist as they choose. And most, if not all, have been in fact decimated or badly marginalized. If the Deaf community focuses on a moral approach, why should the results be any different?

Is this reality of societal machination cold and harsh? Certainly. Is accepting it some kind of failure of moral principle? No. It is what it is. To attach moral judgment to it is individual bias that leads to unproductive flaring of emotional outrage and misses the many opportunities that change affords.

How then to work with it? First, by better understanding it.

Part III: Understanding the Pressures, the Core Principle, the Dominating Impulse, Karl Marx

What is driving the change forces on the Deaf community and what has driven change forces against other minority communities throughout history most often comes down to money and the unending quest for it, nothing more. The history of human society is the history of communities evolving and expanding; confronting, defeating, and absorbing other communities; then losing strength, receding, and dying. Over and over, the key factor in this historical process is economic strength. The Roman Empire was overrun when it became overextended and overleveraged, modern China grows in geographical and cultural influence with every year of near double-digit economic expansion. The American age may be nearing its end because of the nation's financial crises. Simply put, the stronger economic force wins; the weaker one is relegated to the pages of history books. Correspondingly, the sustenance of the Deaf community is a matter not of finding some ethical, moral, or even research-based educational validation but of focusing on practical matters of economy.

This will be a shift. As the Deaf community has developed toward recognition and equality over the past decades, it has not always had to pay heed to economic forces. Consider whence the community emerged. As it took shape, other than in a few isolated communities such as Martha's Vineyard, it was mostly in institutions set up in the margins of society, on the asylum model, supported by consideration and charity. The community as a whole had almost no land, mineral wealth, or other financial resources, nor was it a market to be exploited. Largely left untouched by the demands of free-market capitalism, it grew into something unique in this world. I do not claim to have the authority or ability to describe the Deaf community's unique character but will just say that there is so much that is special there, so much that our chaotic and increasingly anxious modern world would be wise to absorb. Building on this character, through education, legislation, and advocacy, the community has gained ever more measures of respect and equality (leading eventually, as we saw, to the recognition of deaf persons and persons with disabilities as equal members of society and the passage of the ADA). Its relationship with larger society has emerged from one of charity to one of equality.

Herein returns the crux of the issue: economics. Equality is not just a right but also a responsibility; when you expect to achieve it, you are also expected to pay an equal share of the bill. Economic forces do not care about the particulars of your condition—almost everyone has or feels they have an unfair condition. Nor do economic forces care about the beauty you created out of hardship—almost everyone seeks to feel special about themselves and their own struggle. In this world, during these times, people generally care most about themselves and their bottom line. We should constantly remind ourselves that, as Karl Marx famously said, "The soul of history is economic" (Rorty, 2000).

As an example, to return to the earlier discussion of cochlear implants, although people are still researching and debating their efficacy, the most inarguable reasons for their rapid spread are economic ones. First, as stated before, they diffuse the cost of educating deaf children from the state to the district, family, insurance, and assorted professionals. Second, they are financially supported by industries and lobbies—implant companies, medical research companies, surgeons, and so on—with enormous economic strength and stake in their success. What might does moral argument, however sterling, have in the face of that?

If the Deaf community wants to thrive in the new century then it must obtain more economic strength. To obtain more economic strength, it must focus its educational institutions more directly on that task. The record of minority communities that have thrived through history backs up the strategy of pursuing financial solutions and not moral victories. Furthermore, that record offers compellingly similar templates applicable to the Deaf community's efforts. The next section will describe one such minority community's successes.

Part IV: The Jewish Example, Crisis Into Opportunity, the Economic Virtue of Cultural Pragmatism

Although the circumstances and history could hardly be more different, the long effort of the Jewish people to maintain their culture is a fascinating and possibly instructive parallel to the Deaf community's effort for continued survival and relevance.

The Jewish people have successfully maintained their community in precarious surroundings for more than 4,000 years. Judaism's history is filled with existential crises brought on by its regular status as a minority population in the midst of hostile majority populations. And when the Jews were able to reside in their area of origination and majority status, currently known as Israel, they were caught in military, religious, and social crossfire between European, African, and Asian societies.

Max Dimont, in his influential work *Jews, God, and History* (from which this section draws heavily), posits the counterintuitive thesis that this constant crossfire and crisis is what has enabled the Jewish community to survive so long (Dimont, 2004). Unstable realities forced the Jews to find new ways to sustain themselves. They succeeded—and not only succeeded but prospered. Nearly every tragedy or crisis the community sustained strengthened their economic situation in the end.

> A people in exile, banished from its homeland, produces no culture, but gradually either dies out through assimilation, or stagnates by reverting to a nomadic existence. This has been the history of all other exiled peoples. The Jews were the only exception. (Dimont, 2004, p. 116)

How? The key to Jewish survival was that in every hostile environment they faced, Jews created and developed areas of economic strength. The precariousness of their situation forced the Jews to constantly innovate and find new ways to sustain themselves with and within other societies. Crisis leading to innovation, innovation leading to economic strength, economic strength leading to survival—this process played out again and again. In the Middle Ages, for example, exiled from their homeland, scattered throughout Europe and the Middle East, facing vast odds, the Jews thrived by developing an entirely new industry—international banking. International banking and lending did not exist in any way, shape, or form until the Jews, who were excluded from many other forms of enterprise by laws and prejudice, created it. Then they used it to gain economic wealth and, through that wealth, power to sustain their culture.

In time, this concentration of wealth and power led to problems of its own, and the Jews were often forced to relinquish their gains and restart somewhere else. Regardless, the Jewish people continued to thrive across Europe until the Holocaust by developing niche areas for economic security. And whereas other religions lapsed into dogmatic fundamentalism predicated on obeisance and order, Judaic teachers and leaders, surely influenced by their precarious community situations, encouraged flexibility. With this objective view and intellectual flexibility, Jews became skillful assimilators and adapted to fit the diverse larger communities that exile handed them.

> When a civilization was philosophic, like that of the Greeks, the Jews became philosophers. When it was composed predominantly of poets and mathematicians, like that of the Arabs, the Jews became poets and mathematicians. When it was scientific and abstract, like that of modern Europeans, the Jews became scientists and theoreticians. When it was pragmatic and suburban, like the Americans, the Jews became pragmatists and suburbanites. (Dimont, 2004, p. 116)

In the 20th century, other American minority cultures such as African Americans, Asians, and the gay community followed this template and were able to lift their communities from marginalization and powerlessness by, among other things, pursuing opportunities in music and art and using those opportunities to gain economic muscle. Unfortunately, examples of the converse are more common nowadays. All over the globe—from the Amazon, to Africa, to the Pacific Islands—native and minority cultures are pushed aside, oppressed, and ignored as larger economies seek more resources, land, and consumers for their products. These native cultures can make no convincing economic case for their continued existence, and so they are demolished.

The parallels between their situations and the Deaf community's are compelling and instructive. And although it is (to put it mildly) a bit simplistic to compare a thousands-year-old global religious tradition with a small group of historically marginalized individuals that has just recently discovered its cultural voice, it appears inarguable that any community that fails to appreciate the changeability of the times and does not find and nourish compelling economic engines and niches of sustainability will be at the mercy of populations who cannot understand its communal treasures and do not care to. After all, these larger populations are guided by their own economic pressures. The survival of the Deaf community—and by extension of its flagship university—is the Deaf community's responsibility. Following the example of the Jewish people, this does not need to be a burden but can be instead a fantastic opportunity for creative evolution, community empowerment, and individual growth.

Part V: The Way Forward: Philosophical Mindset; Pragmatic Recommendations; Economic Possibilities; Tools, Tactics, and Challenges

If the economic strength of deaf individuals is crucial to the survival of the Deaf community, what steps can Gallaudet University take to foster it?

The community does face challenges unique to itself. The deaf experience perhaps most acutely manifests itself in issues of access, and access is crucial for maximizing opportunities. There are other pressures as well, many recited earlier in this chapter, from spending freezes on deaf education at the state and federal level to the worst economic recession in 80 years. In addition, Gallaudet is under pressure from expanded competition—state and community colleges are more and more taking on the challenge of educating deaf students, as they are, in fact, mandated by the ADA to provide services to any deaf student who asks for them.

Yes, this is a communal crisis, but every crisis is an opportunity. In this spirit, following is a list of suggestions—some already undertaken and bearing fruit—that might help Gallaudet and the Deaf community work toward the economic empowerment that is so crucial to survival.

1. Always put the student first.

Gallaudet University has had twin responsibilities over the years: as a school of higher education and as the center of the national and international Deaf community. At times the two responsibilities have blurred, especially as, for years, a large percentage of employment opportunities for students were within the Deaf community itself. But it must be clear now that the first and foremost duty at Gallaudet is preparing students to gain the skills and abilities to thrive in whatever workplace they choose. All communal responsibilities and requests must be secondary to this.

2. Focus on technology, writing, and social skills for working in the hearing economy.

Classes that prepare students directly for the hearing workplace should be identified, created, and emphasized. The rush of technological progress in the past 2 decades has profoundly changed the workplace and made it more deaf friendly. Business that used to be carried out on the telephone is now done via e-mail and even text messaging. Interpreting services can now be dialed up online, instantly. Caption access real time is now available for conference calls. The newest smart phones carry the capability of dialing up video relay interpreters on the spot. Students should be trained in the latest of these technologies, as they will be crucial to workplace success. Gallaudet could even try to partner with companies producing such technologies to help test and improve them. Also essential is student instruction in business writing and in the people management skills they will need when they reach positions of authority in the hearing workplace.

3. Focus on where modern society is going, not just what deaf people are good at.

"Deaf gain" has recently gained attention in Gallaudet University and the community (Bauman & Murray, 2010). It is a wonderful premise—to identify areas where being deaf creates advantages for the individual. The question is does it go far enough in securing economic power for the Deaf community? The market for deaf-related items is relatively small and not limited to deaf manufacturers. Witness also that advantages are often quickly co-opted, as in the national explosion in baby signing courses—almost all of which are run by hearing people—and in the videophone industry.

A broader focus not just on deaf-advantageous situations but also on careers and industries in which technology and social justice have leveled the playing field and on industries that will be crucial to future society would better serve the deaf workers of tomorrow. Where is the national economy moving? Where is the workforce underrepresented? Where can the Deaf community plug in and thrive? To give one example, because of the health care reform act of 2010, 30 to 40 million more people will shortly be entering the health insurance system—Where are the deaf doctors, nurses, and medical technology specialists? Thankfully, T. Alan Hurwitz, the current president of Gallaudet University, working with other university partners, has recently convened a task force to work on this very issue (Byrd, 2010).

4. Emphasize internships, externships, and exchange programs.

It is most beneficial for deaf and hard of hearing students to be active learners and participatory members of their own community. It is also crucial to prepare these students for the diversity of communities and experiences that are present and shared in the common world. Returning to the example of Jews in Europe, starting in the 1700s they made it a point to instruct students in the language of the nation of residence so that they could succeed in the workforce (Dimont, 2004). Perhaps this concept can go so far as to require Gallaudet students to spend one semester as transfer students at a hearing university for the experience of interacting within the larger hearing community. Paradoxically, this could strengthen the university by making it more appealing to mainstream students while reaffirming how important a community center is.

5. Emphasize community service.

The neighborhoods and municipalities surrounding Gallaudet University have little interest in the university's survival because of the fences, literal and metaphorical, that have kept the university and city apart. There are few ties of commerce, service, and concern between northeast Washington, DC, and Gallaudet. Were the university to close tomorrow, there would be very little outcry from the surrounding public. Gallaudet can take the initiative and become more integrated in the city around it. The university has started moving in this direction with the

6th Street project,[3] and there are many other exciting ways it can further serve the city's residents. Students in DC public schools, seniors in nursing homes, and U.S. military service members returned from the wars in Iraq and Afghanistan along with other local populations have strong interests in the social, academic, auditory, and related therapies that Gallaudet could provide. Students should be encouraged or even required to work with such populations. These types of service partnerships should be formed by Deaf communities across the country. To get others to care about the Deaf community, the Deaf community would benefit by showing how deeply it cares about them.

6. Cultivate political power.

Gallaudet University should continue to build on its recent successful efforts to obtain greater political relevance. It is an arguable fact of our time that financial strength leads to political might. The reverse is also true. Taking more initiative in helping the communities around it will go a long way toward giving the university local political standing. Judiciously putting the university's support behind appropriate national and international causes will have an impact on those levels. But very often in politics—as in all businesses—power comes down to individual relationships. Gallaudet has begun to nourish important contacts with district and national political leaders, and sitting little more than a mile away from the nation's political center, the university has the opportunity to open and nourish so many more such relationships.

7. Focus on advocacy, local and international.

The world stands at the cusp of an exciting new era in equality for persons with disabilities. Perhaps the most stirring moment in Gallaudet University history and definitely the most famous was the Deaf President Now protest of 1988. As noted, this protest became part of a national groundswell for the rights of persons with disabilities, culminating in the ratification of the ADA of 1990.[4] The ADA is now the international gold standard for rights for persons with disabilities. In 2008, the United Nations ratified the Convention on the Rights of People with Disabilities, which is modeled on the ADA. Currently, 145 nations are signatories (United Nations, 2009–2010). By signing the Convention on the Rights of People with Disabilities, these countries pledge to work to legislate equality to their citizens with disabilities, but many have no idea what that equality requires or looks like. Meanwhile, the World Health Organization (2010) estimates that there are around 300 million deaf and hard of hearing people in the world today. More than 90% are now born in the developing world, but most developing countries have a handful of deaf professionals and professionals with disabilities at best and so have no

3. For more information about this exciting project, see Schwartzman (2008).

4. As noted earlier. See note 2.

idea of all that deaf people are capable of. With its standing as the only university for the deaf in the world, its international reputation as a driving force in the push for equality, and its connections with local and national deaf organizations on six continents, Gallaudet University has been an international leader in guiding and supporting efforts to educate leaders and populations in countries as varied as Thailand, Costa Rica, Belize, Malawi, Gabon, Nigeria, and China about what deaf people can achieve . . . But it can always do more.

8. Continue to educate the world about the remarkable abilities and diversity in the Deaf community.

This speaks to directly building on the incredible strides that deaf people have made in the last few generations in gaining rights, visibility, and respect. Speaking or signing, implanted or not, every deaf person has something to contribute to the international community. It is important to constantly remind the world of that via the actions and abilities of Gallaudet students and community members. It is also important to remind deaf people around the world that nothing is "wrong" with them, and they can take pride in their lives, communities, and work and in whatever communication modality they choose.

9. Foster an open and dynamic dialogue about the future of the university and of the community.

Gallaudet University should strive to propagate an environment that respects and even celebrates every form of deafness and every chosen communication modality. It should make sure that emotional reactions never again overwhelm pragmatic agendas. The university must be supremely practical, eschewing the search for and championing of a single position or single truth to instead find ways to work with all positions, with all technological, communicative, and language variations. It should push toward framing the current moment as an economic crisis and not a moral one and not seek great and grand answers but incremental progression. It should push the idea that change is constant and identity will constantly evolve. It should be flexible for the new fields of opportunity that will arise as well as the unknown problems it will surely face.

Conclusion: The Necessary Mind-set

The stressors that the Deaf community, and by extension Gallaudet University, faces are many—demographic, political, technological—but they almost always boil down to the financial. If the community can master that element, it can almost certainly ensure its survival, regardless of what further societal and technological developments are in store. As we have seen, in the historical record there are plentiful examples of other communities facing similar challenges and rising to master them. However, if the Deaf community puts the perpetuation of the Deaf community in one specific form—whatever that may be—above the individual success of its diverse members, there will in all likelihood be no community survival, no university.

To relegate the success of the community's individual members to the backseat is to lose that success. To say that there is one correct way for such a rich and diverse international population is to lose that diversity. To say that one mode of communication—signing or spoken language—holds more truth than any other is to disregard the nobility of all.

To those who worry about losing the community's essence: this is not a death but an evolution. What emerges from the other side of this time of transition may very well be more far ranging, empathic, enriched, and empowering than anything that came before it. The world is connected as it has never been before—a man in China, a child in Alabama, a teacher and class in Uruguay can all watch the same video at the same moment. This is the global community. The challenge for the Deaf community is to become a respected, valued, and even essential part of that community. Having fought for equality and attained it in many respects, the community now must begin to live it, keeping in mind that all people—hearing or deaf, Black or White, male or female, old or young—go through life with the same instinctual wound, the same sense of incompleteness. Accepting that common humanity, cherishing its diversity, empowering its individuals, the Deaf community can use its strengths not just to help itself but also to help all of humankind.

References

Bauman, H.-D. L. (Ed). (2008). *Open your eyes: Deaf studies talking*. Minneapolis: University of Minnesota Press.

Bauman, H.-D., & Murray, J. (2010). Deaf studies in the 21st century: "Deaf gain" and the future of human diversity. In M. Marschark & P. Spencer (Eds.). *Oxford handbook of deaf studies, language, and education* (Vol. 2, pp. 210–225). New York: Oxford University Press.

Byrd, T. (2010, May). A team effort to 'broaden and reform' health care. Retrieved April 8, 2011, from http://pr.gallaudet.edu/family/Article.asp?ID=16356

Deaf and Hard of Hearing Alliance. (2010, May). *Early Hearing Detection and Intervention Act of 2010 introduced in Senate. Legislative updates page*. Retrieved August 2010, from http://dhhainfo.com/updates

Dimont, M. (2004). *Jews, God, and history* (2nd ed.). New York: Signet Classics.

Gallaudet Research Institute, Gallaudet University. (2006, July). *Can you tell me how many deaf people there are in the United States?* Retrieved April 2010, from http://research.gallaudet.edu/Demographics/deaf-US.php

Gallaudet University. 2008. *Visual language and visual learning Website*. Retrieved April 8, 2011, from http://vl2.gallaudet.edu

National Institute on Deafness and Other Communication Disorders. (2009, August). *Cochlear implants*. Retrieved April 2010, from http://www.nidcd.nih.gov/health/hearing/coch.html

North Carolina Office of Educational Services. (2004). *Early intervention in North Carolina*. BEGINNINGS. Raleigh, NC. Retrieved via e-mail March 2010.

Roan, S. (2009, August). Cochlear implants open deaf kids' ears to the world. *Los Angeles Times*. Retrieved August 2010, from http://articles.latimes.com/2009/aug/03/health/he-deaf-children3

Rorty, R. (2000). *Philosophy and social hope*. New York: Penguin.

Schwartzman, P. (2008, October 4). Gallaudet's new aesthetic of openness. The *Washington Post*.

Silva, R. (2005, April). *Audism and Deaf culture*. Retrieved July 2010, from http://www.lifeprint.com/asl101/topics/audism.htm

Soukup, B. J. (2008). *DPN and the civil rights movement*. Retrieved July 2010, from http://dpnnews.com/2008/02/28/%e2%80%9cdpn-and-the-civil-rights-movement%e2%80%9d-by-benjamin-j-soukup-chair-gallaudet-university-board-of-trustee

Treni, K. (2009, April 30). *Listening and spoken language: A crisis of capacity in the public system*. Paper presented in Washington, DC, the U.S. Capitol.

United Nations. (2009–2010). *Enable*. Retrieved June 2010, from http://www.un.org/disabilities

van der Merwe, N., & Clark, M. (2009, August). Let our children hear—and learn to speak. *The Times of South Africa*. Retrieved September 2010, from http://www.timeslive.co.za/opinion/letters/article33699.ece

World Health Organization. (2010, April). *Deafness and hearing impairment fact sheet*. Retrieved August 2010, from http://www.who.int/mediacentre/factsheets/fs300/en/index.html

Zena, M. (2009, February). *Third deaf school closing proposed this summer*. Retrieved July 2010, from http://www.mishkazena.com/2009/02/04/third-deaf-school-closing-proposed-this-summer

CONTRIBUTORS

Benjamin Bahan is a Professor in the Department of American Sign Language and Deaf Studies at Gallaudet University. He is the co-author of the book *Journey into the Deaf World* (1996) and *The Syntax of American Sign Language* (2000). Benjamin has also co-directed and co-scripted the following videos: *Audism Unveiled* (2008) and *A to Z: ABC Stories in ASL* (2010). He currently serves as Executive Editor with Dirksen Bauman and Melissa Malzkuhn of the *Deaf Studies Digital Journal* (DSDJ.gallaudet.edu), the world's first online, peer-reviewed academic and cultural arts journal to feature scholarship and creative work in both signed and written languages.

H-Dirksen Bauman is Professor of Deaf Studies at Gallaudet University where he serves as the coordinator for the master's program in Deaf Studies and Coordinator for the Office of Bilingual Teaching and Learning. He is the co-editor of the book/DVD project, *Signing the Body Poetic: Essays in American Sign Language* (2006) and editor of *Open Your Eyes: Deaf Studies Talking* (2008). Dirksen Bauman is also a producer and co-director of the film *Audism Unveiled* (2008). He currently serves as Executive Editor with Ben Bahan and Melissa Malzkuhn of the *Deaf Studies Digital Journal* (DSDJ.gallaudet.edu), the world's first online, peer-reviewed academic and cultural arts journal to feature scholarship and creative work in both signed and written languages.

John B. Christiansen is Professor Emeritus of Sociology at Gallaudet. He received his PhD in Sociology from the University of California, Riverside, in 1976 and taught at Gallaudet from 1977 until his retirement in 2009. His most recent book is *Reflections: My Life in the Deaf and Hearing Worlds* (2010) He co-authored (with Sharon Barnartt) *Deaf President Now! The 1988 Revolution at Gallaudet University* (1995) and (with Irene W. Leigh) *Cochlear Implants in Children: Ethics and Choices* (2002/2005) He has also written or co-authored dozens of articles and book chapters. A cochlear implant user (on one ear only), when he is not reading or writing he can usually be found riding his bicycle.

Jane Dillehay has been a faculty member of Gallaudet since 1980 and is currently Full Professor in the General Studies program. She has been the Chairperson of the Biology Department and was Dean of the College of Liberal

Arts, Sciences and Technologies for 9 years. She obtained her PhD in molecular biology from Carnegie Mellon University in 1980. Dr. Dillehay has collaborated with researchers from Lawrence Livermore National Laboratories and George Washington University Medical School in studying the mechanisms of eukaryotic DNA repair. Her current research interests are in bioethics and the application of the principles of cognitive psychology to effective pedagogy in science education. She obtained a cochlear implant in September 2008 and is learning to handle the world of sound.

Jill Duncan is Head of Graduate Studies at the RIDBC Renwick Centre for Research and Professional Education at the Royal Institute for Deaf and Blind Children and Conjoint Senior Lecturer in the School of Education, University of Newcastle, Australia. She has had the privilege of learning from Professors Richard and Laura Kretschmer, and Professor Roberta Truax and working alongside Helen Beebe. She is a practicing Teacher of the Deaf and an Auditory-Verbal Therapist.

Maribel Gárate is currently an Assistant Professor in the Department of Education at Gallaudet University. She earned two master's degrees from Gallaudet University—Deaf Education: Elementary and American Sign Language Linguistics. Her PhD is in Deaf Education with a focus on bilingual education. Dr. Gárate has taught Deaf and Hard of Hearing students in both residential and mainstreamed settings. She is actively involved in teaching, training, consulting, and researching about ASL/English bilingual education. She has also conducted training and made presentations on topics related to bilingual methodologies, literacy instruction, and ASL linguistics to teachers and school administrators both nationally and internationally.

Raychelle L. Harris is a faculty member at Gallaudet University in the Department of American Sign Language (ASL) and Deaf Studies where she serves as a coordinator of the masters' program in Sign Language Teaching. She earned her doctorate from Gallaudet University in Deaf Education with a focus on Educational Linguistics. Her dissertation study was about the construction of academic language in a bilingual ASL/English preschool classroom with Deaf teachers and students. As a committed advocate of social justice, Dr. Harris presents and publishes about the ethics of research within Sign Language communities.

Poorna Kushalnagar received her Ph.D. in Developmental Psychology with a focus in Developmental Cognitive Neuroscience at the University of Houston. She is a Ruth L. Kirstein NIH research fellow the University of Rochester School of Medicine and Dentistry. Her research interests focus on translating research to empirically supported interventions that result in improved quality of life outcomes among children and adolescents who are deaf or hard of hearing. She received her first implant in 2008 and second implant in 2009, both with similar experiences.

Raja Kushalnagar has a JD in Law, a LLM in Intellectual Property Law, and recently completed requirements for a PhD in Computer Science at the University of Houston. He is an Assistant Professor in the Department of Information and Computing Studies at the National Technical Institute for the Deaf at Rochester Institute of Technology. His focus is accessible technology for deaf and hard of hearing students in mainstreamed classrooms. He has two implants, a second generation in 1999 and a third generation in 2009, and had very different experiences after each one.

Irene W. Leigh, PhD, a deaf psychologist, has done high school teaching, psychological assessment, psychotherapy, and mental health administration. From 1985 to 1991 she worked at the Lexington Center for Mental Health Services, serving as Assistant Director the last two years. She has been a professor in the Gallaudet University Clinical Psychology doctoral program since 1992 and is currently Chair of the Department of Psychology. In addition to numerous presentations, she has published over 50 articles and book chapters, edited *Psychotherapy with Deaf Clients from Diverse Groups* (1999, 2010), co-authored *Cochlear Implants in Deaf Children: Ethics and Choices* (2002/2005), and *Deaf People: Evolving Perspectives from Psychology, Education, and Sociology* (2004). Her most recent book is *A Lens on Deaf Identities* (2009). She is a Fellow of the American Psychological Association and an Associate Editor for the *Journal of Deaf Studies and Deaf Education.*

Deborah Maxwell-McCaw completed her master's degree at Gallaudet University, and began her career in the mental health field by working at the Lexington Mental Health Center as a Mental Health Counselor providing individual, group and family counseling to deaf students and their families from 1989–1993. A desire for advanced training in psychodynamic therapy led her to pursue doctoral studies at The George Washington University, where she obtained her PhD in Clinical Psychology in 2000. She has been a faculty member in the Department of Psychology at Gallaudet University since 1996. Her current area of research is in the area of deaf identity development across the diverse deaf/hh population and its impact on psychological functioning. Dr. McCaw has been a cochlear implant user since 2006.

Julie Cantrell Mitchiner is an Instructor with the Education Department at Gallaudet University. Julie received a master's degree in Deaf Education with a specialization in Family-Centered Early Education from Gallaudet University. She is currently a doctoral candidate at George Mason University in Education with a specialization in Early Childhood Education and Multicultural/Multilingual Education. Before she started worked as a faculty, she taught preschool at Laurent Clerc National Deaf Education Center with deaf and hard of hearing children for six years. Her research interest is on bilingual education in ASL and English for young deaf and hard of hearing children.

Donna A. Morere, PhD, is a Professor in the Department of Psychology (Clinical Psychology Program) at Gallaudet University. She is also the Neuropsychological Assessment Director for the Early Language Educational Study and Psychometric Toolkit at the Science of Learning Center on Visual Language and

Visual Learning. She received her PhD in Medical (Clinical) Psychology from the University of Alabama at Birmingham in 1989. She maintains a private practice in Clinical Neuropsychology with a focus on deaf children with multiple challenges. She has presented and published on the neuropsychological assessment, reading skill development, and audiovisual processing of deaf individuals. Her current research involves the interaction of cognitive, linguistic, and perceptual process related to academic achievement in young deaf adults and reading skill development in deaf children. She has a son with bilateral cochlear implants.

Debra Berlin Nussbaum is Coordinator of the Cochlear Implant Education Center (CIEC) at the Laurent Clerc National Deaf Education Center at Gallaudet University. She earned her master's degree in Audiology from George Washington University and has worked at the Clerc Center since 1977; first as a pediatric audiologist and since 2000 as Coordinator of the CIEC. She has spearheaded efforts to look at the roles of spoken language and signed language in the education of children who are deaf and hard of hearing. She has developed numerous resource materials and professional training workshops, and speaks nationally and internationally on this topic.

Raylene Paludneviciene is a faculty member with the Department of Psychology at Gallaudet University where she teaches primarily in the undergraduate program. She received her PhD in Clinical Psychology from Gallaudet University and completed a postdoctoral fellowship at the University of Rochester. Dr. Paludneviciene's current research projects include the development of American Sign Language assessment tools. Spurned by the fact that half of her family has cochlear implants, she is also interested in studying the relationship between cochlear implants and the deaf community.

Khadijat Rashid is a Professor in the Department of Business at Gallaudet University. She received her MBA from the University of Maryland at College Park and her PhD in International Relations from American University. She has been a member of the Gallaudet faculty since 1994, including a stint as Chair of the Department of Business. Her focus is primarily on international development and she has served on the boards of the World Deaf Leadership Program and Discovering Deaf Worlds, guiding development projects for deaf communities in developing countries. She was implanted in 2008.

Ellen A. Rhoades, Ed.S., LSLS Cert AVT, a consultant and AV mentor for practitioners, provides training on an international level. She has been recognized with many awards including "Outstanding AV Clinician of the Year" from AVI, "Outstanding Professional of the Year" and "Outstanding Program of the Year" from AG Bell, and the "Nitchie Award in Human Communications" from the League for the Hard of Hearing. In addition to authoring many book chapters and papers for peer-reviewed publications, she co-edited the book *Auditory-Verbal Practice: Toward a Family-Centered Approach*. She served as director on the boards of AVI, AG Bell, and other nonprofit AV centers. In addition to having founded an AV center that she directed, she established and directed three other AV programs over a period of 25 years. Her more than 35 years of experience includes university instructor, AV practitioner, classroom teacher, supervisor, parent-infant coordinator, adult rehabilitation therapist, administrator, fundraiser, marketer, and grant writer. Due to bilateral congenital sensorineural deafness with genetic etiology, Ellen has been a hearing aid user since 1947 and a bilateral cochlear implantee since 1996.

Marilyn Sass-Lehrer is a Professor at Gallaudet University in Washington, DC. She received a master's degree in Deaf Education from New York University and a PhD from the University of Maryland in Early Childhood Education and Curriculum and Instruction. Her research and writing include professional competencies, guidelines for best practice, and family involvement. Dr. Sass-Lehrer is actively involved in national organizations and initiatives that address programs and policies for infants, toddlers, and their families. She is a co-author of *Parents and their Deaf Children: The Early Years* (2003), and co-editor of *The Young Deaf or Hard of Hearing Child: A Family-Centered Approach to Early Education* (2003).

Susanne M. Scott is a Cochlear Implant/Bilingual Specialist at the Laurent Clerc National Deaf Education Center at Gallaudet University. She earned her master's degree in Audiology from Gallaudet University and has worked at Gallaudet University and the Clerc Center since 1980; first as an educational audiologist, then as a clinical educator in the Department of Hearing, Speech and Language Sciences. She joined the Cochlear Implant Education Center in 2003 where she provides content expertise in cochlear implants and ASL/English bilingual education for professionals and families at the Clerc Center and throughout the nation.

Josh Swiller's first book *The Unheard: A Memoir of Deafness and Africa* was a *New York Times* bestseller and received several awards. He has also published articles in the *Washington Post*, the *Washingtonian* magazine, the *New York Times Magazine*, and other national publications and has lectured in over twenty states. Deaf since age four, he received a cochlear implant 30 years later. He graduated from Yale University, received a master's degree in Social Work from New York University, and co-founded Deaf Worldwide Community Advocacy Network (Deaf We Can) an international non-profit that focuses on ensuring the rights and access of the deaf in the developing world. Currently, he works as a special assistant to the chief of staff of Gallaudet. He thanks Brendan U. Stern for his assistance in preparing this chapter.

Joseph Michael Valente is an Assistant Professor of Early Childhood Education at Pennsylvania State University. He is also affiliate faculty in the Disability Studies and Comparative and International Education programs. Dr. Valente is the author of the autobiographical novel and autoethnography *d/Deaf and d/Dumb: A Portrait of a Deaf Kid as a Young Superhero*. Currently Dr. Valente is the co-Principal Investigator of the project Kindergartens for the Deaf in Three Countries, funded by the Spencer Foundation. He received his BA from Bates College and PhD from Arizona State University. To learn more about his work, please see http://joevalente.net.

INDEX

Figures, notes, and tables are indicated with f, n, and t following the page number.